Foundation Concepts of

Global Community Health Promotion and Education

Barbara Lorraine Michiels Hernandez, PhD, CHES, CDE
Professor and Health Graduate Coordinator
Eta Sigma Gamma Advisor
Lamar University
Beaumont, Texas

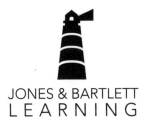

JONES & BARTLETT
LEARNING

World Headquarters

Jones & Bartlett Learning
40 Tall Pine Drive
Sudbury, MA 01776
978-443-5000
info@jblearning.com
www.jblearning.com

Jones & Bartlett Learning Canada
6339 Ormindale Way
Mississauga, Ontario L5V 1J2
Canada

Jones & Bartlett Learning International
Barb House, Barb Mews
London W6 7PA
United Kingdom

Jones & Bartlett Learning books and products are available through most bookstores and online booksellers. To contact Jones & Bartlett Learning directly, call 800-832-0034, fax 978-443-8000, or visit our website, www.jblearning.com.

Substantial discounts on bulk quantities of Jones & Bartlett Learning publications are available to corporations, professional associations, and other qualified organizations. For details and specific discount information, contact the special sales department at Jones & Bartlett Learning via the above contact information or send an email to specialsales@jblearning.com.

Production Credits

Publisher, Higher Education: Cathleen Sether
Acquisitions Editor: Shoshanna Goldberg
Senior Associate Editor: Amy L. Bloom
Senior Editorial Assistant: Kyle Hoover
Senior Production Editor: Renée Sekerak
Associate Production Editor: Jill Morton
Associate Marketing Manager: Jody Sullivan
V.P., Manufacturing and Inventory Control:
    Therese Connell
Cover Design: Kristin E. Parker
Associate Photo Researcher: Sarah Cebulski
Photo and Permissions Associate: Emily Howard
Composition: Toppan Best-set Premedia Limited
Cover Images: Business team on laptop, © Dennis Owusu-
    Ansah/ShutterStock, Inc.; Family talking in kitchen, ©
    Rob Marmion/ShutterStock, Inc.
Printing and Binding: Malloy Incorporated
Cover Printing: Malloy Incorporated

Library of Congress Cataloging-in-Publication Data
Hernandez, Barbara Lorraine Michiels.
    Foundation concepts of global community health promotion and education / by Barbara Lorraine Michiels Hernandez.
        p. ; cm.
    Includes bibliographical references and index.
    ISBN-13: 978-0-7637-8168-2
    ISBN-10: 0-7637-8168-1
    1. Health promotion. 2. Health education. I. Title.
    [DNLM: 1. Health Promotion. 2. Health Education. 3. World Health. WA 590 H557f 2011]
    RA427.8.H64 2011
    613—dc22
                                                                    2010009693
6048
Printed in the United States of America
14 13 12 11 10   10 9 8 7 6 5 4 3 2 1

TABLE OF CONTENTS

PREFACE

This book examines the concepts and content for the global foundations of community health promotion and health education. It investigates the history, terminology, philosophy, theory, ethics, programs, resources, and practice settings. Emerging and reemerging threats to global health are explored, as well as societal influences on health. It addresses professional competencies and preparation, standards, models, theories, careers, technology, and the role of professional associations/organizations on a global basis. Health administrative skills included are hiring, needs assessments and planning, implementing, and evaluating programs. Health literacy, prevention, promotion, protection, access, enhancement, and maintenance are emphasized throughout the book. Interviews on philosophical viewpoints with outstanding health professionals are included along with health practitioners' real-life job descriptions and skills. Cultural aspects of health and administration details are given. This book presents information and answers questions on health, historic figures and events, models and theories used, programs administered, philosophies needed, professional standards, and student career choices. It is an all-in-one comprehensive introductory text with a global viewpoint that includes all standards and entry level and advanced responsibilities and competencies geared to the Certified Health Education Specialist (CHES) competencies. This textbook could be used as a study guide for the CHES certification test.

CHAPTERS

The chapters are organized sequentially so that skills, content, and knowledge from one chapter lead to the next. The chapters address basic conceptual learning, epidemiology, history, theory, strategic plans, philosophies, standards, technology, careers, and future predictions. Basic health concepts and terminology from each chapter are sequential, with each chapter building upon the previous chapters so students have a broad understanding of health content from many diverse areas and see their relationships and connections. Diverse viewpoints are given in some areas so students can make judgments on information. Global resources for diverse careers and health are listed in Appendix C. The e-portfolio section is very timely for students. Because all information could not possibly be included in the content, additional conceptual learning, terms and definitions, relevant Web sites, enhanced readings, and reflective thinking questions are included to broaden the educational learning experience by presenting information beyond the textbook for increased comprehension and synthesis. The conceptual learning section and conceptual terms and definitions should be reviewed after reading the content and summary.

CHAPTER OBJECTIVES

Each chapter addresses specific objectives from the Entry and Advanced Level Health Education Competencies (see Appendix A). In addition, specific objectives are written for each chapter using

Bloom's *Taxonomy of Educational Objectives* (1979) terminology for clarity. The objectives focus on the content and skills that require mastery for prospective health educators. The conceptual terms, base margin definitions, conceptual learning, and relevant Web sites are reviews of chapter information and objectives. The enhanced readings, career concepts, reflective thinking, and conceptual ideas expand the learning experiences for global thought processes. Students should review the objectives before and after reading each chapter to best understand the purpose of the content. Skills mastery should be comprehended by understanding the objectives and applying them.

CONCEPTUAL TERMS AND DEFINITIONS

Important terms are bolded in each chapter to emphasize their importance to the statements. The conceptual terms listed at the end of each chapter are important to review before and after reading each chapter. The conceptual definitions pertinent to each section are included in the base margins. Comprehension of specific health-related terms lends itself to understanding the content of each chapter. After reading each chapter, students should review the meaning of each conceptual term bolded in the chapter, the conceptual definitions in the base margins, the conceptual terms listed at the end of each chapter, and the glossary at the end of the book, and they should apply the terms in the conceptual learning section.

CHAPTER SUMMARY

The bulleted summary at the end of each chapter is a good review of the major health concepts. It should be examined along with the conceptual terms and definitions after reading the chapter. Students should ensure they can interpret and understand each part of the summary thoroughly as well as accompanying details concerning each of the topics delineated in each chapter.

CONCEPTUAL LEARNING

These questions are geared to the objectives, content, summary, and conceptual terms in each chapter. They extend and develop learning outcomes and help students recall, interpret, analyze, synthesize, and extrapolate information.

RELEVANT WEB SITES

The Web sites are links to information that will expand the conceptual learning above and beyond the textbook content and investigate more global health information. Students are encouraged to access each link and evaluate and analyze the contents. These are excellent resources available online for health content, theory, and information pertinent to the profession. Additionally, these resources help students examine how health technological information is presented. It is also recommended that students bookmark these links for use in other courses and research purposes. Students are encouraged to further explore the additional linked Web sites available from these Internet resources since there are too many to list in this textbook.

ENHANCED READINGS

The enhanced readings present supplementary information that is pertinent to the profession. Most are too large to include in the textbook but are recommended so students comprehend and recognize the broader context of health and relevant documents. Pertinent documents are listed that require judgments and analysis of content. Students should explore any further readings listed in the enhanced readings since all cannot be included in this textbook. It also is recommended that students bookmark the links or keep hard copies of these files for further use in other courses and research purposes.

REFLECTIVE THINKING

This section of each chapter actually encourages students to apply what they have learned to real-life situations, use decision making skills, evaluate carefully, and make value judgments.

THOUGHT CONCEPTS

The idea sections help students analyze health in the broader context of the real world and recognize the importance of the profession to society. They should provide thought-provoking responses and discussions.

CAREER CONCEPTS

The career sections in each chapter help students synthesize the skills and responsibilities of health educators and assist in formulating career goals that best suit their interests and background. The different types of careers discussed in these sections and the health practitioners' templates provided in Chapter 8 give examples of possible jobs and real-world job descriptions for students to examine.

ACKNOWLEDGMENTS

This book resulted from years of teaching with supplements and using several textbook sources for a health foundations course. I kept saying to my students that I needed to write a book that covered all of the aspects that they needed to begin their coursework for a health career. I wish to thank all of my students who throughout the years helped me to become a better teacher and gave me ideas on what to include in this book. I want to thank Lamar University for giving me a developmental leave for one semester to work on the book, and I am grateful for that opportunity. Although it took longer to complete, this allowed dedicated time to the book that I would not ordinarily have. My colleagues who have encouraged me throughout the years deserve recognition. They include Sam Coker, Bob Blackburn, Rick Barnes, Ann Severance, Gladys Keeton, Janice LaPointe Crump, and George Strickland. Shoshanna Goldberg, Amy Bloom, Jill Morton, and the whole editorial team and all the staff members at Jones & Bartlett Learning who worked on the book deserve praise. They were always willing to help and were generous with their time and expertise. They did a fabulous job editing this textbook. My family has been an overwhelming support system for me. Acknowledgments go to my husband, who is my rock and my love; my daughter, who is a wonderful mother and smart career woman; and my beautiful and sweet grandchildren, who are such a source of laughter, pride, and joy. Finally, I wish to acknowledge my father. His advice on my first teaching job was immeasurable. He told me to introduce myself to everyone working at the school and express how proud I was to be a part of the team. Today, I realize I automatically established a "social support system" for myself in my first job because of his advice. Writing this book has been an incredible experience and I am grateful for the opportunity. Please give me feedback on this *First Edition*, and I hope it will benefit your course work.

ABOUT THE AUTHOR

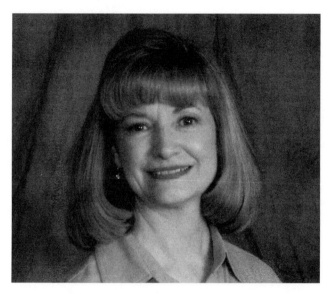

Barbara Lorraine Michiels Hernandez received her PhD from Texas Woman's University and her bachelor's and master's degree from Northwestern State University of Louisiana. She is currently a professor at Lamar University of Texas in the Department of Health and Kinesiology. Previous university teaching experiences were at Northwestern State University of Louisiana, Missouri Southern State College at Joplin, Pittsburg State University of Kansas, and Texas Wesleyan University. Her career includes positions as a university professor, public school teacher, dance educator, artistic director, and executive director for the National Dance Association. She is a widely published journal and book author as well as author of many technology publications and online courses, a presenter, and a reviewer for professional journals. Barbara is a Certified Health Education Specialist and a Certified Dance Educator. Her research areas are women's health, teacher certification and standards, health histories and dancer's health. She was inducted as a Research Fellow for the Research Consortium of the American Alliance for Health, Physical Education, Recreation and Dance in 2009. Dr. Hernandez is a member of Eta Sigma Gamma and founded the Delta Omicron chapter at Lamar University. Her professional service activities have been at the international, national, state, and local levels.

CHAPTER 1

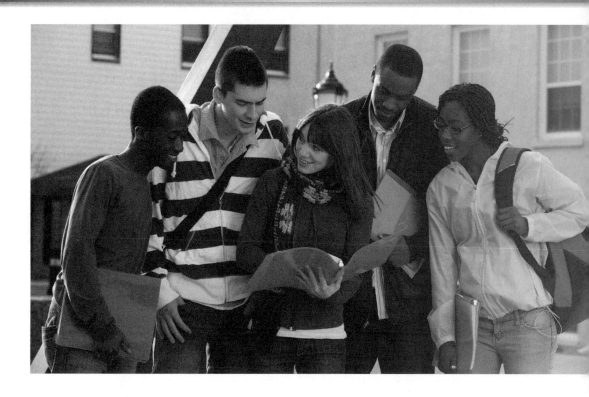

Underlying Concepts of the Health Education and Promotion Profession

OBJECTIVES AND ASSESSMENTS

This chapter meets the following National Commission for Health Education Credentialing, Inc., Society for Public Health Education, and American Association for Health Education Responsibilities and Competencies for Entry Level and Advanced Level Health Educators.* The learner will:

6. Serve as a health education resource person.
7. Communicate and advocate for health education.

This chapter meets the following learning objectives. The learner will:
1. Examine and discuss the functions of medical and health governmental/nongovernmental agencies, professional associations, and organizations.
2. Construct definitions and demonstrate the concepts of health literacy, prevention, promotion, protection, access, enhancement, and maintenance.
3. Define and apply basic health education terms, disease terms, epidemiological terms, and surveillance rates.
4. Compare and summarize the current health status, risks, protective behaviors, determinants, and leading causes of diseases and death in the world and the United States.
5. Evaluate corresponding health education programs for Healthy People 2010 and review the objectives of Healthy People 2020.
6. Compare national, state, and local laws, policies, and regulations affecting community health.

Source: Reprinted with permission of NCHEC.

    National Commission for Health Education Credentialing, Inc. (NCHEC), Society for Public Health Education (SOPHE), & American Association for Health Education (AAHE). (2006). *A competency-based framework for health educators-2006*. Whitehall, PA: NCHEC.

INTRODUCTION

As changes in health occur throughout the globe, there is a need for professional health educators to effect change and make a positive difference. Through planning appropriate health programs, the population can learn to manage disease symptoms, improve nutrition levels, perform prescribed physical activity, function more effectively in daily life, contribute to the well-being of their community, and experience a much higher **quality of life**.

The job of a health educator relates to constructive, optimistic changes for society. It is a respected profession, though still not completely understood. Not only is prevention a focus for health educators, but health promotion, literacy, and protection can reduce disease in populations. Access to health services, maintaining health, and enhancing current health are services offered by health promotion activities carried out by health educators. You do not have to be diagnosed with a disease to benefit from health programs.

The old saying that "an ounce of prevention is worth a pound of cure" still holds true today. Health educators are constantly searching for health prevention and promotion programs that benefit good health in populations. Health educators effect changes in health every day. It is an honored profession and is more relevant today in a global world.

As we scan the globe, we see an imperfect world that needs to come together and prepare for health emergencies and promote healthier lives for all people. This is the job of health education specialists, and you will learn about the characteristics of the profession and the elements that define it. The health professional conducts health condition studies; researches trends; establishes controls for endemics, emerging, and reemerging diseases; and assesses conditions and lifestyles that are determinants of health problems. A health educator works in understanding and advocating for positive changes in social, political, regulatory, policy, and environmental factors that are health determinants.[1]

Improving global health is a responsibility for all to pursue. The nations of the world must work together and share the burden of threats to health since inevitably they affect all humans. The factors that determine health such as economics, healthcare access, social factors, education, safety factors, and many others are controlled in many countries by laws or policies that affect health. Health practitioners advocate for changes in practices and policies that affect health.

With economic globalization and free trade agreements, cooperation among nations needs to be solidified when discussing how these global changes affect health. Global agreements and policies that solidify and combine efforts for improved health are a necessity in this world that is becoming borderless. This book hopes to communicate the skills performed on a daily basis by health education professionals and illustrate how this profession contributes to a healthier global society through cooperative efforts and solutions.

> **Career Concept**
>
> *Are you good at multitasking, and do you enjoy wearing many hats? If so, you might be a good health administrator, sales person, or employee in a professional/technical health organization.*

Quality of life: A person's sense of satisfaction with his or her life and environment. This concept includes all aspects of life that affect health including rights, values, benefits, beliefs, and conditions.

HEALTH AND WELLNESS CONCEPTS

The definition of health needs to be considered before defining the health education profession. For most people, they consider health to be the status of one's physical well-being. But today, we know that many factors influence a person's health. Health is "a state of balance between the body, mind, and spirit."[2] According to the the **World Health Organization (WHO)** in 1947, **health** is "a state of complete physical, mental, and social well-being and not merely the absence of infirmity."[3] Within the context of health promotion, health has been considered a means to an end, expressed as a resource permitting people to lead an individually, socially, and economically productive life. The WHO said that health is a resource for life and is a very positive concept emphasizing social and personal resources and physical capabilities.[4] When contemplating what they prize most in life, most individuals will almost unanimously state that their health is a precious commodity.

Wellness is a more comprehensive version of health. Wellness is a strategic focus on health that balances the many dimensions of a person's life. Wellness is achieved by increasing and adopting health-enhancing conditions and behaviors rather than minimizing conditions of illness or disease. It is also an active process of positive health choices, decisions, and lifestyles by individuals that affect the quality and duration of human life.

Wellness concepts, according to Insel and Roth, refer to quality of life measures that encompass the many dimensions of health as physical, emotional, intellectual, spiritual, interpersonal and social, and environmental; they also address planetary wellness.[5] In addition to these wellness concepts, occupational wellness receives more emphasis today and must be included in this list.[6] Thus, physical health is not the only factor affecting the health of people today; many dimensions affect health. Some equate holistic health with wellness as being the health of the whole person, including physical, mental, emotional, and spiritual domains. This concept is that the body, mind, and spirit are in sync with one another and provide balance within these holistic components.[7] Wellness extends the concept of health to everything in a person's life that affects his or her health whether in a large or small way.

HEALTH EDUCATOR CONCEPTS

A **profession**, according to the Merriam Webster dictionary is "a calling requiring specialized knowledge and often long and intensive academic preparation."[8] A **health educator** works "to

---

World Health Organization (WHO): The directing and coordinating authority on health for the United Nations that promotes health development, security, systems, research, partnerships, and performance.
Health: "A state of complete physical, mental, and social well-being and not merely the absence of infirmity" (WHO, 1947).
Wellness: An active process of positive health choices, decisions, and lifestyles by individuals that affects the quality and years of human life.
Profession: A type of employment requiring specialized learning and training.
Health educator: A professionally prepared educator who develops, implements, and evaluates policies, procedures, interventions, systems, and appropriate educational strategies conducive to the health of individuals, groups, and communities for prevention of disease and adverse health conditions.

encourage healthy lifestyles and wellness through educating individuals and communities about behaviors that promote healthy living and prevent diseases and other health problems."[9] A professionally prepared health educator serves in a variety of roles and uses appropriate educational strategies and methods. The development of policies, procedures, interventions, and systems conducive to the health of individuals, groups, and communities is a main goal of the profession.

Examples of practice settings for health education and application include, but are not limited to, medical care settings, colleges and universities, schools, public health departments, nonprofit organizations, private business,[9] communities, work sites (e.g., business, industry, and school), rehabilitation centers, professional associations, governmental agencies, environmental agencies, mental health agencies, and professional associations. See Chapter 8 for more information on the different careers available. A health educator works in prevention, promotion, literacy, protection, and access to services to preserve, maintain, and enhance healthy lifestyles in communities. This pursuit involves assisting individuals and communities to adopt healthy behaviors. Health educators collect and analyze data; identify community needs; plan, implement, monitor, and evaluate programs designed to encourage healthy lifestyles, policies, and environments; and administer programs and resources for health.

The health profession is considered a helping profession. Health educators are not medical health personnel. Health educators do not diagnose, treat, prescribe, medicate, or perform surgery. They work with people before a health crisis and intervene after a health crisis. The programs facilitated by health educators before a person needs medical care are to help prevent and promote health, literacy, protection, and access to health services. Once disease strikes, the medical profession takes over. After rehabilitation and sometimes during rehabilitation, health educators continue promoting and protecting health; preventing further damage; improving literacy; and advocating access, maintenance, and enhancement of the health status—all in an effort to create lives and healthy places for all people. The profession is emerging, and the purpose of the profession is not always understood; however, many jobs are facilitated by health education specialists.

A **Certified Health Education Specialist (CHES)** has met required health education qualifications, including earning an appropriate health degree and passing a competency-based exam. The exam is administered by the National Commission for Health Education Credentialing, Inc. This organization mandates that continuing education requirements are necessary to maintain the national credential for health educators.[10] This credentialing is available for health education graduates and professionals.

DISEASE CONCEPTS

Health educators must understand the disease causation cycles. **Communicable diseases** (also called infectious diseases) are caused by some specific biological agent or toxic products that are transmitted from an infected person, animal, or inanimate reservoir to a susceptible host.

Certified Health Education Specialist (CHES): A specific credentialing available to qualified health educators requiring academic qualifications and testing requirements administered by the National Commission for Health Education Credentialing, Inc.
Communicable diseases: Infectious diseases caused by some specific biological agent or toxic products that are transmitted from an infected person, animal, or inanimate reservoir to a susceptible host.

Non-communicable diseases (also called chronic diseases) cannot be transmitted from an infected host to a susceptible host; they are instead caused by lifestyles and inherited predispositions.

Until the 1950s, the emphasis was on the control of infectious diseases in the United States. In the first half of the 20th century, a combination of public health measures and medical care interventions helped bring infectious diseases under control in the United States. The current status of health education is a focus on chronic disease and diseases related to lifestyle choices. Chronic degenerative diseases with a behavior and lifestyle component emerged as the leading causes of death in the United States.[7] However, in countries with poverty and lack of access, many infectious diseases still flourish.

Health behaviors are important **health indicators** in people today. Therefore, the study of current disease rates is important for health educators to help predict the changes necessary to help reduce morbidity, disability, and mortality in a particular population when planning programs.

Inherited, environmental, and behavioral influences can all provoke disease and health **risk factors**. Health disease risk factors can be modifiable, semi-modifiable, and non-modifiable, meaning that some may appear with previous disposition and some may not. Examples of *non-modifiable* health disease risk factors—or those factors we cannot normally change—include race, gender, heredity, age, income, education, healthcare access, environment, and disability.[5] *Semi-modifiable* health disease risk factors are those affected by community, society, group, policy or law, and government interventions. They include environment, access to health care, income, ethnicity, culture, and education. Examples of *modifiable* health disease risk factors—or those that can be changed by the person through lifestyle changes, education, or environmental changes—include riskful behaviors and habits, stress, alcohol abuse, insufficient nutrition, inadequate exercise, smoking, and lack of self-literacy.[5]

The **Communicable Disease** or **Infection Model** is a triangle that depicts the interaction of the agent (disease), host (person), and environment (the setting in which the disease may flourish). This is the triangle effect of the infection model interacting to cause an infectious disease in a new person through a disease-causative agent (infection). The process begins when an agent as a vector (living organism) or fomite (inanimate objects with a vector) enters the host. The environment is desirable for infection to take place. Once infected, the host can communicate it to others via a vector or fomite or even a reservoir. A reservoir is an inanimate object where the vector may multiply. Thus, the vicious cycle of the infection continues. See **Figure 1–1** for the model.

The **Multi-causation Communicable Disease Model** describes when diseases are caused by more than one factor or a combination of factors such as behavior choices, lack of medical care, exposure,

---

Noncommunicable diseases: Chronic diseases caused by behavior, lifestyles, and inherited predispositions and not transmitted from an infected host to a susceptible host.

Health indicators: The statistics or health data that describe health problems and identify trends that help decision makers set priorities and improve global health when designing, implementing, and evaluating health education programs used as health indices.

Risk factors: Inherited, environmental, and behavioral influences capable of provoking disease and unwellness. Health disease risk factors can be modifiable, semimodifiable, and nonmodifiable.

Communicable Disease or Infection Model: A triangle depicting how the agent (disease), host, and environment interact to cause an infectious disease in a new person.

Multi-causation Communicable Disease Model: A model that describes when diseases are caused by more than one factor or a combination of factors such as behavior choices, lack of medical care, exposure, environment, or social circumstances.

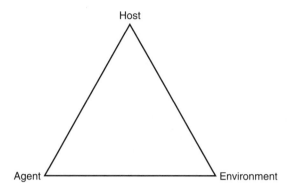

FIGURE 1-1   Communicable Disease Model

environment, or social circumstances. When there are multiple causes, there can be multiple problems finding solutions or cures. Thus, the multi-causation model may need to be treated differently than a single disease-causative agent (see **Figure 1–2**). The **Chain of Infection Model** shows how diseases are spread as pathogens enter the human reservoir, exit, transmit through the portal of entry, and establish the disease in a new host. **Figure 1–3** demonstrates how a single disease agent is transmitted.

HEALTH STATUS CONCEPTS

For the sake of clarity, a modification of **health status categories** may be helpful. Health status is the current state of a person's health, normally including healthy, afflicted, or death. Of course, individuals can move across this continuum, trying to avoid death by improving their health status through treatment options, new discoveries, and behavior and lifestyle changes (unless they have a non-curable or non-reversible illness or disability). We will use a fourth category—non-healthy—to explain the difference between healthy and afflicted. Health status of humans is categorized as:

1. *Healthy*: No sign or symptom of disease, illness, injury, or disability
2. *Non-healthy*: Infected with disease, illness, or injury
3. *Afflicted*: Disabled, impaired, or dependent as result of disease, illness, or injury
4. *Death*: No longer living as a result of an affliction or combination of afflictions

---

Chain of Infection Model: A model that shows how diseases are spread as pathogens enter the human reservoir, exit, transmit through the portal of entry, and establish the disease in a new host.
Health status categories: Healthy, nonhealthy, afflicted, and death.

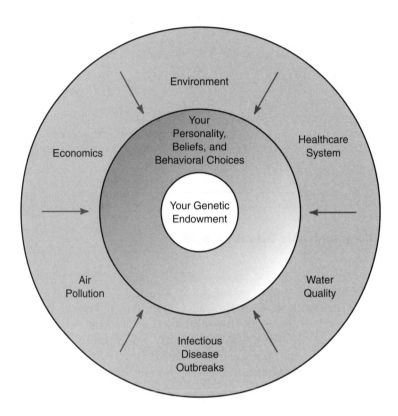

FIGURE 1–2   Multi-causation Disease Model

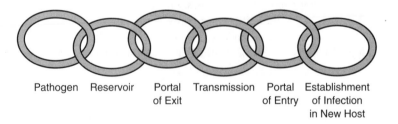

FIGURE 1–3   Chain of Infection Model

CONCEPTS OF HEALTH EDUCATION AND
COMMUNITY HEALTH PROMOTION

Health Education

Health education is a multi-dimensional term that encompasses skills from a variety of disciplines. **Health education** is a combination of planned learning experiences based on proven research theories and models that provide individuals, groups, and communities the needed skills, knowledge, and opportunities to make informed and meaningful health decisions. According to the WHO, "Health education comprises consciously constructed opportunities for learning involving some form of communication designed to improve health literacy, including improving knowledge, and developing life skills which are conducive to individual and community health."[11] According to the Report of the 2000 Joint Committee on Health Education and Promotion Terminology, "Health Education is any combination of planned learning experiences based on sound theories that provide individuals, groups, and communities the opportunity to acquire the information and skills needed to make quality health decisions."[12(p99)] Health education is used in community promotion programs and school health programs.

Comprehensive School Health Education is when formal health education is given as a core curriculum subject in the public schools. Every student in grades K–12 should have the opportunity to participate in comprehensive and coordinated health education as a core curriculum subject. The Comprehensive School Health Program is the part of the coordinated school health program that includes the development, delivery, and evaluation of planned, sequential, and developmentally appropriate instruction, learning experiences, and other activities designed to protect, promote, and enhance the health literacy, attitudes, skills, and well-being of students, pre-kindergarten through grade 12 by certified teachers trained in the subject matter.[13] The content is derived from the **National Health Education Standards**.[14]

The **Coordinated School Health Program** is a set of organized policies, procedures, and activities. When effectively coordinated, they can protect, promote, and improve the health and well-being of students, faculty, and staff, and improve a student's ability to learn. The eight components of a coordinated school health program are 1) comprehensive school health education, 2) school health services, 3) a healthy school environment, 4) school counseling, psychological and social services, 5) physical education,

---

Health education: A combination of planned learning experiences based upon proven research theories and models that provide individuals, groups, and communities the needed skills, knowledge, and opportunities to make informed and meaningful health decisions.

Comprehensive School Health Education: The identified content areas that are recommended as part of the core curriculum in health education in the schools K–12.

National Health Education Standards: Model standards written by the Joint Committee on National Health Education Standards for the health education core curriculum in grades K–12.

Coordinated School Health Program: The eight components determined as part of a planned, sequential, and integrated school health program that meets the health/safety needs of students grades K–12 according to the National Center for Chronic Disease Prevention and Health and the Centers for Disease Control and Prevention.

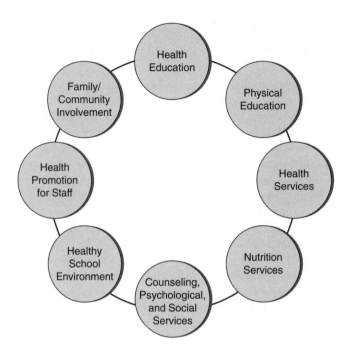

FIGURE 1–4   Coordinated School Health Program Model

Source: Courtesy of the Centers for Disease Control and Prevention, Department of Adolescent and School Health, 2007. Used with permission.

6) school nutrition services, 7) family and community involvement in school health, and 8) school site health promotion for staff.[13] See the Coordinated School Health Program model in **Figure 1–4**.

Health in education is when planned learning experiences within a school system mandate interdisciplinary and curriculum integration programs to make connections with health concepts within other disciplines when there is no formal mandated health curriculum. It takes the form of parallel instruction between two subject areas: (1) cross-disciplinary instruction (i.e., two or more subject areas addressing a common theme), also called curriculum infusion; or (2) a collaborative effort or independent teacher approach where learning focuses on relationships between subject areas.

Formal mandated Comprehensive School Health Education as a core curriculum subject and Coordinated School Health Programs must be enforced using the National Health Education Standards[14] (see Appendix D), the Centers for Disease Control and Prevention's (CDC's) Characteristics of Effective Health Education Curricula and Division of Adolescent and School Health DASH program,[13] and the CDC's Health Education Curriculum Analysis Tool.[15] School Health Advisory Councils (SHAC) are resource consultants to the district and should be mandated for all states and school districts so healthy schools become a reality. SHAC provide expertise and input, and each school district must establish one in every school. SHAC assist in developing objective policies in accordance with community needs. The committee involves school personnel, community health agencies, families, media, healthcare workers, religious and community leaders and organizations, and students. Schools provide a mechanism by which many agencies work together for the well-being of young people.[13] A School Health Education Coordinator should also be mandated for every school district. They are certified health professionals at the state, district, or school district level who manage, coordinate, implement, and evaluate the coordinated school health program and comprehensive school health curriculum.

A state certified, qualified health educator (preferably with CHES credentials) must be hired to implement the Comprehensive School Health Education Curriculum.[13] Too often, school districts assign non-health personnel to teach health or include it in the physical education program with no specific time requirement. While integrating health concepts into physical education is a good practice, a separate health education class taught by a certified health educator is needed.

The **Youth Risk Behavior Surveillance Survey (YRBSS)** monitors priority health risk behaviors and the rates for young people and adolescents. The YRBSS includes a national school-based survey conducted by the CDC and state, territorial, tribal, and local governments.[16] Examining the results can also help schools use research and successful research-based programs within the curriculum.

Health Promotion

Health promotion is the process of enabling people to improve their health by increasing control over the determinants of health. Health education is used in health promotion. The WHO describes health promotion as "a process that enables people to increase control over their health and subsequently, to improve their health."[4] It is a comprehensive social and political process that involves a combination of educational, political, environmental, regulatory, or organizational mechanisms that support the skills and capabilities of individuals' actions and conditions of living. It is directed toward making social, environmental, and economic conditions conducive to the health of individuals, groups, and communities.[11]

Using public policy, laws and regulations to improve health are dealt with carefully. Not mandating too many health behaviors is a balancing act between accepting and promoting health. That is why research and statistics are necessary to back up efforts for regulating health in societies. The Ottawa Charter identified three basic strategies for health promotion: advocacy, enabling, and mediating.[4] The advocacy creates the essential conditions for health. The enabling helps all people achieve their full health potential. The mediating is between the many different interests in society in the pursuit of health. The strategies have five priority areas for health promotion, including building healthy public policy, creating supportive environments for health, strengthening community action for health, developing personal skills, and reorienting health services.[11]

Youth Risk Behavior Surveillance Survey (YRBSS): A telephone survey of randomly selected adolescents about risk factors, preventive health, and access to services and insurance; it monitors priority health-risk behaviors and the rates for young people and adolescents in the United States.

Health promotion: The process of enabling people to improve their health by increasing control over the determinants of health.

Healthy Lifestyles

Every health educator must carry forth the concept of a healthy lifestyle. Healthy behavior patterns maximize quality of life and decrease susceptibility to negative health outcomes. **Quality of life (QOL)** is when a person acquires a sense of satisfaction with his or her life and environment. This concept, according to the WHO, includes all aspects of life that affect health, including rights, values, benefits, beliefs, and conditions.[11] A strategy for a person with disease is to assess his or her quality of life at different times of the day on a 1–10 scale or a pain scale. In arthritis patients, this helps indicate the times of day when pain is more intense and less intense. Perhaps a global quality of life scale should be applied to countries to help demonstrate the areas that need change and to shed light on health problems that may potentially be solved. It could also indicate strengths in countries so less healthy nations could look at the strategies used by healthier nations.

Healthy Communities

The **Healthy People** initiative sets national health goals aimed at eliminating health disparities and improving the quality of life for all Americans. Healthy People 2010 is built on initiatives pursued for more than two decades.[17] The 1979 Surgeon General's Report, Healthy People, and Healthy People 2000: National Health Promotion and Disease Prevention Objectives established national health objectives. These objectives served as a template for providing states, communities, professional organizations, and others with a premier plan. *Healthy People 2010* was a document written by health experts and presents a vision for the future to bring change and improved health to all people in the United States. Healthy People 2010 was developed through a broad consultation process utilizing scientific knowledge and was designed to measure programs over time. Meeting the objectives of Healthy People 2010 represents a challenge to put prevention into practice by choosing healthy behaviors for healthy lifestyle choices. Healthy People 2020 proposed objectives are now being disseminated for comment. The results should be available soon. The additional proposed categories are listed here under the Healthy People 2010 categories that will remain:[17]

1. The leading health indicators defined by Healthy People 2010 are physical activity, overweight and obesity, tobacco use, substance abuse, responsible sexual behavior, mental health, injury and violence, environmental quality, immunization, and access to health care. The first goal of Healthy People 2010 is to increase quality and years of healthy life. It is meant to help individuals of all ages increase life expectancy and improve their quality of life. The second goal is to eliminate health disparities among different segments of the population. The nation's progress in achieving the two goals of Healthy People 2010 was monitored through 467 objectives in these focus areas. These statements helped frame the overall purpose of each focus area. The final results of Healthy

---

Quality of Life: Program Goal: The final aim of a health program that raises the level of health in communities and groups as evidenced by the data collection, epidemiological statistics, and/or statistical computations.
Healthy People 2010 and 2020: A continuous government program led by health experts to present a vision for the future and bring change, prevent disease, and promote improved health to all people in the United States.

People 2010 are being calculated, and the proposed *Healthy People 2020* document will be final-ized in the near future.[17]

2. There are 28 focus areas for Healthy People 2010 that contain a concise goal statement and 38 focus areas proposed for Healthy People 2020. The additional proposed focus categories to Healthy People 2020 are early and middle childhood, genomics, global health, health information technology (added to health communication), healthcare association infections, hearing and other sensory or communication disorders (separated from vision and hearing), weight status (changed from nutrition and overweight), older adults, quality of life and well-being, and determinants of health.[17]

A *healthy community* is described by the United States Department of Health and Human Services in the *Healthy People 2010* document as one that continuously creates and improves both its physical and social environments, helping people to support one another in aspects of daily life, and to develop to their fullest potential.[17] *Healthy places* are those designed and built to improve the quality of life for everyone living, working, learning, and playing in that community. Healthy communities and places are defined by a collective body of individuals identified by geography, common interests, concerns, characteristics, or values. Every person in a healthy place, as a community, must be free to make healthy choices within a variety of available, accessible, and affordable options. A simpler definition of community is the people or persons in a given geographic location that share something in common, such as locale, city, experience, interest, or school district.[18]

Within a healthy community, participation and involvement of the members is important. Active participation can help people assume ownership and responsibility to apply and maintain the programs and/or services developed.[19] Engaging the population in positive changes in behavior and environments through many diverse actions are important. When people accept responsibility for not only their health but also the health of others, positive actions can determine how quickly change can occur. Policy changes are ways to advocate for the greatest overall effect on health. Working together, communities can effect and advocate healthy changes.

Community Health Education is a theory-driven process with the main objectives of promoting health and preventing disease within populations. It is used in community- and school-based health programs facilitated by health educators. The field of Community Health Promotion requires many concepts and skills for appropriate practices with measurable outcomes for lifestyles and communities. Communities are homes for people. The Coordinated School Health Program ensures proper health instruction in grades K–12 along with cooperative efforts from all other health-related aspects in the schools. It includes community-based initiatives to reinforce and promote these life skills. Protecting and improving the health of a community by involving the participants and by continued education beginning at a young age in school health are the best ways to effect quantitative change in improving a higher quality of life for all. Involved participants in effective health programs result in positive community actions. Health education and promotion activities involve health literacy, prevention, promotion, protection, and access for maintaining and enhancing health status resulting in healthy places for all people. Health educators are recognized as an integral part of health promotion outcomes that promote healthy life skills and behaviors in communities and schools with quality programs.

Health Literacy

The WHO in 1998 stated that health literacy "represents the cognitive and social skills which determine the motivation and ability of individuals to gain access to, understand and use information in ways which promote and maintain good health."[11(p10)] Health literacy is the capacity of an individual to obtain, interpret, and understand basic health information and services. The individual possesses the competence to use this information and services in ways that are health enhancing. Health literacy can enable an individual to address the personal, social, and cultural factors that affect positive health.[11] It provides the knowledge, skills, and confidence to take action for improving community and individual health by changing personal lifestyles and living conditions. By improving access to health information and the ability to use the information effectively, health literacy can lead to empowerment for communities and individuals. Health literacy is self-education and an important component of health education. Everyone should be a critical consumer of health information and knowledgeable in using health information resources, including technology.[7] All educational materials (print and media) must be planned with the intended audience's literacy level in mind.

Health education in schools is a vital part of this literacy effort. Health education, if mandated globally in the core curriculum subjects in school systems around the world, could have a huge impact on promoting health. It could offer health skills and information beginning in childhood and encourage healthier behaviors earlier in life. If this program strategy was enacted, its benefit to the health of future generations worldwide would most assuredly be supported and statistically validated. Hubbard and Rainey found that comprehensive health education instruction that includes standards-based texts can assist in developing health literacy.[20] Literacy-appropriate materials are necessary when instructing in the education, community, and global setting.

Health Prevention

Some authors refer to disease prevention or **health prevention** efforts, but the term *prevention* alone is used in this text because more is involved than just preventing disease. It means practicing beneficial health behaviors. Prevention includes actions and interventions designed to identify risks and reduce susceptibility or exposure to health threats before the onset of disease. This includes not engaging in risky behaviors and preventing negative effects from interfering with all aspects of the wellness concepts and health paradigm. Prevention is accomplished by reducing health risk factors, performing healthy behaviors, and alleviating disease to support, preserve, and restore health.[11]

There are four basic types of **prevention**. Generally, three are listed, but other authors agree that a primordial prevention category is necessary. The four types are described as follows:[21]

- *Primordial prevention*: Knowledge of the social, economic, and cultural living patterns that contribute to increased risk of disease

---

Health prevention: The practice of beneficial health behaviors, actions, and interventions designed to identify risks and reduce susceptibility or exposure to health threats before the onset of disease.
Prevention types: The four types of prevention: primordial prevention, primary prevention, secondary prevention, and tertiary prevention.

- *Primary prevention*: Detection and treatment of disease in early stages
- *Secondary prevention*: Protection against progress and recurrence of disease
- *Tertiary prevention*: Alleviation of the effects of disease and injury

Primordial prevention involves predisposition to disease due to outside factors, risk factors, and/or inherited traits (e.g., genetic testing could determine a risk, which could then possibly be prevented through existing medical interventions and/or social change); primary prevention is to reduce incidence (e.g., immunizations), secondary prevention is to reduce prevalence (e.g., screenings), and tertiary prevention is to reduce impact (e.g., rehabilitation).[21,22]

Prevention is planning for and taking measures to forestall the onset of disease or other health problems before the occurrence of undesirable health events, or taking measures to reduce disease reoccurrence. Health restoration is when a person has regained his or her health status to the degree before disease onset. It can be accomplished with numerous means, the greatest of which is proper medical care, treatment, and rehabilitation for curable diseases. All types of prevention cover measures to reduce risk factors. These are actions that undermine the progress and reduce consequences of diseases if risk or risk factors are established and combated. Risk factor reduction efforts and beneficial health behaviors can help reduce the probability of disease risks, disease disability, and debilitating health conditions for individuals, groups, or communities.[11]

Health Protection

Health protection is when a person or community has in place available health shields enabling a high quality of life. It involves the traditional beliefs of physical and mental protection as well as spiritual and/or religious adherence.[2] Protection offers a home or community where safeguards are deliberately put in place that contribute to a healthy lifestyle and environment. Defining the shields necessary is not always easy and usually requires behavior and/or environmental changes. Defining what are healthy practices and reducing or eliminating unhealthy practices is not always easy. According to the CDC, "Healthy places are those designed and built to improve the quality of life for all people who live, work, worship, learn, and play within their borders—where every person is free to make choices amid a variety of healthy, available, accessible, and affordable options."[23(p1)]

The health protection shield is similar to the moat of a castle. It is like an invisible circle of particular health behaviors, community, environmental interventions, and laws and practices that safeguard people and communities. They are put in place to continuously arm against negative health effects and promote a high quality of life. In reality, a lot of these are voluntary practices, but policy and education can promote this concept. Environmental quality laws, safety laws, and food quality laws and regulations are example of protective factors. The CDC has created a set of four overarching Health Protection Goals. These are supported by goals and objectives. The goals are healthy people in every state of life, healthy people in healthy places, people prepared for emerging health threats, and healthy people in a healthy world.[23] These goals are essentially health shields that, when enacted, protect human health.

> **Health protection:** Health shields or traditional beliefs that a person or community has in place to provide physical and mental protection and spirituality, enabling a high quality of life.

Healthcare Access

Access to quality health care and disease control tools such as clinics, medical personnel, drugs, vaccines, and diagnostics is a critical health determinant of populations. There is general agreement that equitable access to health technologies needs improvement, but there is a lack of consensus on what access actually means. Health educators need to determine how it can be measured and apply knowledge to identify and forge relationships between access and the outcomes of health.[1] Access applies to such factors as healthcare delivery systems, including availability and location of services, health insurance coverage and benefits, and understandable language.[2] Barriers to health are numerous, but the greatest is the cycle of poverty (see **Figure 1–5**).[2(p110)]

Health Enhancement and Maintenance

Health enhancement and maintenance are integral parts of continuing the work of health education, even when programs may no longer be available in communities. **Health maintenance** is the everyday way that people attempt to stay well and include proper clothing, food, healthcare access, and social support.[2] **Health enhancement** is extraordinary measures taken to continuously improve one's health.

The concept of empowerment or social action is very important for health education, enhancement, and maintenance.[11] There are three types of health empowerment: delegated, enabled, and assumed empowerment. *Enabled* empowerment involves bringing about some beneficial action and is the most common reference used, *delegated* empowerment involves transferring power from one group or person to another; and *assumed* empowerment involves taking power through self-actualization.[24] When skills and ways of life are institutionalized or embedded in lives and communities, the people will continue to advocate and become caretakers for themselves and their communities. The Community Tool Box (CTB) defines **institutionalization** as "...the active process of establishing your initiative—not merely continuing your program, but developing relationships, practices, and procedures that become a lasting part of the community."[18,p.1A,Ch.1,Sec.5] The CTB also states that empowerment should be part of evaluation and should aim "to assess the effort's worth while improving the community's desire and ability to take care of its own problems."[18]

Thought Concept

What does the saying "health is wealth" mean?

Access: The availability of quality health care and disease control tools including clinics, medical personnel, drugs, vaccines, and diagnostics; it is a critical health determinant of populations.
Health maintenance: The everyday way that people attempt to stay well, including such considerations as proper clothing, food, shelter, healthcare access, healthful environment, and social support.
Health enhancement: Extraordinary measures taken to continuously improve one's health.
Institutionalization: The organizational factors that address rules, regulations, policies, and informal structures that can restrict or support the behaviors recommended.

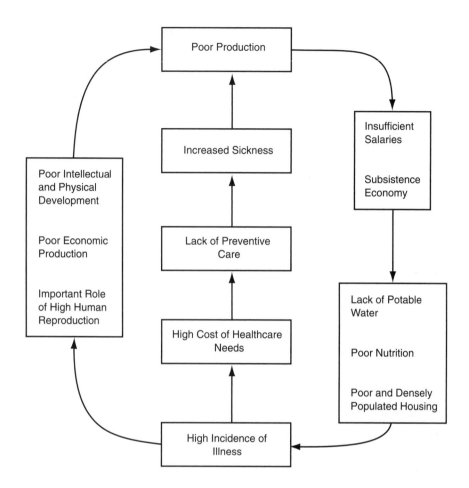

FIGURE 1–5   The Cycle of Poverty

Source: Reproduced from Spector, R. E., Cultural Diversity in Health and Illness, 7th ed. © N/A.
Electronically reproduced by permission of Pearson Education, Inc., Upper Saddle River, New Jersey.

HEALTH DETERMINANTS, EPIDEMIOLOGY, AND STATISTICS

The WHO lists several factors that define disease,[25] saying that a disease is any dysfunction in any of
the body systems characterized by symptomatology, etiology, course and outcome, treatment response,
linkage to genetic factors, and linkage to interacting environmental factors. **Epidemiology** is the study

Epidemiology: The study of the distribution and disease transmission in humans including descriptives, statistics, causes, rates, risks, trends, and problem solving.

of disease transmission in humans including descriptives, statistics, causes, rates, risks, trends, and problem solving. Last described it as "...the study of the distribution and determinants of health related states or events in defined populations, and the application of this study to control health problems."[22(pp55–56)] Epidemiology provides the basis for disease prevention activities and identification of disease transmission and origins in society. Epidemiological information defines individual, population, and/or physical environmental risks.

Epidemiology uses social classifications (such as socioeconomic status) to study human disease but mainly investigates disease and health in populations.[11] It also looks at health risks for diseases. **Social-behavioral epidemiology** examines the behavioral components to lifestyle-related diseases and infectious diseases such as sexually transmitted diseases.[21] It is a study of biological, cultural, and social phenomenon for analysis. Chronic diseases could also fall under the purview of social-behavioral epidemiology, considering that epidemiologists are tracking and studying these non-infectious, lifestyle-related diseases and are studying behavior and lifestyle characteristics that increase or reduce risks for certain chronic diseases. Perhaps a better term is simply behavioral epidemiology, which covers chronic and infectious disease patterns, inherited diseases, and the relationship to all factors involved in a person's lifestyle and behaviors.

Health statistics refers to the data collection techniques that rely upon **health indices**, or indicators, to design, implement, and evaluate health education programs. Statistics collect and compare international, national, state, and local health data as a way to describe health problems, identify trends, help decision-makers set priorities, and improve global health.[25] The WHO is the international component for collecting global health information statistics. This organization collects disease statistics globally and alerts countries to epidemiological events and/or crises. The WHO generates the World Health Report, which is an authoritative annual report that assesses the health of the world and makes recommendations for improvement.[26]

National statistics for the United States are collected and reported by the National Institutes of Health (NIH) and the CDC. The NIH's mission is to provide for medical and behavioral research and promotes "science in pursuit of fundamental knowledge about the nature and behavior of living systems and the application of that knowledge to extend healthy life and reduce the burdens of illness and disability."[6(p1)] It comprises 27 institutes and centers. In addition, the NIH provides leadership and financial support for researchers in states and the world and is the nation's medical research agency. The NIH is part of the U.S. Department of Health and Human Services (USDHHS). Thus, it is the primary U.S. federal agency that conducts and supports medical research. NIH scientists institute strategies to prevent disease and address the causes, treatments, and cures for diseases. They also contribute to important medical discoveries for improving people's health and reducing mortality. As the leading public health agency in the United States, the CDC uses science for all factors that affect the nation's health. The CDC's major health concerns today are the interaction between people and their environ-

---

Social-behavioral epidemiology: The study of biological, cultural, and social phenomena for analysis.
Health statistics: The data collection techniques used for health indices or indicators in groups.
Health indices: The statistics collected to compare international, national, state, and local health data as a way to describe health problems.

ments. The CDC is committed to achieving true improvements in people's lives by accelerating health impact and reducing health disparities.[27]

For state population demographics and vital statistics in the Unites States, there are state, county, and city data centers and agencies for access to current statistics. The CDC and NIH also contribute to the state statistics data collection. Rates of both communicable and non-communicable diseases are recorded and documented systematically as **surveillance** efforts. Surveillance efforts are important for reducing mortality, morbidity, and disability. These collected rates are also important for trend analyses and for determining epidemics, and other disease patterns. **Etiology** agents are the causes of diseases. The purpose of surveillance is to document total diseases in geographic areas, communicate disease necessary interventions, identify disease changes, identify new emerging diseases, track disease patterns and risk factors, and provide laboratory services for isolating these etiology agents.[21]

The **determinants of health** are very closely related to the health statistics, since most ultimately determine the health of an individual. These are the personal, social, economic, and environmental factors that determine health status.[11] Determinants of health precipitate a new direction for focusing on the basics of shelter, education, safety, food, income, secure economic systems, resources, social justice, equity, and policies affecting social determinants of health.

Spector[2] says that **cultural components** and other major factors are very significant health determinants. She defines **culture** as "Non-physical traits, such as values, beliefs, attitudes and customs, that are shared by a group of people and passed from one generation to the next."[2(p358)] It consists of learned experiences (socialization) by which people learn how to see and interpret their environment. Heritage consistency includes culture, ethnicity, and religious background, which also affect health. Factors affecting these three concepts are social organization, communication, space, time, biological variations, and environmental control. **Acculturation**, or adapting to another culture, also affects health status.[2] Sometimes detrimental compromises for health are made in acculturation or improved health results from immersion into a culture with more beneficial health practices. Some health determinants are presented in **Figure 1–6**.

Measurement and Rates

Rates are measures of an event, disease, or condition that determines health or health status in a population along with time specifications. The WHO is the definitive world reporting agency for disease- and

---

Surveillance: Systematic recording and documenting of rates of both communicable and noncommunicable diseases.
Etiology: The study of disease causes.
Determinants of health: The personal, social, economic, and environmental factors that determine health status, focusing on the basics of health maintenance.
Cultural components: The behavioral components of lifestyles and learned experiences (socialization) that determine how people learn to see and interpret their environment.
Culture: The learned experiences (socialization) and knowledge people gain through their environment.
Acculturation: The process of adapting to another culture.
Rates: Measures of an event, disease, or condition that determine health or health status in a unit of population along with time specification.

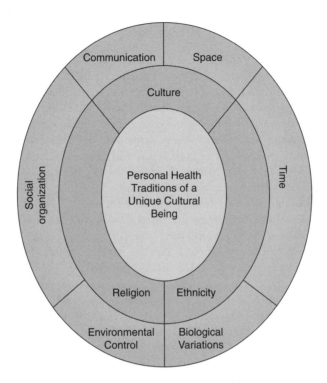

FIGURE 1–6   Personal Health Traditions of a Unique Cultural Being

Source: Reproduced from Spector, R. E., Cultural Diversity in Health and Illness, 7th ed. © N/A. Electronically reproduced by permission of Pearson Education, Inc., Upper Saddle River, New Jersey.

other health-related statistics on an annual basis. It studies the cause, or etiology, of the disease and gathers data on disease outbreaks. These basic demographic and health characteristics of populations provide the scores used for determining the relevant rates and ratios for the world, nations, and cities, and also determine disease patterns. Formulas and ratios are used for determining the rates. Rates are collected in two ways, enumeration and registration. Enumeration is done by taking a census of a population, usually every decade. Registration is the continuous, permanent, and mandated recording of the occurrences and characteristics of vital events.[28]

The WHO has been instrumental in helping to adopt methods, norms, and guidelines for gathering health statistics. It also promotes analyzing, reporting, and interpreting data and information. These statistical rates collected can help monitor and evaluate health trends, risks, and diseases and the impact of health-related interventions. The WHO promotes developing basic health data systems worldwide and the coordination and cooperation of information systems and services throughout the world.[29]

The Life Expectancy (LE) rate is based on age-specific death rates. These indicate the average number of years of life at a particular age for people.[30] Life Expectancy at Birth (LEB) rate compares

TABLE 1-1 CRUDE RATES			
Name of Rate		**Definition of Rate**	**Multiplier**
Crude birth rate	=	$\dfrac{\text{Number of live births}}{\text{Estimated midyear population}}$ ×	1,000
Crude death rate	=	$\dfrac{\text{Number of deaths (all causes)}}{\text{Estimated midyear population}}$ ×	1,000

the progress of health status between gender and population groups.[30] The Years of Healthy Life (YHL) rate measures life years without any disease, injury, or disability, while the Years of Potential Life Lost (YPLL) rate measures premature mortality when the age of 75 years is subtracted from the age at death.[30]

Mortality rates are death or fatality rates due to disease or injury, and most are expressed in populations per 100,000. Excess mortality rates are the differences between the number of deaths in a group and the number of expected deaths with the general population. Crude morality rates are not good indicators of risk because they are generalized rates. Adjusted crude rates are better indicators. However, age, birth, and disease-specific rates are significant indicators. These adjusted rates refer to total population rates that are statistically adjusted for a certain population subgroup, for a particular disease (i.e., disease-specific rates), or for certain characteristics such as age, gender, race, or community (i.e., cause-specific rates). **Relative risk** is a measure of the association between exposure and outcome. It is reported as an identified risk factor for that outcome (disease or injury).[21] Rates are measurement instruments that provide statistical data useful for determining health program needs. **Tables 1–1** and **1–2** show how different disease rates are calculated.

Community rates are very specific indicators for measuring health and health status for people in a given area. It is always a good idea to look at the global rates and country rates for overall rates, but specific area rates give individual health indicators for specific areas. For example, in the United States, health educators examine state, county, and city rates to get a clear picture of risk for certain diseases. These city or community rates are very important for targeting risk factors. Formulas have been developed for the most commonly used vital and health statistics.[28]

The following list describes the types of rates commonly used in measuring disease, illness, and accident occurrence in humans:

- Mortality rates measure the number of deaths from a certain disease or illness or accident.
- **Morbidity rates** measure the number of persons infected with a disease or illness or accident.
- **Incidence rates** measure new case numbers of people infected with a disease or illness or accident in a specified time.

Mortality rates: Measures of death due to disease or injury; most are expressed in populations per 100,000.
Relative risk: A measure of the association between exposure and outcome.
Morbidity rates: The number of persons infected with a disease or illness.
Incidence rates: The new case numbers of people infected with a disease or illness in a specified time.

TABLE 1–2   SAMPLE RATES IN EPIDEMIOLOGY

Rate		Definition		Multiplier	Examples
Age-specific death rate	=	$\dfrac{\text{Number of deaths, 15-24}}{\text{Estimated midyear population, 15-24}}$	×	100,000	79.2/100,000
Infant mortality rate	=	$\dfrac{\text{Number of deaths under 1 year of age}}{\text{Number of live births}}$	×	1,000	6.76/1,000
Neonatal mortality rate	=	$\dfrac{\text{Number of deaths under 28 days of age}}{\text{Number of live births}}$	×	1,000	4.5/1,000
Cause-specific death rate	=	$\dfrac{\text{Number of deaths (diabetes mellitus)}}{\text{Estimated midyear population}}$	×	100,000	24.8/100,000
Age-specific, cause-specific death rate	=	$\dfrac{\text{Number of deaths, 15-24 (motor vehicles)}}{\text{Estimated midyear population}}$	×	100,000	26.1/100,000

- **Prevalence rates** measure the number of community cases of a disease, illness, or accident existing at a given time. These rates include all causes of a specific disease, illness, or accident among a specific group of people in a specified time.
- **Point prevalence** measures the number of disease, illness or accident cases existing in a defined population at a defined point in time.
- **Endemic rates** measure the number of disease, illness, or accident cases that occur in a population regularly.
- **Epidemic rates** measure large numbers of disease, illness, or accident cases not normally expected in a population. These are usually given within 6 to 12 month ratios.
- **Pandemic rates** measure the number of disease, illness, or accident outbreaks over a very large geographic area.
- Natality rates measure birth rates.
- Cases measure the number of health related events as morbidity and mortality.
- Incidence rates measure the number of new disease, illness, or accident cases within a given time.

Prevalence rates: The number of community disease cases existing at a given time.
Point prevalence: The number of active disease cases existing in a defined population at a defined point in time.
Endemic rates: Large numbers of disease cases that occur in a population regularly.
Epidemic rates: Large numbers of disease cases not normally expected in a population.
Pandemic rates: Disease outbreaks over a very large geographic area.

TABLE 1–3   INCIDENCE, PREVALENCE, AND ATTACK RATES

Name of Rate	Definition of Rate
Incidence rate	$= \dfrac{\text{Number of new health-related events or cases of a disease}}{\text{Number of people exposed to risk during this period}}$
Prevalence rate	$= \dfrac{\text{Total number of all individuals who have an attribute or disease at a time}}{\text{Population at risk of having the attribute or disease at this point or period of time}}$
Attack rate*	$= \dfrac{\text{The cumulative incidence of infection in a group observed during an epidemic}}{\text{Number of people exposed}} \times 100$

*Attack rates are usually given as a percentage.

- Annual incidence rates measure the number of new disease, illness, or accident cases occurring within a specific year.[28]
- Sporadic rates measure that number of disease, illness, or accident cases that appear irregularly.
- Attack rates are special incidence rates calculated for a single disease, illness, or accident outbreak and expressed as a percentage.
  See **Table 1–3** for examples of some standardized formulas used for determining these rates. However, there is no universal system globally for how these disease, illness, or accident statistics are collected, reported, or formulated among nations, making it difficult to report worldwide disease information accurately.

Disability measures are expressed in terms of healthy life rate loss and survival rates. The Disability-Adjusted Life Years (DALY) or Years Lived with Disability (YLD) indicates the number of years a person is afflicted with a disabling condition. This measure is used to express the burden of living with disability. One DALY is equal to one lost year of life. A fairly new measure is Disability-Adjusted Life Expectancy (DALE) or healthy life expectancy. It is estimated from the life tables and adjusted with estimates for disability and other non-fatal health outcomes to indicate the healthy survival rate for those living with a disability.[30]

National Health Surveys and Data Collection

Several groundbreaking surveys and data collection centers had an impact on the health of the United States as a result of the National Health Survey Act of 1956.[31] This act provided for a continuing survey and studies to secure current, accurate statistical information on the amount, distribution, and effects of disease and disability in the United States. The act sparked new and additional surveys and data collection, including the following:

1. The National Health Interview Survey by the National Center for Health Statistics (NCHS), which consisted of a telephone survey on health and behaviors[32]
2. The National Health and Nutrition Examination Survey (NHANES), which collected data through direct physical exams as well as clinical and lab tests
3. The National Vital Statistics System, which consisted of intergovernmental data sharing on vital and health statistics
4. The National Health Care Surveys, including The National Hospital Discharge Survey (NHDS) and The National Hospital Ambulatory Survey (NHAMCS), which surveyed hospital and clinical practices
5. The National Immunization Survey, which gives estimates of childhood vaccination rates recommended by the Advisory Committee on Immunization Practices (ACIP)[31]
6. The Behavioral Risk Factor Surveillance System and the Youth Risk Factor Behavior Surveillance System, which consisted of a telephone survey of randomly selected adults and adolescents about risk factors, preventive health, and access to services and insurance[16]

Each survey brought about empirical standardized data on physical, clinical, and psychological research based on the health of Americans. Medical and health practitioners and educators used these results to effect positive changes in disease prevention and control efforts, risk factor surveillance data, hospital care and discharge policies, and ultimately, health status. The National Health Care Surveys provided vital information to healthcare policy makers and researchers. This information is used in decision making and influences the quality of health care, the use of healthcare resources, and disparities in healthcare services provided to populations in the United States.[31]

Health and wellness are used interchangeably but have different meanings. Health is the status of a person's body, mind, and spirit. Wellness concerns the choices a person makes which that affect a high quality and quantity of life. Healthy lifestyles affect Healthy Communities. A health educator's job is health education. A health educator works towards the primary concepts of health, including prevention, promotion, literacy, protection, and access to services to preserve, maintain, and enhance healthy lifestyles in healthy communities.

Comprehensive School Health Education (CSHE) is the content curriculum, and Coordinated School Health Programs include everything in the school that affects the students' health. The Healthy People initiative began in the 1970s and has continued to set national health goals aimed at eliminating health disparities and improving the quality of life for all Americans.

Health statistics are collected in many different ways. Some examples of types of rates used include mortality, morbidity, incidence, and prevalence.

HEALTH APPLICATIONS

There is an even more pressing need for health professionals and health educators today. The Alma-Alta Conference advocated primary health care for all, with solidarity and participation as priorities. Social justice and the right to better health for all was reiterated at this international conference.[26] Primary health care is paramount in addressing new health challenges to improving and maintaining health. World health gaps have widened, and cultural and health disparities remain unchecked in many countries, including the United States. Social, democratic, and epidemiological transformations, along with globalization, urbanization, and aging populations pose challenges not anticipated many years ago.[26]

The World Health Report recommends a response to the challenges of a changing world and narrowing the gap between aspirations and reality. The report recommends that all countries secure healthier communities through public policy reforms, universal coverage reforms with access and service protection, service delivery reforms centered on people's needs and expectations, and leadership reforms centered around more effective government and more active participation of the stakeholders.[26]

It is difficult to determine the 10 leading causes of death in the world because the data collection systems are different. The World Health Organization makes a concerted effort to publish the statistics they are able to collect[26] (see **Table** 1–4). The list also differs depending on the income of a particular country and other variables. A standardized global data collection system is needed. The world faces many health challenges, including poverty, control of infectious and chronic diseases, and the threat of chemical terrorism. Coalitions and world health organizations should continue to work together for data collection, to advocate for improved health of all populations, and to try to solve as many health, social, and environmental problems as possible for the benefit of all humans. [26] Health education needs global implementation so every school system from beginning to end will include health in the school curriculum. Such programs will promote health literacy, healthier nutrition intake, life skills, and safe and healthy lifestyles earlier in life when habits are formed.

The world and the United States are becoming increasingly diverse. In developed countries, the population is living longer, and in many countries, minority population groups are growing. Meeting the health needs of these multicultural populations that differ from the norm requires cultural sensitivity and competence in dealing with the customs, values, and beliefs of other cultures and communities. Cultural sensitivity refers to respect and tolerance. Cultural differences, beliefs, traditions, and community ideologies often interfere with communication between minority groups and health educators and healthcare practitioners. These differences should be viewed as sources of identifying likenesses and understanding similarities with social support and connections across cultures and communities.[7] **Cultural competence** is the ability to work with other cultures with sensitivity, effectiveness, and respect for their differences. It is the responsibility of all health educators to become culturally sensitive and competent when working in communities. Another responsibility is helping to bring about social and organizational change for health programs, policies, interests, and populations.

The United States faces many individual, community, and group societal health challenges. The epidemic of overweight and obesity, brought on by lifestyle choices of physical inactivity and poor diet, is a huge challenge to our nation's health.[33] The leading causes of death (according to the NCHS) in the United States today are mainly chronic diseases brought on by lifestyle choices (see **Figure** 1–7). Political, social, economic, educational, and ethical issues arise when these serious health problems are combated.[7] Individual decision making is vitally important for people's health in supportive, healthy communities. These healthy communities are defined by their health education efforts in prevention, promotion, protection, literacy, enhancement, maintenance, and access for all citizens.

Cultural competence: The ability to work with other cultures with sensitivity, effectiveness, and respect for their differences.

TABLE 1-4   THE TEN LEADING CAUSES OF DEATH
Differences in High-Low Economic Countries and All Countries (Worldwide)

	High Economic Countries	Middle Economic Countries	Low Economic Countries	All Countries
Coronary Heart Disease	1	2	2	1
Stroke and Other Cerebrovascular Diseases	2	1	5	2
Lower Respiratory Infections	4	4	1	3
Chronic Obstructive Pulmonary Disease	5	3	6	4
Diarrheal Diseases	N/A	N/A	3	5
HIV/AIDS	N/A	N/A	4	6
Tuberculosis	N/A	9	7	7
Trachea, Bronchus, Lung Cancers	3	5	N/A	8
Road Traffic Accidents	N/A	6	N/A	9
Prematurity and Low Birth Weight	N/A	N/A	10	10
Alzheimer and Other Dementia	6	N/A	N/A	N/A
Colon and Rectum Cancers	7	N/A	N/A	N/A
Diabetes Mellitus	8	10	N/A	N/A
Breast Cancer	9	N/A	N/A	N/A
Stomach Cancer	10	8	N/A	N/A
Hypertensive Heart Disease	N/A	7	N/A	N/A
Malaria	N/A	N/A	9	N/A
Neonatal Infections	N/A	N/A	8	N/A

Scale of 1–10 (1 being the highest cause of death).
Source: Adapted from World Health Organization, The Top Ten Causes of Death, Fact Sheet no. 310, Retrieved Jan 26, 2009, from http://www.who.int/mediacentre/factsheets/fs310/en/index/htm

Ethnographic and qualitative approaches to community health have shown the importance of improved social determinants to increased health and well-being. The role of educating the public and policy makers needs to be implemented. Supporting public action policy for health is paramount to improving a higher quality of life. More political engagement and health associations advocating action on health determinants issues are needed. Equitable distribution of wealth and progressive tax policies are a necessity. Health advocates today must be political to achieve a healthier, more progressive world

- Number of deaths: 2,426,264
- Death rate: 810.4 deaths per 100,000 population
- Life expectancy: 77.7 years
- Infant mortality rate: 6.69 deaths per 1,000 live births

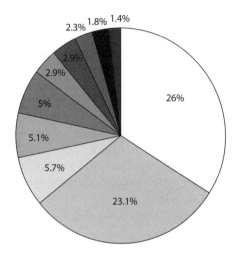

Number of deaths for leading causes of death:

- Heart disease: 631,636 = 26%
- Cancer: 559,888 = 23.1%
- Stroke (cerebrovascular diseases): 137,119 = 5.7%
- Chronic lower respiratory diseases: 124,583 = 5.1%
- Accidents (unintentional injuries): 121,599 = 5%
- Diabetes: 72,449 = 2.9%
- Alzheimer's disease: 72,432 = 2.9%
- Influenza and pneumonia: 56,326 = 2.3%
- Nephritis, nephrotic syndrome, and nephrosis: 45,344 = 1.8%
- Septicemia: 34,234 = 1.4%

FIGURE 1–7   Leading Causes of Death in the United States, 2006
Source: Modified from Centers for Disease Control and Prevention, National Center for Health Statistics, Deaths: Final Data for 2006. http://www.cdc.gov/nchs/fastats/deaths.htm

with equal opportunity for all. Health educators can address health determinants in practice. Shaping health policies with positive changes means conveying education programs and knowledge transference to all policy makers who affect health determinants. Raphael in 2008 stated that health professionals need to look back and look forward to a new focus since political, economic, and social forces differ by country, region, and community.[34] Health and disease patterns are a global problem, and global statistical data are necessary to understand and interpret smart solutions with progressive, problem-solving health programs. Good health must be viewed and promoted by all governments as a basic human right for everyone throughout the globe.

SUMMARY

- Many factors other than physical ones affect health. Wellness is a broad concept enveloping all the aspects of a person's life that influence health.
- A health educator is a trained professional who encourages prevention and promotion of health through programs.

- Communicable diseases are transmitted from person to person, while non-communicable diseases are caused by lifestyle choices and inherited traits. Some disease risk factors are modifiable, and some are non-modifiable.
- The communicable disease model and multi-causation model explain disease transmission in humans.
- Health status is measured in four categories ranging from healthy to death.
- Healthy communities are results of appropriate health literacy, prevention, promotion, protection, access, enhancement, and maintenance.
- Health education refers to the process of transmitting health knowledge to enable a desirable quality of life.
- Comprehensive School Health Education incorporates the National Health Education Standards and is the inclusive element of Coordinated School Health programs.
- CHES is a designation for the profession.
- The YRBSS monitors health behaviors in young people.
- Healthy People is a government effort that provides a vision for health in the United States.
- Epidemiology is the study of disease and health determinants. Rates refer to statistical measures of health or health status or accidents (unintentional injuries) and are reported in many different ways, including morbidity and mortality.
- National health surveys convey important health information for designing health prevention and promotion programs.

CONCEPTUAL TERMS

Quality of life
World Health Organization (WHO)
Health
Wellness
Profession
Health educator
Certified Health Education Specialist (CHES)
Communicable diseases
Non-communicable diseases
Health indicators
Risk factors
Communicable Disease or Infection Model
Multi-causation Communicable Disease Model
Chain of Infection Model
Health status categories
Health education
Comprehensive School Health Education
National Health Education Standards
Coordinated School Health Program
Youth Risk Behavior Surveillance Survey (YRBSS)

Health promotion
Healthy People 2010 and 2020
Health prevention
Prevention types
Health protection
Access
Health maintenance
Health enhancement
Institutionalization
Epidemiology
Social-behavioral epidemiology
Health statistics
Health indices
Surveillance
Etiology
Determinants of health
Cultural components
Culture
Acculturation
Rates

Mortality rates
Relative risk
Morbidity rates
Incidence rates
Prevalence rates

Endemic rates
Epidemic rates
Pandemic rates
Cultural competence

REFLECTIVE THINKING

You are a health educator in the public schools. The state mandates immunizations for all enrolled students. However, there is a waiver in place for religious reasons; a note from a student's church leader is an accepted reason for the student to not receive the required immunizations. You are informed by your principal that a student in your school contracted measles and one student is not immunized for religious reasons. Laws preclude releasing the students' names to the teachers or parents, but the fact that there has been an occurrence of measles is reported to the proper authorities, and all students and teachers are monitored due to the threat of contracting the disease. The parents of the unimmunized child still refuse to immunize their child once informed of the health threat. One of the teachers in your school recently found out she is pregnant. What are the disease transmission risks and other health risks for the students, teachers, administrators, and staff? What is the role of the principal in enforcing health measures in the school and/or providing recommendations to the students, teachers, parents, and community? What are the requirements (considering agencies and legal responsibility) for the principal in reporting this communicable disease?

CONCEPTUAL LEARNING

1. Differentiate between communicable diseases and non-communicable diseases. List the disease trends in developed and underdeveloped countries regarding these two types of diseases.
2. Examine and explain the differences in disease transmission in humans using the Communicable Disease Model and the Multi-causation Communicable Disease Model. Give an example of a disease caused by each model.
3. Compare these different rates: Life Expectancy (LE), Life Expectancy at Birth (LEB), Years of Healthy Life (YHL), and Years of Potential Life Lost (YPLL). What factors influence life expectancy at birth? How does disability affect the years of healthy life and years of potential life lost?
4. Explain age-specific rates, cause-specific rates, and disease-specific rates. Distinguish between the age-specific rates and gender-specific rates for life expectancy. What are the health implications of identifying these rates?
5. Compare and contrast the worldwide traditional indices of health status including the mortality and morbidity rates from the WHO's data. Find the latest data publication of the leading causes of death and work backward until you have a five-year period or trend chart.
6. Differentiate between the following measurement rates: incidence, prevalence, endemic, epidemic, pandemic, and sporadic.

7. Demonstrate how each of the following rates is calculated: excess mortality rate, crude morality rate, adjusted crude rate, Disability-Adjusted Life Years (DALY) or Years Lived with Disability (YLD), and Disability-Adjusted Life Expectancy (DALE). Create your own definition of the following concepts: health literacy, prevention, promotion, protection, enhancement, maintenance, and access.

9. List and define at least five basic professional concepts and five practice settings of the health education profession.

10. In your own words, define and summarize the terms community health, health education, and health educator. Cite three examples in professional references that back up your definition of health education. Revisit your definitions at the end of the course to see if you want to revise your definitions.

11. Differentiate between three specific health determinants in populations. Prioritize the importance of each health determinant on a scale of 1 to 10, with 10 being the most important determinant of health.

12. Summarize the importance of the 1979 Surgeon General's report entitled *Healthy People: The Surgeon General's Report on Health Promotion and Disease Prevention*. Identify three specific provisions of this report. Identify the latest *Healthy People* report, and relate the goals, the number of priority areas, and the categories and number of objectives.

13. Research two of the following national health surveys. Evaluate each and give examples of how they impacted health in the United States. Surveys include the National Health Interview Survey by the National Center for Health Statistics (NCHS), National Health and Nutrition Examination Survey (NHANES), Youth Risk Behavior Surveillance Survey (YRBSS), National Hospital Discharge Survey (NHDS) by the NCHS, and National Hospital Ambulatory Survey (NHAMCS).

14. Construct your own definition of a health educator and the term "community health wellness." Revisit your definitions at the end of the course to see if you want to revise or change the definitions.

15. Defend the use of the Certified Health Education Specialist (CHES) credential in the health profession. Discuss two examples of how it has improved the profession.

16. Discuss prevention factors (against disease) within your own community. List and explain at least three significant risk factors for disease in your community. What strategies could be used in a health program to reduce these risk factors?

17. List the four categories of prevention and relate a specific example of each.

REFERENCES

1. Oswaldo Cruz Foundation. (2006). *Equitable access to health care and infectious disease control—concepts, measurement and interventions*. Conference News No 19, United Nations Research Institute for Social Development (UNRISD). Retrieved January 15, 2009, from http://www.unrisd.org

2. Spector, R. E. (1996). *Cultural diversity in health and illness* (4th ed.). Stanford, CT: Appleton and Lange.

3. World Health Organization. (1947). *Constitution of the World Health Organization*. Chronicle of the World Health Organization. Geneva, Switzerland: Author.

4. World Health Organization. (1986). *Ottawa charter for health promotion*. Geneva, Switzerland: Author. Retrieved February 20, 2010, from http://www.who.int/healthpromotion/conferences/previous/ottawa/en/

5. Insel, P. M., & Roth, W. T. (2008). *Core concepts in health* (10th ed.). New York: McGraw-Hill.

6. National Institutes of Health. (2008, November). *About NIH and occupational health.* Retrieved February 20, 2010, from http://www.nih.gov/about/index.html#mission

7. Teague, M. L., Mackenzie, S. L. C., & Rosenthal, D. M. (2007). *Your health today: Choices in a changing society.* New York: McGraw-Hill.

8. Merriam Webster Online Dictionary. (2009). *Profession.* Retrieved February 20, 2010, from http://www.merriam-webster.com/dictionary/profession17

9. United States Department of Labor, Bureau of Labor Statistics. (2010–2011 ed.). *Occupational outlook handbook, health educators.* Retrieved January 15, 2009, from http://www.bls.gov/oco/ocos063.htm

10. National Commission for Health Education Credentialing, Inc. (2002). *Main menu.* Retrieved February 20, 2010, from http://www.nchec.org/

11. World Health Organization. (1998). *The WHO health promotion glossary.* Retrieved February 20, 2010, from http://www.who.int/healthpromotion/about/HPG/en/index.html

12. Joint Committee on Health Education and Health Promotion Terminology. (2001). Report of the 2000 Joint Committee on Health Education and Health Promotion Terminology. *American Journal of Health Education, 32*(2), 89–103.

13. Centers for Disease Control and Prevention. (2007). *Healthy youth and characteristics of effective health education curricula.* Retrieved February 20, 2010, from http://www.cdc.gov/HealthyYouth/index.htm

14. The Joint Committee on National Health Education Standards. (2007). *National health education standards: Achieving excellence* (2nd ed.). Atlanta: American Cancer Society.

15. Centers for Disease Control and Prevention. (2009). *Health Education Curriculum Analysis Tool (HECAT).* Retrieved February 20, 2010, from http://www.cdc.gov/HealthyYouth/HECAT/index.htm

16. National Center for Chronic Disease Prevention and Health Promotion Data and Statistics. (2008). *YRBSS: Youth Risk Behavior Surveillance System.* Retrieved February 20, 2010, from http://www.cdc.gov/HealthyYouth/yrbs/index.htm

17. United States Department of Health and Human Services. Office of Disease Prevention and Health Promotion. (2000). *Healthy People 2010* (2nd ed.). Retrieved February 20, 2010, from from http://www.healthypeople.gov/default.htm

18. Kansas University Work Group on Health Promotion and Community Development. (2005). *The community tool box.* Lawrence, KS: University of Kansas. Retrieved February 20, 2010, from http://ctb.ku.edu/en/tablecontents/

19. Green, L., & Kreuter, M. (2005). *Health program planning* (4th ed.). New York: McGraw-Hill.

20. Hubbard, B., & Rainey, J. (2007) Health literacy instruction and evaluation among secondary school students. *American Journal of Health Education, 48*(6), 332–337.

21. Buckingham, R. W. (2001). *A primer on international health.* Boston: Allyn & Bacon.

22. Last, J. M. (1995). *A dictionary of epidemiology* (3rd ed.). New York: Oxford University Press.

23. Centers for Disease Control and Prevention. (2008). *Designing and building healthy places.* Retrieved February 20, 2010, from http://www.cdc.gov/healthyplaces

24. Tai-Seale, T. (2001). Understanding health empowerment. *The Health Educator, 33*(1), 23–29.

25. World Health Organization. (2008). *10 facts on the global burden of disease.* Retrieved February 20, 2010, from http://www.who.int/features/factfiles/global_burden/en/

26. World Health Organization. (2008). *The World Health Report 2008 primary health care, now more than ever.* Geneva, Switzerland: Author.

27. Centers for Disease Control and Prevention. (2008). *Goals.* Retrieved February 20, 2010, from http://www.cdc.gov/osi/goals/index.html

28. Basch, P. F. (1990). *Textbook of international health.* New York: Oxford University Press.

29. World Health Organization. (2007, March). *International classification of disease.* Retrieved March 20, 2010, from http://www.who.int/classifications/icd/ICDrevision.pdf

30. World Health Organization. (2006, September 4). *Country health information systems.* Retrieved March 15, 2010, from http://www.who.int/healthinfo/systems/en/

31. United States Department of Health and Human Services, Centers for Disease Control and Prevention, National Center for Health Statistics. (2009, February 24). *Surveys and data collection systems.* Retrieved February 20, 2010, from http://www.cdc.gov/nchs/surveys.htm

32. United States Department of Health and Human Services, Centers for Disease Control and Prevention, National Center for Health Statistics. (2001, March 15). *National Health Interview Survey, 1997*. Retrieved February 20, 2010, from http://www.cdc.gov/nchs/nhis.htm

33. National Center for Health Statistics. (2007). *Health, United States 2007 with chart book on trends in the health of Americans* (Table 31, Chart 1). Hyattsville, MD, Washington, DC: U.S. Government Printing Office.

34. Raphael, D. (2008). Getting serious about the social determinants of health: New directions for public health workers. *Promotion and Education, 15*(3), 15–20.

ENHANCED READINGS

National Cancer Institute and National Institutes of Health. (August, 2004). The health communication process model. *Making health communication programs work—a planners guide*. United States: Department of Health and Human Services, National Cancer Institute and National Institutes of Health. Available at: http://cancer.gov/pinkbook
See:

1. Introduction
2. Overview: The Health Communication Process
3. Appendix E: Glossary

RELEVANT WEB SITES

Texas Association for Health, Physical Education, Recreation and Dance. (2009). *Texas Association for Health, Physical Education, Recreation and Dance (TAHPERD)*. Available at: http://www.tahperd.org/
See: Position Statement on Health Terminology

World Health Organization (WHO). (1998). *The WHO health promotion glossary*. Available at: http://www.who.int/healthpromotion/about/HPG/en/index.html

Smith, B. J., Tang, K. C., & Nutbeam, D. (1996). *WHO health promotion glossary: New terms*. Health Promotion International. First online published, 1–6. Available at: http://www.who.int/home-page/

United Nations. (2009). *United Nations millennium development goals*. Available at: http://un.org/millenniumgoals/

Centers for Disease Control and Prevention. (2009). *Designing and building healthy places*. Available at: http://www.cdc.gov/healthyplaces

Public Health Agency for Northern Ireland. (2009). *Improving your health and wellbeing*. Available at: http://www.publichealth.hscni.net

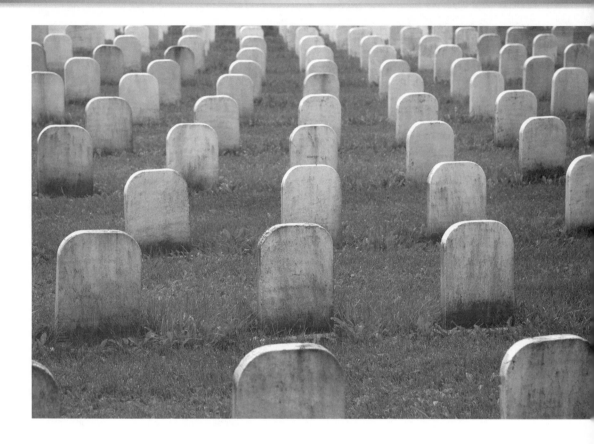

CHAPTER 2

Global Health Surveillance and Epidemiological History

OBJECTIVES AND ASSESSMENTS

This chapter meets the following National Commission for Health Education Credentialing, Inc., Society for Public Health Education, and American Association for Health Education Responsibilities and Competencies for Entry Level and Advanced Level Health Educator competencies.* The learner will:

1. Assess individual and community needs for health education.
7. Communicate and advocate for health and health education.

This chapter meets the following learning objectives. The learner will:
1. Construct a time line of the history of global health education and promotion.
2. Identify past and future societal changes impacting the health education practitioner, including biostatics, environmental factors, health threats, quarantine, sanitation, and immunizations.
3. Choose and examine global, national, state, and local laws, policies, and regulations affecting health throughout the ages.
4. Select a WHO global health education program and judge the health effects.
5. Construct examples of global health education needs, services, environments, surveillance, and security efforts.

INTRODUCTION

The planet today is more globally oriented, with travel easily occurring between countries, alliances are forged, health programs are shared, and coalitions are formed to create a more stable health infrastruc-

---

Sources: Reprinted with permission of NCHEC.

National Commission for Health Education Credentialing, Inc. (NCHEC), Society for Public Health Education (SOPHE), & American Association for Health Education (AAHE). (2006). *A competency-based framework for health educators-2006*. Whitehall, PA: NCHEC.

ture. Preparedness for community health emergencies has never been more crucial. The threat of bioterrorism and mutating diseases continues to be foremost in the minds of health professionals. Terrorists deliberately releasing harmful biological elements (including diseases) into the environment is a constant world threat. Although there are cures for infectious diseases, we know that many underdeveloped, impoverished countries do not have access to these medical resources, and diseases flourish and can mutate into more virulent disease agents or resist current medical treatments.

Tragic events of the past, including the HIV/AIDS and other disease epidemics, the environmental and health aftereffects of the September 11th terrorist attacks in New York City, the countless deaths of children who have not received **immunizations** or who live in severe poverty conditions, and the worldwide spread of illness due to a lack of resources and health access, prove that there is still work to perform as health professionals. The concept of all health being local, pertaining to a specific population, can only serve a few. Global concepts of community health promotion and education must include international emergency preparedness, address current health problems, and promote coalitions among all governments for a common goal.

We live in a borderless society that is very different from many past health concerns. **Demographic trends** are changing and resulting in increased diversity within communities. These demographic statistics collected on population size and geographic distribution—including population growth, fertility and contraception, mortality, migration, ageism, and urbanism—are changing constantly. There has never been a more pressing or urgent need for community and public health educators to pursue global improvements and solutions to health problems throughout the world. Coming together to present health information, collecting and disseminating appropriate statistics, promoting successful programs, and sharing resources creates a climate of a health cultural change.

It is to this end that health educators play a prominent role in effecting global health change. New efforts and solutions are necessary. This profession can substantially influence health prevention, promotion, literacy, protection, maintenance, enhancement, and access efforts on a global basis.

> ### Career Concept
>
> *Do you want to impact thousands of people and make a difference in people's lives? You might like to be a health educator in a school or enjoy working in a philanthropic organization.*

GLOBAL HEALTH

International health is a term used when talking about relationships between states and governments; thus the term "global health" is preferred. **Global health** refers to worldwide cooperation and interaction

---

Immunization: The active exposure of a certain disease element in a person to illicit an immune response; it is commonly given in the form of a vaccination.

Demographic trends: Statistics collected on population size and geographic distribution including population growth, fertility and contraception, mortality, migration, ageism, and urbanism.

Global health: Health initiatives that involve worldwide cooperation and interaction across national borders. It extends to relations beyond governments to include individuals and groups within societies advocating for the protection of communities, countries, and the globe to deter health and disease risks through preventive medicine, health education, communicable disease control, sanitary measures, and environmental controls.

across national borders, and it extends to relations beyond governments to include individuals and groups within societies.[1] Global health is the science of protecting and improving the health of entire populations, communities, neighborhoods, etc., through education, promotion of healthy lifestyles, and research for disease and injury prevention. Globalization links our health more closely to one another than ever before. The rapid movement of people across borders means a disease can travel from a remote location to an urban city faster than ever before. Public and community health professionals analyze the effect of health on genetics, personal choice, and the environment to develop protective health programs.

Global health achievements resulted in healthcare equity, improved quality of life, and accessibility. These changes caused increased life expectancy, reduction of infant/child mortality, and the elimination and/or reduction of many communicable diseases. Health leaders continue to strengthen their roles as advocates for improved population-based health in an international and global community. The aim is to prevent problems from happening or reoccurring and to limit **health disparities**.[2] Global health means protecting and improving the health of a community through preventive medicine, health education, communicable disease control, sanitary measures, and monitoring of environmental hazards.[3] Protecting one community helps protect other communities in close proximity and deters health and disease risks to other communities, countries, and the globe.

AREAS OF GLOBAL HEALTH

Areas of global health are **environmental health, biostatistics, behavior science/health education**, epidemiology, health services administration/management, maternal and child health, nutrition, international/global health, public health laboratory practices, public health policy, and public health and health education practice. A brief description of each area follows:[4]

- *Environmental health* studies the impact of our surroundings on our health. It encompasses these areas: air quality, food protection, radiation protection, solid waste management, hazardous waste management, water quality, noise control, environmental control of recreational areas, housing quality, and vector control. Environmental health is a very relevant field today. Many health educators are focusing on jobs in this field because of the increase of environmental risks to society.
- *Biostatistics* identifies health trends through the application of statistical procedures, techniques, and methodology, leading to life-saving measures. Biostatistics support epidemiology.

Health disparities: Discrimination against certain people concerning their health needs, limiting prevention, promotion, protection, literacy, and access for all.
Environmental health: The impact of our surroundings on our health.
Biostatistics: Method of identifying health trends through the application of statistical procedures, techniques, and methodology that lead to life-saving measures.
Behavior science/health education: A focus on ways to encourage healthy choices in humans by developing communitywide education programs that promote healthy lifestyles to prevent disease and injury, and by researching health issues.

- *Behavioral science/health education* focuses on ways to encourage healthy choices in humans, including the development of communitywide education programs that promote healthy lifestyles to prevent disease and injury, and research of health issues.
- *Epidemiology* is the science of investigating the causes of disease, health risks, determinants, and how the spread of disease occurs. Epidemiologists determine the causes of disease or injury, the risks, and the populations at risk, and they try to prevent further incidences. This field also includes the study of health statistics and interpreting them for communities. This helps identify increased health risks and determine disease patterns and **disease trends**. Biostatistics are used in conjunction with epidemiology.
- *Health services administration* is the management of the human and fiscal resources to deliver public health services. Priorities are often difficult to determine with limited resources.
- *Maternal/child health* involves the use of advocacy, education, and research to improve public health delivery systems for women, children, and families.
- *Nutrition* examines how food and nutrients affect the health and lifestyle of populations.
- *International/global health* addresses global health concerns among different cultures. Global public health needs go beyond national boundaries.
- *Public health laboratory* practices test biological and environmental samples to diagnose, prevent, treat, and control infectious diseases.
- *Public health policy* involves advocating for the public's health through legislative action at all levels.
- *Public health and health education practice* is a field involving many disciplines and the application of public health principles.

OVERVIEW OF THE EVOLUTION OF MEDICINE, HEALTH, AND EPIDEMIOLOGY

Historically, lifestyle has been the most important health determinant for humans. For as long as humans have inhabited this planet, they have struggled to protect themselves against adversity within their environment. Lifestyle refers to the practices, environment, and actual survival of mankind. The main objective is to preserve life and prevent death. Early factors affecting health included adequate food, **sanitation**, water, and housing. As civilizations evolved, additions included income, employment, education, and safety.[1] Population, movement, politics, war, and technical developments all relate to the health status of a country or region.

As civilizations developed, new health concerns emerged including considerations such as water distribution systems, sewage systems, and ample supplies of food and water for growing populations, which in turn brought further concerns for vectorborne (e.g., malaria) and waterborne diseases (e.g.,

---

Disease trends: Disease patterns that determine increased health risks in humans.
Sanitation: A health measure concerned with international trade and health risks that led to measures for disease notification and handling of infected travelers and goods. This resulted in the first International Sanitary Regulations.

cholera). Epidemics or contagious diseases occurred. Then, as medicine and epidemiology developed, many contagious diseases were eradicated in the more prosperous countries.[5]

Socioeconomics has always been a health determinant. News headlings constantly remind us that we live in a world where many communicable diseases have cures available for those with means. The health consequences as a result of poverty are adverse. Poverty contributes greatly to communicable diseases and unhealthy societies in many parts of the world even today.[1] Lack of resources, economics, and the basic health needs of food, water, shelter, and adequate medical care contribute to the vicious cycle of poverty and communicable diseases.

One hundred years ago, infectious diseases such as cholera, plague, yellow fever, diarrhea, influenza, malaria, pneumonia, and tuberculosis ravaged civilizations and threatened health. They dominated entire regions and spread in pandemics. Little could be done to halt their progression until there were major advances in preventive medicines and cures for infectious diseases. The first half of the 20th century brought new drugs, preventive environmental practices, and new vaccines. These advances helped industrialized countries, which had reliable access to them, to eliminate and/or decrease the infectious disease threats. These landmark efforts in public health in modern times promoted efforts to prevent, control, and cure infectious diseases.[5]

Third-world or developing countries still suffer from infectious diseases, diarrheal diseases, lack of basic human needs, extreme poverty, lack of immunizations, lack of access to health services, and poor, inadequate natural resources.[1] Poverty and malnutrition affect every country's health. Poverty is usually caused by a lack of resources in medical care, insurance, and education. Malnutrition is directly related to poverty. Poverty is related to deaths due to preventable diseases, especially in young children and women. Just as improvements in hygiene and standards of living in the more prosperous parts of the world altered the conditions that once allowed communicable diseases to flourish,[5] increased resources and improved economics can shift the pendulum of the poverty and disease cycle in today's less developed societies.

In developed or industrialized countries today, new diseases and strains emerge as chronic diseases, caused by lifestyle and behavior choices. These changes are new challenges to developed countries.[6] Developed countries' health problems today include obesity, atherosclerosis, high blood pressure, and coronary heart disease—all chronic, noninfectious diseases.[1] **Genetic health determinants** or inherited health traits also play a great role in risk factors for certain diseases.

Buckingham cites two criteria to consider when looking at the health of a country: infant mortality rate (IMR) and the population size. He states that infant mortality is the single most important determinant of the health status of a nation, although population size is also notable. Population and demographic trends have a direct correlation with resources; more people means more natural resources consumed. These two issues are related to the different spectrums of poverty—diseases that occur due to a lack of resources in poverty-stricken nations and diseases attributable to lifestyle in developed nations.[5]

Even though many communicable diseases have cures, the resources are not always available in all countries. Global health and epidemiology faces many different challenges due to these and other circumstances. Their evolution, however, provided answers for many problems. Schoenbach cited many

---

Genetic determinants: These are inherited health traits that play a great role in risk factors for certain diseases in humans.

categories in the evolution of epidemiology, including advances in public health knowledge and practice, advances instigated by military wars, and scientific progress.[7(p17)] He also included factors that affect each other and global health including history of health and disease, history of ideas and concepts, history of methods, and history of knowledge gained through these concepts and methods. A time line of the major events in the history of health and epidemiology is included in **Table 2–1**.

GLOBAL HEALTH HISTORY

Early Civilizations: BC

In the beginning of mankind, the earliest health practices were probably associated with rites, herbs, and possibly religion, but these went unrecorded.[8] Early recorded concepts of health are very closely tied to religion.[9] There is evidence in 8000 BC that prehistoric medicine practiced the first surgical procedure, or trephining.[10] In 2000 BC, Ancient Egyptian medicine developed a systematic method of treating diseases.[7] In Egypt, over 3000 years ago, there was evidence of a pustular eruption similar to smallpox in the mummified head of Ramses V, who died in 1157 BC. Smallpox is probably mankind's oldest known disease.[11] In 400 BC, Hippocrates and other Greek writers drew links to environmental factors as disease causation, and the Romans associated plumbism with wine from lead-glazed pottery.[12,7] The first codes and laws were developed between the 5th and 1st centuries BC in Mesopotamia, Egypt, India, and Europe. Water use, waste disposal, agriculture, and physician healing first began. Trade and travel routes increased, spreading infectious and contagious diseases, and the threat of new diseases occurred.[5]

1–1100 AD

Separating people with disease from the healthy population is an ancient practice. There are both biblical and Koranic references to the isolation of lepers.[9] China established a policy in the 7th century of detaining sailors and foreign travelers infected with the plague.[5] Evidence suggests that smallpox existed in some parts of Asia and China by about the year 50 AD and that smallpox spread to parts in Europe and western Africa in the 10th century.[11] Galen formulated the first medical theories based on scientific experimentation in 100 AD. The plague occurred in three epidemics—one in 543, another in 1348, and another in 1664. The era from 500 AD to 1500 AD is known as the spiritual era. Disease epidemics during this period included smallpox, diphtheria, measles, influenza, tuberculosis, anthrax, and syphilis.[8]

1100–1400 AD

In 1100 AD, university medical schools were first established in Europe.[10] In 1334, Petrarch introduced the concept of comparison and of a clinical trial.[7] The Bubonic plague epidemic occurred in Europe in 1347.[5] The term **quarantine** was used by health officials in the 14th century when people coming from

---

Quarantine: The mandatory isolation of people infected with a disease or arriving from countries with certain diseases.

TABLE 2–1	TIME LINE FOR THE HISTORY OF HEALTH AND EPIDEMIOLOGY
Date	**Event**
Antiquity	Concepts of health closely tied to religion (e.g., Old Testament)
ca. 8000 BC	Prehistoric medicine
ca. 2000 BC	Ancient Egyptian medicine
ca. 400 BC	Greek writers draw links to environmental factors (e.g., Hippocrates); Romans associate plumbism with wine from lead-glazed pottery
7th century	China quarantines for plague
1334	Petrarch introduces the concept of comparison and indeed of a clinical trial
1347	Bubonic plague epidemic in Europe
1603	John Graunt writes *Bills of Mortality* and the "law of mortality"—the first life table, giving the probability of dying at each age
ca. 1700	Bernardino Ramazzini, "Father of Occupational Epidemiology"; also breast cancer discovered in nuns
1706–1777	François Bossier de Lacroix (known as Sauvages) systematic classification of diseases ("Nosologia Methodica")
1708	Forerunner of U.S. Public Health Service started at Merchant Marine Hospital
1747	James Lind scurvy experiment
1775	Percival Pott scrotum cancer findings
1796	Edward Jenner develops cowpox vaccination against smallpox
1787–1872	Pierre Charles Alexandre Louis (1787–1872), the "Father of Epidemiology" creates *La methode numerique LaPlace*; Poisson, the birth of statistics
1834	William Farr, William Guy, William Budd (all students of Louis) found the Statistical Society of London
1837	Horace Mann, Secretary of Massachusetts Board of Education (U.S.) annual report for mandatory hygiene instruction in schools
1847	Ignaz Semmelweis (Vienna) discovers transmission and prevention of puerperal fever
1849	John Snow discovers waterborne transmission of cholera
1850	Epidemiological Society of London established
1851	John Grove on the nature of epidemics (presented the germ theory); first International Sanitary Conference
1866	Cholera epidemic in London; Oliver Wendell Holmes and George Shattuck, Jr., (and Shattuck's student, Edward Jarvis) found the American Statistical Society
1870	Beginning of the era of bacteriology

TABLE 2–1 *(Continued)*

Date	Event
1887	The Hygienic Laboratory, forerunner of the National Institutes of Health, is created within the Marine Hospital Service in Staten Island, NY
1900	Yule notion of spurious (i.e., nonsubstantive) correlations, confounding ("Simpson's paradox")
1914–1918	Joseph Goldberger studies pellagra
1918	American Child Health Association established (U.S.) and advocates good decision-making behaviors; Sally Jean Lucas (director) coins term health education
1920	Split between U.S.-organized medicine and physicians interested in public health (the latter were interested in national health insurance; public health concern vs. individual concern); key issue only now being revisited today
1929–1931	The Ohio Research Study (U.S.) uses student health needs and interests to design curriculum; conducted by Delbert Oberteuffer
1930s	Emphasis on eating healthier foods and fluoridation of drinking water in the United States
1937	Austin Bradford Hill writes *Principles of Medical Statistics*
1942	Office of Malaria Control in War Areas (in U.S.; became Communicable Disease Center [CDC] in 1946, Center for Disease Control in 1970, Centers for Disease Control in 1980, and Centers for Disease Control and Prevention in 1992)
1946	World Health Organization (WHO) created
1947	WHO Epidemiological Information Service
1948	John Ryle becomes first chairman of social medicine at Oxford; observed that physicians have curiously little concern with prevention
1949	First U.S. Office of Education Conference for undergraduate professional preparation of students majoring in health (Washington, DC)
1950s	Emphasis on motor vehicle safety in the United States
1950–1970	Epidemiology successes in fluoride, tobacco, blood pressure and stroke, coronary heart disease risk factors, toxic shock syndrome, Legionnaire's disease, Reye's syndrome, endometrial cancer and exogenous estrogens
1951	International Sanitary Regulations
1962	The National School Health Education Study by Elena Sliepcevich identifies student knowledge and needs and results in K–12 comprehensive health curriculum
1965	Medicare and Medicaid enacted in the United States
1969	International Health Regulations enter into force

(Continues)

TABLE 2–1	*(Continued)*
Date	**Event**
1970	Family planning programs in the United States
1974	Bureau of Health Education (became the Center for Health Promotion) established by the CDC/Lalonde Report from Canada
1978	The National Task Force on the Preparation and Practice of Health Educators established in Bethesda, MD, at conference
1979	Healthy People U.S. and Health Objectives for the Nation established as result of Surgeon General's report; eradication of smallpox
1980	Office of the Director of Heath Information and Promotion in Washington DC responsible for Healthy People's implementation
1985	*A Framework for the Development of Competency Based Curriculum for Entry Level Heath Educators* first published in the United States
1988	U.S. Institute of Medicine Report of the Committee for the Study of the Future of Public Health: Public health system is in "disarray" with AIDS, injuries, teen pregnancies, Alzheimer's disease; National Commission for Health Education Credentialing Inc. established in the United States; first exam administered 1990
1991	Cholera epidemics in Latin America; Joint Committee on Health Education Terminology updated and expands 1973 report on health terminology
1995	Conference on Health Education in the 21st Century addresses partnering effort for priorities of the profession
1996–1997	Graduate competencies for health educators accepted, Dallas, Texas
1997	Standard Occupation Classification Policy Review committee approves occupation of Health educator; finalized in 1998 for collecting U.S. statistics
2000	Code of Ethics for Public Health and Health Professions adopted in the United States; life expectancy is 76.9 years in the United States
2003	Severe acute respiratory syndrome (SARS) outbreak
2004	Avian influenza
2005	WHO adopts International Health Regulations
2007	International Health Regulations enter into force
2009	Swine flu (H1N1) epidemic; Healthy People 2020 proposal released
2010	Haiti earthquake and Chile earthquake–global action plans by WHO and PAHO

Source: Adapted from *Understanding the Fundamentals of Epidemiology: An Evolving Text*; Victor J. Schoenback, http://www.epidemiolog.net, 2000, used with permission; World Health Organization, 2007;[5] Insel, P. M., & Roth, W. T., 2008;[6] Hayden, J., 2000.[17]

plague-infested areas were isolated. The port of Ragusa, under the control of the Venetian Republic (1397), required the isolation of people arriving from plague countries. Other Mediterranean ports followed suit, and these public health measures became international over the following centuries. These quarantine measures did not contain the infectious diseases. The term quarantine was an Italian word for "forty," because patients were held for a period of 40 days.[13]

1500s AD

In the 1500s, Vesolius (1543) published the first study of human anatomy.[10] The 1600s brought about John Graunt's *Bills of Mortality* (1603) and the "law of mortality" describing the relationship of morbidity and mortality in man. This was the first life table on the probability of dying at a given age.[7,12,14] Some consider him the first biostatistics pioneer by compiling vital statistics.[12] The laws formulated an attempt to construct the "laws of epidemics." He is recognized as the first person to use quantitative methods to describe population vital statistics.[7,12,14] The contagium vivum theory (a forerunner of the germ theory that infection is caused by a living organism) was a generalization of the observed facts that diseases might be caused by contagia viva (e.g., smallpox, measles, and cholera).[14] Thus, physicians in Europe visiting plague victims wore protective clothing, including a mask and a beak containing strong smelling herbs (see **Figure 2–1**). By 1674, **Anton van Leeuwenhoek**, a Dutch scientist, discovered and identified **bacteria**.[10] Bacteria are microorganisms, some of which are pathogenic and cause infectious diseases including fatal bacterial diseases.

1600s AD

In the 1600s, England obliged all London-bound ships to wait at the mouth of the River Thames for at least 40 days to help prevent the plague from spreading across Europe. The attempt failed, and the plague devastated England until 1666.[5] Other diseases in European nations at this time included smallpox, malaria, and the plague. Smallpox, measles, and other diseases spread to the colonists in the New World of the Americas and the Native American Indians.[8]

1700s AD

The 1700s brought about more changes. Industrialized growth caused unsafe and unsanitary conditions, especially in the workplaces.[8] Smallpox spread to the Americas in the 16th century.[11] Bernardino Ramazzini's work earned him the title "Father of Occupational Epidemiology," and he was also noted for his research on breast cancer. The systematic classification of diseases, called "Nosologia Methodica" by Francois Bossier de Lacroix (known as Sauvages), was established from 1706–1777.[7] By 1708, the

---

Anton van Leeuwenhoek: A Dutch scientist who discovered and identified bacteria in 1674.
Bacteria: Groups of microorganisms, some of which are pathogenic and cause infectious diseases including fatal bacterial diseases.

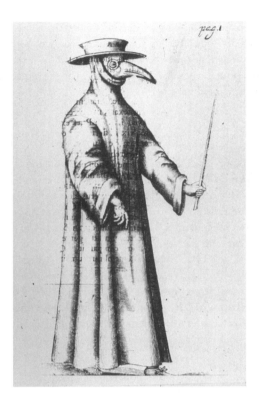

FIGURE 2–1   Illustration of a Doctor During the Plague   From the 14th century, European doctors visiting plague victims wore protective clothing, a mask, and a beak containing strong-smelling herbs.

United States Public Health Service was started at the Merchant Marine Hospital.[15] James Lind performed his experiment (1747) on the etiology and treatment of scurvy. He demonstrated that citric acid fruits cured the disease.[14]

Percival Pott revealed his scrotum cancer findings in 1775.[7] From 1787 to 1872, Pierre Charles Alexandre Louis of France, the "Father of Epidemiology," used statistical methods and compared groups of people in observational studies. This resulted in "la methodenumerique LaPlace."[7,14] Poisson initiated the birth of statistics with a distribution system to describe the occurrence of rate events or the sampling distribution of isolated counts, with a continuum of time or space. This system was used in modeling person–time incidence rates.[16] Municipal boards of health were established in the United States in 1799, but diseases such as cholera, typhoid, and smallpox occurred along with a yellow fever epidemic in Philadelphia in 1793.[8]

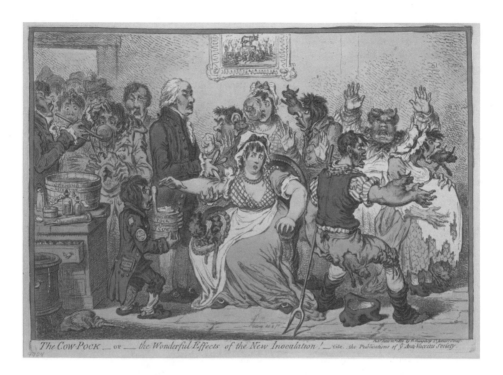

FIGURE 2–2 Caricature of a Vaccination Scene   In this cartoon, the British satirist James Gillray caricatured a vaccination scene at the Smallpox and Inoculation Hospital. The image shows Edward Jenner vaccinating frightened young women and cows emerging from different parts of their bodies. The cartoon was inspired by the controversy over the inoculation against smallpox.

In the 18th century, smallpox killed every 7th child born in Russia and every 10th child born in France and Sweden. **Dr. Edward Jenner** was an English physician and saw that patients exposed to cowpox, a related but milder disease, seemed immune to smallpox. Subsequently, Jenner developed the successful cowpox vaccination against smallpox in 1796. He inoculated an 8-year-old farm boy with cowpox virus, observed the reaction, and inoculated him with the smallpox virus. The boy did not develop the disease, Jenner's new procedure was widely accepted, and the smallpox death rates fell rapidly[5,7,8] (see **Figure 2–2**).

Edward Jenner: An English physician who successfully gave the first cowpox vaccination against smallpox in 1796.

1800s AD

The era of 1850–1900 became known as the bacteriologic time.[8] In 1834 William Farr, William Guy, and William Budd (all students of Pierre Charles Alexandre Louis of France) founded the Statistical Society of London.[7] They acted as sanitary physicians in the 1800s and continued epidemiologic studies in the field.[14] In the United States in 1837, Horace Mann, the Secretary of the Massachusetts Board of Education, called for mandatory hygiene instruction in schools in his annual report.[17] Peter Panum investigated the 1846 measles outbreak on the Faroe Islands, using classic epidemiologic techniques. Investigations on the transmission of cholera, typhoid fever, and puerperal fever forged new understandings in the ability to reduce the spread of major infections.[7,14] Ignaz Semmelweis of Vienna discovered the transmission and prevention of puerperal fever in 1847. This disease, often called childbed fever, is contracted by women after childbirth or miscarriage (or abortion) and is an infection called septicaemia resulting from genital tract sepsis.[7,12]

Physician **John Snow's** observation in 1849 resulted in the subsequent achievements in preventing waterborne transmission of cholera. His famous work during the 1854 cholera epidemic in London was based on years of recording outbreaks and debates on the cause of the disease.[12,14] He mapped the locations of homes of those who had died in the London epidemic. He noted clusters of cases around a particular water pump. As soon as Snow persuaded the authorities to disable the handle to the well, the cholera case numbers and deaths declined. Snow's demonstration that cholera was associated with polluted water was a rebuttal of the "miasma" theories or transmission through poisonous vapours.[5,7,14,18] In 1851, John Grove presented the germ theory on the nature of epidemics.[7] Improvements in sanitation in the United Kingdom reduced the threat of cholera. However, endemic diarrheal disease from other causes was not solved. London constructed a new sewage system in the 1880s.[19]

William Budd published his studies of contagious typhoid fever as person-to-person transmission from 1857–1873.[14] In 1862, **Louis Pasteur**, a French chemist and microbiologist, proposed the germ theory, or biogenesis theory. He and his colleagues did experiments and disproved the theory of spontaneous generation. He is also credited with pasteurization of milk for sanitary purposes. In London, the Registrar's General's Office was formed in 1836, and the Epidemiological Society of London was established in 1850. William Farr, at the Registrar's General's Office, developed the concept of mortality surveillance.[7,14] Pasteur and Koch's remarkable study from 1850–1900 proved that diseases are caused by certain bacteria or living organisms.[8,12] **Robert Koch**, a German physician, advanced the theory of specific disease agents or the relationship between a microorganism and a disease. His first demonstration was with the anthrax bacillus in 1876.[8,12]

The first International Sanitary Conference was held in 1851.[5] Oliver Wendell Holmes, George Shattuck, Jr., and Edward Jarvis founded the American Statistical Society in 1866. The beginning of

---

John Snow: A physician who discovered the waterborne transmission of cholera in 1854.

Louis Pasteur: A French chemist and microbiologist who in 1862 proposed the germ theory or biogenesis theory disproving the spontaneous generation theory. He is also credited with pasteurization of milk for sanitary purposes.

Robert Koch: A German physician who advanced the theory of specific disease agents or the relationship between a microorganism and a disease. His first demonstration was with the anthrax bacillus in 1876.

the era of bacteriology began in 1870.[7] Gerhard Armauer Hansen discovered the bacillus that causes Hansen's disease, *Mycobacterium leprae*, in 1873. In 1878, the first Federal Quarantine Act was passed, and the U.S. Congress appropriated funds to investigate the origin and causes of epidemic diseases, especially yellow fever and cholera.[3]

The Hygienic Laboratory, a forerunner of the National Institutes of Health (U.S.), is created in the Marine Hospital Service in Staten Island, NY in 1887.[7] Milk pasteurization began in the U.S. in 1890.[8] In 1893, a new Quarantine Act in the U.S. strengthened the Quarantine Act of 1878 and repealed the act establishing the National Board of Health.[3] In 1898, Marie and Pierre Curie discovered radium for cancer treatment in France.[10] In 1894, Hansen's disease patients were transferred to Carville, Louisiana, which became the USDHHS hospital where diagnosed patients were quarantined in the United States.[15,20]

1900s AD

The 1900s are known as the modern era. However, as McKenzie et al. stated, influenza, pneumonia, tuberculosis, typhoid fever, malaria, diphtheria, noninfectious diarrhea, pellagra, rickets, vitamin deficiencies, poor dental heath, and gastrointestinal track infections were prominent.[8] Major towns and cities along the eastern seaboard of the United States had passed quarantine laws by this time. These laws were enforced only when there were epidemics.[5] Also at this time, Yule developed the notion of spurious (nonsubstantive) correlations that confounded Simpson's paradox.

Sigmund Freud developed the psychoanalytic method for treatment of mental illness in the 1900s.[10] By 1900, Major Walter Reed of the United States said that yellow fever was carried by mosquitoes. Thirty-eight states in the United States had state health departments established.[8] The Pure Food and Drug Act of 1906 was passed in the United States. From 1914 to 1918, Dr. Joseph Goldberger discovered the cause of pellagra, a disease that results from a diet deficient in niacin and disproved that the disease was carried by germs. This disease killed many poor Southerners.[3]

The American Child Health Association was established in the United States in 1918 and advocated good decision-making behaviors. In the same year, the director, Sally Jean Lucas, coined the term health education.[17] Also at that time in the United States, the Chamberlain-Kahn Act provided for a venereal disease study.[3]

In 1920, a split between U.S. organized medicine and physicians interested in public health took place. The physicians were interested in national health insurance, while public versus individual health concerns were key issues that continue to be reviewed to this day. In 1928, **Alexander Fleming**, a Scottish medic, pharmacologist, and bacteriologist, discovered the antibiotic penicillin.[7] In the United States, the Ohio Research Study, conducted by Delbert Oberteuffer, used student health needs and interests to design curriculum from 1929–1931.[17] In the United States, on August 14, 1935, Title VI of the Social Security Act passed, authorizing the funding for health grants to the states for investigat-

---

Alexander Fleming: A Scottish medic, pharmacologist, and bacteriologist who discovered the antibiotic penicillin in 1928.

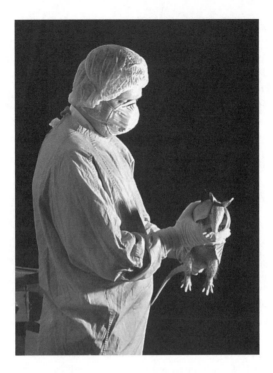

FIGURE 2–3   The Armadillo Controversy and Hansen's Disease

ing disease and sanitation problems.[3] The *Principles of Medical Statistics* was published by Austin Bradford Hill in 1937.[7]

Promin (and later dapsone) was discovered as a "cure" for Hansen's disease in endemic Louisiana in 1941 at the Carville leprosarium, a U.S. Public Health Service hospital and now a world-renowned research center (discussed further in Chapter 4). The armadillo was the first animal model or prototype used for Hansen's disease in this hospital's research (see **Figure 2–3**). Multidrug therapy (dapsone, rifampicin, and clofazimine) was discovered in 1981, and the disease is now under control thanks to its effectiveness. Hansen's disease is still a problem in some nations where treatments are not available due to lack of resources and access.[15,20]

The Office of Malaria Control in War Areas was created in 1942. In the United States, the Communicable Disease Center (CDC) was established in 1946, subsequently becoming the Center for Disease Control in 1970, the Centers for Disease Control in 1980, and the Centers for Disease Control and Prevention in 1992. In 1946, the World Health Organization (WHO) was created, and in 1947, the WHO Epidemiological Information Service began.[5] Also, in 1947, John Ryle became the first chairman of social medicine at Oxford. He observed that physicians seemed to have little concern with prevention.[7] In 1949, the first U.S. Office of Education Conference for undergraduate professional preparation of students majoring in health was held in Washington DC.[17] The Framingham Study of 1949 pioneered research investigating heart disease risk factors.[12]

Smallpox was still endemic in almost every country in the world when the 20th century began. In the 1950s, an estimated 50 million smallpox cases occurred globally each year, resulting in about 15 million deaths.[11] In the 1950s, **Dr. Jonas Salk**, an American medical researcher, developed the first safe and effective polio vaccine.[8,14]

In 1962, in the United States, the National School Health Education Study was conducted by Elena Sliepcevich. This investigation identified student knowledge and needs that resulted in K–12 Comprehensive School Health Education curriculum.[17] Medicare (to provide elderly patients with health care) and Medicaid (to provide economically deprived patients with health care) were established in the United States in 1965.[3,17] In 1966, the Division of Environmental Health Sciences was established at the NIH for research on the biological, chemical, and physical effects of environmental agents.[3] By 1967, access to smallpox immunizations increased, and these mortality and morbidity statistics fell to 10–15 million cases and 3 million deaths.[11] By 1969, the **International Health Regulations (IHR)** were enforced.[5]

The 1970s brought about many epidemiological changes. In 1974, in the Lalonde Report from Canada, Schoenbach listed many epidemiology research endeavors that impacted history, including fluoride use, ill effects of tobacco, blood pressure and stroke, cardiovascular heart disease risk factors, toxic shock syndrome, Legionnaire's disease, Reye's syndrome, endometrial cancer, and exogenous estrogens.[7]

Also in the 1970s, scientists investigated viruses as the possible cause of cancer.[10] In the United States in particular, there were many significant developments in the 1970s. By 1974, the Bureau of Health Education (now the Center for Health Promotion) was established by the CDC.[17] In 1977, the **World Health Assembly** of WHO held a conference that set a new level of health to be achieved by all people; subsequently in 1978, in Alma Alta, Soviet Union (formerly the U.S.S.R.), a primary health-care declaration was adopted.[8] Globally, the 10-year eradication campaign in 1967 (certified in 1979) helped eradicate smallpox.

The National Task Force on the Preparation and Practice of Health Educators was convened and established at the Bethesda, Maryland, conference in 1978.[17] Of great significance in 1979, the Healthy People program and Health Objectives for the Nation were established as a result of the report by the United States Public Health Service at the Office of the Surgeon General and Health Promotion.[21] The Office of the Director of Heath Information and Promotion in Washington DC was responsible for the implementation of Healthy People 1979.[17] This effort continues today and is updated periodically. Each target area is measured over a 10-year period to assess progress. Healthy People provided a basis

---

Jonas Salk: An American medical researcher who developed the first safe and effective polio vaccine in the 1950s.
International Health Regulations: Global rules adopted and enforced by WHO in 2005 that provide a framework for member states to respond to events that threaten national, state, and global security.
World Health Assembly: The decision-making body for WHO on health issues, budget, management, and administration.

for tracking health status, risks, and services for both individual actions and large-scale changes, such as the environment and health care.[5]

The 1980s saw many significant developments in the United States. In 1981, the 34th World Health Assembly adopted a global strategy to ensure that by the year 2000 all health resources would be distributed so essential healthcare services would be available to everyone.[22] A Framework for the Development of Competency Based Curricula for Entry Level Heath Educators was first published in 1985. In 1987, a Commission on the Human Immunodeficiency Virus Epidemic was appointed by the U.S. President.[3] The National Commission for Health Education Credentialing, Inc., was established in the United States in 1988.[17] Then, in 1988, the U.S. Institute of Medicine Report of the Committee for the Study of the Future of Public Health was published. The public health system was said to be in "disarray," with health threats including AIDS, injuries, teen pregnancies, and Alzheimer's disease.[7]

Cholera is still a major health risk throughout the world. In 1991, cholera emerged in Latin America after more than a century's absence. Africa, Asia, and Europe had a pandemic 30 years earlier. Seafood contaminated by the ships off the coast of Peru was blamed as the contaminant.[23] In addition to human suffering and death, the outbreak provoked panic, disrupted social and economic structures, threatened population development and infrastructure in affected populations and countries, and led to extreme and unnecessary international reactions.[24] European Union countries, the United States, and countries neighboring Peru imposed trade and travel restrictions. Losses from tourism, embargoes to trade, damage and lost production attributable to cholera-related illnesses, and death were estimated to cost affected areas as much as $1.5 billion.[5,24,25]

In the United States, 1991 marked two major developments. The National Center for Human Genome Research in the United States announced the start of the framework map of the human genome.[3] Also, the Vaccine Research Center in the United States was established to focus on searching for a vaccine against HIV/AIDS.[3]

Credentialing in the United States became a reality for health educators in the 1990s. The first exam of the National Commission for Health Education Credentialing, Inc., for the designation of Certified Health Education Specialist (CHES) was administered in 1990.[17] In 1991, the Joint Committee on Health Education Terminology was updated and expanded from the previous 1973 report on health education terminology.[17]

In recent years, the most serious outbreak of plague occurred in India in 1994. It was reported to WHO, as required by the IHR, and international media attention took hold. The outbreak resulted in huge economic consequences for India. Many countries overenforced the measures set out in the IHR (established in 1969) and imposed unnecessary travel and trade restrictions. Within two months, the plague outbreak was brought under control, but it cost India a record trade deficit.[26] Since then, smaller, unrelated bubonic plague outbreaks in Algeria, the Democratic Republic of the Congo, Malawi, and Zambia occurred.[5]

Globally, in 1995, the **International Sanitary Regulations** were published.[5] In the United States, professional priorities, graduate competencies, and the approved occupation of health educators was accomplished. In 1995, the *Conference on Health Education in the 21st Century* was held, and it addressed

---

International Sanitary Regulations: Worldwide regulations on the containment of epidemics within territories.

partnering efforts for priorities of the profession.[17] Then, in 1996–1997, Graduate Competencies for Health Educators were accepted in Dallas, Texas.[17] Finally, in 1997, the *Standard Occupation Classification Policy Review* committee approved the official occupation of health educator. This was finalized in 1998 for the purpose of collecting U.S. statistics on the profession.[27] A landmark effort resulted in the adoption of the **Code of Ethics for the Health Profession** in 1997 in the United States.[17]

2000s AD

The *Code of Ethics for the Health Profession* in 1997 in the United States resulted in the adoption of the unified *Code of Ethics* in 2000.[17] In 2000, a study in the United States demonstrated the use of a nasal spray flu vaccine to protect against the three strains of influenza and a flu strain not covered by the vaccine.[3] The September 11, 2001, terrorist attacks in the United States on the World Trade Center and the Pentagon intentionally threatened the health and safety of citizens. The intentional distribution of anthrax (*Bacillus anthracis* spore) through the U.S. postal system in 2001 made bioterrorism a constant threat. These two events were biological, environmental, and mental threats for many U.S. citizens. In 2003, in the United States, *Project BioShield* began at the National Institutes of Health to help protect the public from weapons of bioterrorism.[3]

A new global health outbreak, Severe Acute Respiratory Syndrome (SARS), occurred in 2003.[5] Then in 2004, another outbreak, the Avian influenza began to spread.[5] A study in the United States in 2004 found that women taking estrogen alone as hormone replacement therapy had no increased risk of coronary heart disease but did have increased risk of stroke.[3] The WHO adopted and enforced the IHR in 2005.[5] Managed by the WHO, these are global rules by the member states to regulate national, state, and **global health security**.

Progress in preventing HIV and sexually transmitted diseases contended with legal and extralegal restrictions on discussion about sex, and in particular, anal sex.[7] In 2005, the Annual Report to the Nation on the Status of Cancer by national organizations (1975–2002) said that cancer was declining in the United States.[3]

In 2005, two natural disasters severely affected part of Louisiana, Mississippi, and Texas in the United States within a few months. Hurricane Katrina devastated New Orleans, surrounding areas, and the Mississippi gulf coast in August, causing horrifically unhealthy and unsanitary conditions for the people who decided to stay or had no financial resources to leave (see **Figures 2–4** and **2–5**). Emergency response systems and resources did not even have time to complete addressing this disaster before the next, Hurricane Rita, hit the coastal areas of southwest Texas and southwest Louisiana in October, bringing havoc to the people in the area. The resources were tapped, and the focus shifted to a new area while the first storm residents were still in dire needs of basic necessities and health care. Emergency response systems began planning after Hurricane Katrina and Rita devastated many areas and felt they were prepared.

Code of Ethics for the Health Education Profession: A document outlining the ethical standards of conduct and rights and protection of human subjects in health research, teaching, and programs.
Global health security: Monitoring and preventing acute public health events that endanger the collective health of populations living across geographic regions and international boundaries.

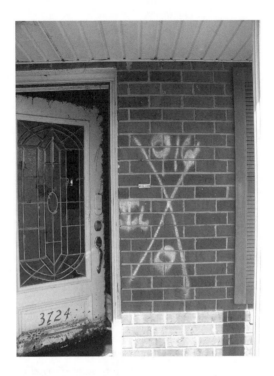

FIGURE 2–4   Hurricane Katrina Damage, 2005, Louisiana   This house was inspected and marked by the National Guard with an X. The top of the X, shows "0 16" for the date inspected, or October 16th; the bottom shows "0" (for the number of occupants at the time inspected); the left shows the name of the National Guard unit inspecting the home; the right side is empty but was used only for recording the number of deceased occupants found at the time of the inspection (none recorded).

The response systems plans were put to use in 2008, when Hurricane Ike devastated the coastal areas of east Texas again. The response teams did a much better job of evacuating victims and assuring resources for those who left. City governments, school systems, and emergency response systems enacted even more measures after these three devastating natural disasters in a very short period of time.

The author was a victim of Hurricanes Rita and Ike, and family members were victims of Hurricane Katrina. The disorder and stress for families and the health challenges they faced during this devastation are unimaginable. The evacuations and dependence on others for basic necessities took its toll on many families. A family member died shortly after losing the family home and all material possessions to Hurricane Katrina, and a friend's husband in ill health succumbed after evacuating from Hurricane Ike. As well, the stresses of having to rebuild or repair, the hassles with insurance companies or lack of

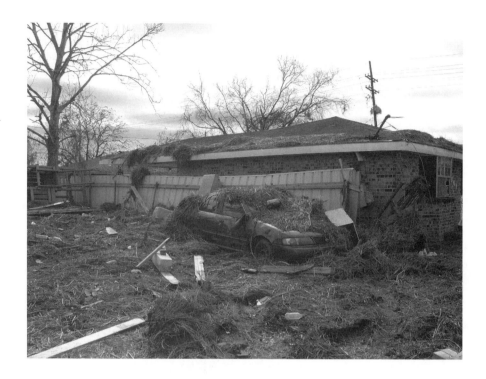

FIGURE 2–5   Hurricane Katrina Damage, 2005   Marsh grass left by flooding in Chalmette, Louisiana.

insurance, unethical contractors, lack of resources, and loss of jobs and income caused many people to relocate and build their lives all over again.

Families and family structures were separated in many cases, children were forced to attend other school systems, and rebuilding community infrastructures was a long and arduous process. Even for returning families, many basic necessities were unavailable. There were distribution centers, but most were not centrally located and were depleted quickly. Gas for transportation was scarce, many cars left behind were ruined, and transportation to these services was impossible for some. Electrical power, water, and sewage systems were nonexistent for months. Businesses such as grocery stores, drugstores, gas stations, and department stores were unavailable for many months, and for some, they were non-existent or demolished. Hopefully, city, county, and state authorities are better prepared for back-to-back natural disasters in the future (B. Hernandez, pers. comm., July 21, 2009).

Because of the Iraq war, many service men and women are accessing mental health services and showing signs of post-traumatic stress disorder, increasing the need and access for mental health. Physical disabilities and post employment options are another factor as a result of the war that need addressing.

In the United States, *Healthy People 1979* resulted in *Healthy People 2000* and was revised and updated due to data collections, leading to *Healthy People 2010* and the proposed *Healthy People 2020*. *Healthy People 2010* is a government public health initiative that seeks to prevent unnecessary disease and disability and to achieve a higher quality of life for all Americans. Each target area is measured over a 10-year period to assess progress. *Healthy People 2010* provided a basis for tracking health status, risks, and services for both individual actions and large-scale changes, such as the environment and health care. This government effort proposed two broad national goals: (1) increase quality and years of healthy life and (2) eliminate health disparities among Americans. The *Healthy People 2010* progress in achieving these U.S. goals is monitored in 28 focus areas through 467 objectives. Many objectives focus on interventions designed to reduce or eliminate illness, disability, and premature death. Each objective has a target for specific improvements to be achieved by the year 2010. *Healthy People 2020 objectives* are now in the proposal stage and the full document will be released soon.[28]

Thought Concept

How does studying the history of health keep us from repeating past mistakes?

In 2009, the Swine Flu (H1N1) became one of the first worldwide influenza virus pandemics and a health risk for many. Resources for the vaccine made significant progress, though the pandemic continued into 2010. In 2010, two earthquakes devastated Haiti and then Chile, causing deaths and destruction in many cities and leaving many homeless and without basic necessities. Worldwide relief efforts were not adequate to keep up with the huge numbers of people and areas affected.

THE FUTURE OF HEALTH BEYOND 2000 AD

Health disparities that are still present in the world today include not having access to health services or discrimination against certain people concerning their health needs. Providing safe drinking water and proper hygiene remains a huge challenge in developing countries. Globally, currently 1.1 billion people lack access to safe water, and 2.6 billion people lack access to proper sanitation. Older children and adults (especially women) are in poor health and miss opportunities for education and productivity; approximately 4,500 children under 5 years of age die every day from easily preventable diseases such as diarrhea.[5] Infant mortality rates are high in many countries from preventable diseases and problems, lack of prenatal care, and lack of access to health services. Migrant health is on issue in many countries and other humanitarian crises. **Table 2–2** shows life expectancy at birth in selected countries.

Since the eradication of smallpox was certified in 1979, there are serious concerns that some countries and terrorist groups may be storing smallpox and other viruses to use as weapons. Smallpox is a significant public health concern in terms of the deliberate release of the virus to cause harm, almost 30 years after its successful eradication.[29] The potential of a bioterrorist attack is causing major health concerns in many countries.[29] WHO reported in 2005 that chemical agent misuse could undo one of the greatest public health achievements in the 21st century.[29] Work is under way on a new and safer vaccine against smallpox, to be produced in huge quantities if immunization against a terrorist release is necessary.

TABLE 2–2 WHERE DO YOU WANT TO LIVE? HEALTH STATUS MORTALITY: LIFE EXPECTANCY IN SELECTED COUNTRIES

Country	Life Expectancy at Birth (Years)
Lowest Life Expectancies	
Guinea-Bissau	46.5
Chad	46.5
Mali	45.5
Rwanda	45.5
Mozambique	45
Burundi	44.5
Democratic Republic of the Congo	44.5
Somalia	44
Cote d'Ivoire	44
Equatorial Guinea	43
Afghanistan	42
Lesotho	41.5
Malawi	41
Angola	40
Sierra Leone	38.5
Highest Life Expectancies	
Greece	84.5
Japan	82.5
Monaco	81.5
Iceland	81
Australia	80.5
Canada	80.5
Sweden	80.5
Switzerland	80.5
Israel	80
New Zealand	80

(Continues)

TABLE 2–2 *(Continued)*	
Country	**Life Expectancy at Birth (Years)**
Norway	80
Singapore	79.5
Netherlands	79.5
United States of America	78.5
Luxembourg	78.5
Cyprus	78.5

Source: Adapted from WHO, 2007, http://www.who.int/whosis/whostat2007/en/index.html

GLOBAL COOPERATIVE SURVEILLANCE EFFORTS 1800S THROUGH PRESENT DAY

By the end of the 19th century, dozens of international and global conferences on disease control were held. The founding of the World Health Organization (WHO) in 1946 and the International Sanitary Regulations (1951) were significant international health events. The likelihood of pandemics is still a threat to public health security.[5] Global surveillance efforts include the epidemiologic collections and monitoring of disease rates in humans.

Some diseases are still thriving in developing countries. Resources and responses are limited, so they could still spread internationally. European leaders of the mid-19th century began to cooperate in controlling the spread of infectious diseases from one nation to another.[25] From the mid-1850s to 1900, 10 International Sanitary Conferences were convened. Twelve European countries or states were involved and worked on containment of epidemics within their territories. The inaugural 1851 conference in Paris lasted six months. It was important because it established that health protection was an international subject.[5]

During the 1880s, some South American nations signed the first set of international public health agreements in the Americas. These agreements covered yellow fever, which was endemic in much of the region, as well as cholera and the plague, which were found among the huge numbers of European immigrants. The first International Sanitary Convention on cholera was signed in 1852. In 1897, the 10th International Sanitary Conference was held, focusing on plague. From these conferences, important new policies were signed into action. Some requirements were the telegraphic notification of first cases of cholera and/or plague. In 1902, 12 countries attended the first International Sanitary Convention of the American Republics in Washington DC. This conference resulted in the creation the Pan American Sanitary Bureau (now the Pan American Health Organization). The European counterpart, the Office International d'Hygiène Publique (OIHP), was established in 1907 and based in Paris.[30]

The First World War brought in its wake the loss of many lives, with epidemics compounding the "war deaths." Diseases included typhus in Russia and cholera, smallpox, dysentery, and typhoid in the Ottoman Empire. These epidemics were the basis for the League of Nations Health Organization (LNHN), spawning from the newly created League of Nations. In 1920, the LNHN formed an epidemic commission for helping countries afflicted with epidemics. In 1951, WHO adopted a revised version of the International Sanitary Regulations of 1892. The approach included measures at border posts to help prevent the spread of infectious diseases, including cholera, plague, smallpox, typhoid fever, and yellow fever, through international borders. The IHR (1969) mandated that member states report disease outbreaks.[5]

Recent events demonstrated the urgent need for a revised set of regulations. The events required greater disease coverage and measures to stop the spread of disease across borders based on epidemiological evidence. The IHR, first issued in 1969, were revised in the 1990s. Authorities looked at the changes in the human world, the microbial world, the natural environment, and human behavior, determining that a new public health response was needed that did not severely impact trade and traffic. An agreed code of conduct was required, and the IHR (2005) responded with a new code for international health security.[31] The IHR were first issued in 1969 and were revised in the 1990s. The WHO gathered resources from more than 140 technical partners from more than 60 countries. The resulting **global network** has kept the international community constantly alert to outbreaks and responses. The response by the partners has provided rapid international multidisciplinary technical support and response for outbreaks in extreme environments. Mechanisms for stockpiling and rapidly distributing vaccines, drugs, and specialized investigation and protection equipment have been established for hemorrhagic fevers, influenza, meningitis, smallpox, and yellow fever.[5]

The WHO continues to strengthen specialized surveillance networks for dangerous pathogens, such as dengue, influenza, and plague. The surveillance network developed by the Global Polio Eradication Initiative supports surveillance of other vaccine-preventable diseases, including measles, meningitis, neonatal tetanus, and yellow fever. This network supports surveillance and response activities for avian influenza, Ebola, Marburg hemorrhagic fever, SARS, and yellow fever. The polio network plans and monitors immunization campaigns and also responds to outbreaks of meningitis and yellow fever. It responded during the Southeast Asia tsunami (December 2004) and the Pakistan earthquake (October 2005). Once polio eradication was completed, there continued to be network investment in the international surveillance and response to outbreaks of vaccine-preventable diseases. Epidemiological surveillance, laboratory facilities, preparedness planning, communication, information management systems, and intersectional collaboration help ensure the highest possible global security measures for health. This effort requires that international ports, airports, and land crossings collaborate with the WHO and member states in preparation for future public health emergencies.[5]

INTERNATIONAL PREPAREDNESS FOR CHEMICAL/BIOLOGICAL THREATS AND EMERGENCIES

The World Health Assembly Resolution WHA55.16, published in 2002, encourages strengthening surveillance systems, emergency preparedness, and response for the release of chemical agents, biological

---

Global networks: Electronic intelligence-gathering tools that provide a safety net for detection of events not otherwise reported.

agents, and radio nuclear materials that could have global public health consequences.[32] The World Health Assembly is the decision-making body for the WHO on health issues, budget, management, and administration. Many countries have limited capacities to detect and respond to these incidents. The WHO established the **Chemical Incident Alert and Response System (ChemiNet)** in 2002 to operate as an alert and response system for communicable diseases. In 2006, this system was extended to other environmental health emergencies. ChemiNet is designed to use early detection, assessment, and verification of outbreaks. It prevents the disruption of environmental health services and provides rapid and effective response to event detection, response, and recovery.[5]

Chemical incidents, such as that in Bhopal, India, brought attention to such occurrences. Preventive measures and a good chemical emergency plan involve all stakeholders. Detection of outbreaks caused by chemical releases includes 24-hour poison centers, like the one in the United States, as a part of public health surveillance systems. Because environmental chemicals once released can cross international borders, the United Nations Economic Commission for Europe (UNECE) Convention on the Transboundary Effects of Industrial Accidents initiated an international agreement to coordinate international preparedness and response.[33] These bioterrorism threats are a constant threat to nations worldwide.

GREATEST GLOBAL PUBLIC HEALTH ACHIEVEMENTS

The WHO cites three sources as the greatest global contributions in the evolution of public health: the 1) plague and quarantine, 2) cholera and sanitation, and 3) smallpox and immunization.[5] Quarantine, sanitation, and immunizations to control these devastating diseases were hugely successful health initiatives with dramatic results, reducing epidemics in populations worldwide. The early response to quarantine and, in time, sanitation efforts, sophisticated medicines, vaccinations, and other efforts helped to contain most infectious diseases. Immunizations and smallpox successfully eradicated diseases in countries where the resources and access were available. In addition, early reporting and notification of incidence, prevalence, attack rates, and crude rates assisted in the implementation of early response and reversal efforts for health disease threats.

Schoenbach states that these developments "are only a few of the myriad influences on the evolution of public health and epidemiology." He continues that with "changing demography, economics, transportation, commerce, technology, organizations, politics, wars the entire health care delivery system has been transformed through the rise of managed care organizations."[7(pp22–23)] Changing diseases and afflictions through the centuries, including hunger, infections, malnutrition, reproductive disorders, chronic diseases, environmental and occupational diseases, violence and injury, health care and pharmaceuticals, mental health, aging, and different disease patterns, have dominated health efforts at different

---

Chemical Incident Alert and Response System (ChemiNet): An alert and response system for communicable diseases and other environmental health emergencies.
Greatest Public Health Achievements in the World: Three achievements cited by the WHO in 2007 that have influenced public health in the greatest capacity, including plague and quarantine, cholera and sanitation, and smallpox and immunization.

times. Developing scientific knowledge and technology changes understanding of diseases and approaches to studying it. The introduction of the Pap smear in the 1940s revolutionized our approach to cervical cancer. Development of coronary angiography enabled visualizing of atherosclerosis as well as coronary artery spasm. The development of microscopy, the stethoscope, electrocardiograms, culture techniques, biochemistry, cytology, computers, angiography, radioimmunoassay, DNA probes, expanding social and political consciousness such as the hygienic movement, social democracy, the health promotion movement, and minority health initiatives were huge health achievements for humankind.[7]

There is an increased demand for epidemiology and public health (e.g., the Lalonde Report). Expanding social organization and investment in public health resources increase the opportunities for epidemiologic research and application. These efforts include hospitals, vital statistics systems, health surveys, research findings, disease registries, insurance systems, record systems, and computerized databases.[5] These changes demand new paradigm shifts and a call for consolidated global health networks to progress towards better health in the future.

TEN GREATEST HEALTH ACHIEVEMENTS IN THE UNITED STATES

The CDC in 1999 named the 20th Century's Ten Great Public Health Achievements in the United States.[34] These achievements are responsible for increasing the life span of populations because of public health initiatives and, to a smaller degree, medical advances. Since 1900, the average life expectancy for Americans has increased by approximately 30 years.[2]

Replication of these achievements in other countries where each achievement is still lacking is recommended and may lead to improved health.

Vaccination

Populationwide vaccinations resulted in the eradication of smallpox and polio (in the Americas) and control of measles, rubella, tetanus, diphtheria, haemophilus influenzae type b, and other infectious diseases in the United States and other parts of the world.

Motor Vehicle Safety

Motor vehicle safety and regulations contributed to large reductions in motor vehicle-related deaths. These improvements included safer highways, vehicle engineering safety efforts, and safety behaviors such as the use of safety belts, child safety seats, motorcycle helmets, and decreased drinking and driving. Many of these changes were a result of laws or policy enforcements.

Safer Workplaces

Work-related health problems were significantly reduced. Coal workers' pneumoconiosis (black lung), silicosis, severe injuries, and deaths related to mining, manufacturing, construction, and transportation decreased. Safer workplace practices resulted in about a 40% reduction in fatal occupational injuries.

Control of Infectious Diseases

Infectious disease control resulted from clean water and better sanitation. Reduction of typhoid and cholera, two major causes of illness and death early in the 20th century, resulted from improved sanitation. Tuberculosis and sexually transmitted diseases were reduced following the discovery of antimicrobial therapy.

Decline in Chronic Diseases

A decline in deaths from coronary heart disease and stroke resulted from risk factor modification. Blood pressure control improved with access to early detection and better treatment. Death rates for coronary heart disease has decreased by more than 50% since the 1970s.

Safer and Healthier Foods

Safer and healthier foods resulted from increases in nutritional content and decreases in microbial contamination since 1900 in the United States. Establishing food-fortification programs and identifying essential micronutrients almost eliminated major nutritional deficiency diseases such as goiter and rickets.

Healthier Mothers and Babies

Since 1900, healthier mothers and babies are a result of the availability of better maternal and neonatal medicine. Better hygiene, good nutrition, antibiotics, access to healthcare services, and technology advances resulted in decreased infant and maternal mortality rates.

Family Planning

Contraceptive and family planning access and services changed the social and economic roles of women. Family planning resources provided significant health benefits, including smaller family size, longer interval between the birth of children, counseling, and screening. It also resulted in fewer infant, child, and maternal deaths. Barrier contraceptives helped prevent unplanned pregnancies and reduced the transmission of HIV/AIDS and sexually transmitted infections.

Fluoridation of Drinking Water

Fluoridation of drinking water began in 1945. Fluoridation benefits everyone by preventing tooth decay and tooth loss in adults regardless of socioeconomic status or access. Fluoridation reached an estimated 144 million persons in the United States in 1999.

Recognition of Tobacco Use as a Health Hazard

Tobacco was recognized as a health hazard in 1964, resulting in changes in the promotion of smoking and reduction of exposure to environmental tobacco smoke. The initial Surgeon General's report prevented health risks of smoking and millions of smoking-related deaths. The prevalence of smoking among adults decreased.[34]

GLOBAL HEALTH SECURITY

Global health security impacts economic or political stability, trade, tourism, access to goods and services, and demographic stability. It includes acute public health events that endanger the collective health of populations living across geographic regions and international boundaries. Approximately 40 diseases have been discovered that were unknown a generation ago. WHO has verified more than 1,100 epidemic events in the past five years.[5] In addition, infectious diseases that have persisted for thousands of years still pose threats on a global scale. Genomic epidemiology, an emerging science, is the management and prevention of common diseases through understanding the molecular origin of disease. Studies of many people from different populations across the globe facilitate policies for handling shared resources and data, guidelines for releasing a person's private health information, and international policies and solutions for large-scale collaborative research efforts. Genomic epidemiology efforts include identifying and screening for genetic risk factors, profiling populations, forming appropriate strategies, and storing research via "biobanks." These security efforts are aimed at protecting epidemiological personal characteristics from unauthorized use as sabotage and recriminatory efforts.[31]

Global health security embraces a wide range of issues, including weather-related events, infectious and noninfectious disease monitoring and **surveillance**, health consequences of human behavior, natural catastrophes, and man-made disasters.[5] Major issues for global health are biosafety, biosecurity, and bioethics, all of which warrant secure policies and handling for public health and safety.[31]

The IHR of 2005 and World Health Assembly resolution WHA55.16 published in 2002 provided a framework to respond to events that threaten global public health security.[31,32] In the globalized world of the 21st century, enforcing border controls is not enough. Based on stopping diseases spreading through control measures at international borders, the IHR (1969) offered a legal framework for the notification and response to cholera, plague, relapsing fever, smallpox, typhus, and yellow fever, but compliance was very inconsistent.[5]

From 1996 to 2005, the IHR (1969) was revised to address the control of emerging and reemerging infectious diseases, the global transit of diseases, and exchange of animals and goods that may carry infectious agents. WHO is now authorized through the IHR (as of 2005) to take information sources other than official notifications and to seek verification of such information from the country.[31] Reputable sources of information are critical in maintaining public awareness and support of prevention and control measures. The sudden emergence of SARS in 2003 was an example of how an infectious disease posed a serious threat to global public health security.[5]

Surveillance Rates: This is the epidemiologic collections and monitoring of disease rates in humans.

A new issue is managing the recent immediate communication modes that have the potential to cause panic. The revised regulations, called the IHR (2005), were enforced in June 2007 to provide a legal framework for reporting significant health risks identified in national boundaries and the measures to stop their international spread.[31] The IHR (2005) defined an emergency as an event that could spread internationally or might require a coordinated response internationally. Mandatory notification is required in a single case of a disease that threatens global public health security. The first list of diseases included "public health emergency of international concern," and the second list included a "disease" that allows for the IHR (2005) inclusion of accidental or intentional release of pathogens, chemical agents, or radio-nuclear materials.[31] The diseases on the first list requiring mandatory notification are smallpox, poliomyelitis, human influenza, and SARS. The secondary list of diseases includes those capable of international spread through its release. These diseases are: cholera, pneumonic plague, yellow fever, viral hemorrhagic fevers (Ebola, Lassa, and Marburg), West Nile fever, and others.[31]

Many of these events are automatically picked up by the Global Public Health Intelligence Network.[35] This electronic intelligence-gathering tool provides a safety net for detection of events not otherwise reported. The inclusion of public health emergencies other than infectious diseases provided comprehensive, global public health security. The IHR (2005) introduced a set of "core capacity requirements" that all countries must meet to detect, assess, notify, and report the events covered by the IHR. Collaboration between member states helps build and strengthen global public health security.[31]

Throughout history, the challenge of infectious disease outbreaks and other health emergencies caused death on unprecedented levels and threatened global health security. The risks of new disease outbreaks and/or chemical agent release are increased today, so global surveillance effort and response systems are vital. However, there is always the threat of a new microbial agent or adaptation. Human demographics, behavior, economic development, land use, international travel and commerce, climate and ecosystem changes, poverty, conflict, famine, and **bioterrorism threats** (i.e., the deliberate release of infectious or chemical agents) have heightened this risk of epidemics today. International measures to prevent the spread of infectious diseases should be continued in the 21st century.[5]

GLOBAL HEALTH PARADIGM CHANGE

Health initiatives emerged around the globe and have had many positive changes through the centuries. Individually focused health programs are encouraged. However, a new paradigm change is the idea of global health. Global health is concerned with protecting the health of entire populations and is still emerging. Health evolution through the centuries saw many new discoveries, cures, diseases, preventive techniques, and health concerns. Health professionals prevent problems from happening and/or reoccurring through planning, implementing educational programs, developing policies, administering services, conducting research, and evaluating results. Health education is concerned with healthcare equity, quality, and access, as well as preventing health disparities. Culturally and scientifically competent health education is a must along with addressing the pervasive poverty issues even in developed countries. Besides global cooperative efforts, the future of the global health enhancement and mainte-

---

Bioterrorism threats: A public health threat to deliberately release infectious or chemical agents; such threats have heightened the risk of epidemics today.

nance of humans relies on prevention, promotion, protection, literacy, and access for all. Health educators play a huge role in continuously improving the spectrum of global health and planning for emerging new issues.

SUMMARY

- Global health monitoring is necessary for prevention and protection of disease elements. Areas of global health include environmental health, biostatics, behavior science/health education, epidemiology, health services administration/management, maternal and child health, nutrition, international global health, public health laboratory practices, public health policy, and health education practice.
- Lifestyle is an important health determinant.
- The earliest records of treatment for disease had religious connotations.
- As civilizations progressed, separating the diseased from the healthy, or quarantine, became the norm.
- John Graunt was a biostatistics pioneer who compiled vital statistics.
- Poisson related the idea of health and disease rates using statistical data.
- Jenner was successful with smallpox immunizations.
- The 1800s–1900s marked the bacteriological era, and epidemiological studies were stated by many health scientists. Disease transmission studies were started.
- The modern era of the 1900s still dealt with contagious diseases and quarantine, but other factors such as diet and behavior were studied. The WHO and epidemiological surveillance began in 1947.
- Health insurance, school health, and prevention methods in the United States are promoted.
- Many countries collected disease statistics and passed regulations to prevent transmission. Developing countries are still struggling with basic health necessities such as clean water.
- A pandemic is still a possible global public health threat. The World Health Assembly in 2002 encouraged strengthening surveillance, emergency preparedness, and response systems for the release of chemical, biological agents, and radionuclear materials. These measures make the reaction to global health security a paramount issue for all countries.
- While most contagious diseases are curable, not all countries and people have the resources. New diseases and adaptations are another global threat. Noncommunicable diseases are on the rise in developed countries.
- The health evolution through the centuries has seen many new discoveries, cures, diseases, preventive techniques, and health concerns. Global health is concerned with prevention, protection, promotion, enhancement, literacy, maintenance, and access for the health of entire populations.

CONCEPTUAL TERMS

Immunization
Demographic trends
Global health
Health disparities
Environmental health

Biostatistics
Behavior science/health education
Disease trends
Sanitation
Genetic determinants

Quarantine
Anton van Leeuwenhoek
Bacteria
Edward Jenner
John Snow
Louis Pasteur
Robert Koch
Alexander Fleming
Jonas Salk
International Health Regulations
World Health Assembly

International Sanitary Regulations
Code of Ethics for the Health Education
    Profession
Global health security
Global networks
Chemical Incident Alert and Response System
    (ChemiNet)
Greatest Public Health Achievements in the
    World
Surveillance Rates
Bioterrorism threats

REFLECTIVE THINKING

You are in a restaurant and go to the restroom. While in the restroom, you observe one of the food service employees leave the restroom without washing her hands. What is your obligation as a future health professional or a practicing health professional? Should you tell the management, or should you ignore what you saw? Discuss why hand washing after using the restroom is required for food service employees to protect the public. What diseases could be spread by neglecting this sanitary practice? Select and discuss other sanitation measures that restaurant employees are required by law to practice. Defend the local health department's role in inspecting restaurants. Discuss the measures taken by local health departments when there are restaurant sanitation violations or disease occurrences.

CONCEPTUAL LEARNING

1. Review examples of religious connotations in the earliest records of treatment for disease.
2. Categorize the new pandemic threats to global health security for the year 2000 and beyond.
3. List and analyze three reasons why countries that have discovered cures cannot solve communicable disease transmissions.
4. Analyze the theory behind the method of quarantine.
5. Construct a time line of the era of 1800–1900, and examine the bacteriological and epidemiological developments.
6. Explain the modern era of the 1900s, and focus on the reason for the examination of lifestyle factors as causes of diseases.
7. Examine and compare two (international, national, state, or local) laws, policies, or regulations affecting community health.
8. Briefly classify and list examples of the following health determinants: genetic determinants, physical environment, and social environment.
9. Compare and contrast the progress made during the first half of this century and that made in the second half of the century, with specific reference to personal health behaviors.
10. Discuss one new disease or epidemiological trend that is occurring within global networks, society at large, demographics, economics, and politics.

11. List three of the greatest risks to international global health today, and discuss how and why they occurred. Discuss the measures that are in place to prevent global health crises today.
12. State three of the greatest achievements in global public health, and assess why they are important today.
13. Discuss WHO's role in global health, prevention, advocacy, and action plans.
14. Explain the relationship between smallpox, polio, and immunizations; cholera and sanitation; and the plague and quarantine.
15. Evaluate the International Health Regulations (IHR).
16. Classify and summarize the achievements of Snow, Jenner, Salk, Koch, Fleming, Pasteur, and Leeuwenhoek.
17. Discuss why surveillance efforts are also important for chronic disease prevention.
18. According to most indicators, global health progress has been made in the 21st century due to public health initiatives. Compare the value of healthy places and these public health initiatives, including medical care access and immunizations, sanitation, protection of the environment, safe living conditions, quarantine, and determination of health risks as contributors to this progress.
19. Defend the aims of global health in prevention, reoccurrence, and limiting health disparities
20. Classify the areas of environmental health, and identify how each plays a role in disease prevention efforts.
21. Trace the development of public health in the world to present day. Design a chronology of events including any significant reports, establishment of organizations, political events, external factors that influenced the pace of development, major breakthroughs and discoveries that influenced health, the role of WHO, expansion of programs, epidemiological success, and the role and importance to health education influenced by public health personnel in the field.
22. Compare the status of global health statistics to U.S. health statistics today.

REFERENCES

1. Buckingham, R. W. (2001). *A primer on international health*. Boston: Allyn & Bacon.
2. Turncock, B. J. (2004). *Public health: What it is and how it works* (3rd ed.). Sudbury, MA: Jones and Bartlett Publishers.
3. National Institutes of Health. (2009). *NIH history highlights*. United States: Office of Health and Human Services. Retrieved March 20, 2010, from http://history.nih.gov/exhibits/history/index.html
4. Association of Schools of Public Health and Pfizer Public Health. (2009). *What is public health?* Retrieved February 22, 2010, from http://www.whatispublichealth.org/impact/achievements.html
5. World Health Organization. (2007). *Evolution of public health security. Global public health report in the 21st century* (pp. 1–14). Geneva, Switzerland: Author.
6. Insel, P. M., & Roth, W. T. (2008). *Core concepts in health* (10th ed.). New York: McGraw-Hill.
7. Schoenbach, V. J. (2000). *Understanding the fundamentals of epidemiology: An evolving text*. Retrieved January 20, 2009, from http://www.epidemiolog.net
8. McKenzie J. P., Pinger, R. R., & Lotecki, J. E. (2008). *An introduction to community health* (6th ed.). Sudbury, MA: Jones and Bartlett Publishers.
9. Catholic Biblical Association of Great Britain. (1966). *The Holy Bible*. (Trans.). Camden, NJ: Thomas Nelson and Sons.
10. World Book Encyclopedia. (1981). *Medicine* (vol. 13). Chicago, IL: Worldbook Childcraft International.
11. Fenner F., Henderson, D. A., Arita, I., Jezek, Z., & Ladnyi, I. D. (1988). *Smallpox and its eradication*. Geneva, Switzerland: World Health Organization.

12. Friis, R. H., & Sellers, T. A. (1996). *Epidemiology for public health practice*. Gaithersburg, MD: Aspen Publications.
13. Porter, R. (1997). *The greatest benefit to mankind: A medical history of humanity, from antiquity to the present*. London: HarperCollins.
14. Lillenfield, D. E., & Stolley, P. D. (Eds.). (1994). *Foundations of epidemiology* (3rd ed.). New York: Oxford University Press.
15. Furman, B. (1984). *A profile of the United States Public Health Service, 1798–1948*. Washington, DC: U.S. Government Printing Office. DHEW Publication (NIH), *73*(369), 308–311.
16. Last, J. M. (1995). *A dictionary of epidemiology* (3rd ed.). New York: Oxford University Press.
17. Hayden, J. (Ed.). (2000). *The health educator specialist: A study guide for professional competencies* (4th ed.). Whitehall, PA: The National Commission for Health Education Credentialing, Inc.
18. Davey, S. G. (2003). Behind the Broad Street pump: Etiology, epidemiology and prevention of cholera in mid-19th century Britain [commentary]. *International Journal of Epidemiology, 31*, 920–932.
19. Cairncross, S. (2003). Water supply and sanitation: Some misconceptions [editorial]. *Tropical Medicine and International Health, 8*, 193–195.
20. Hernandez, B. L. M., Vengurlekar, R., Kelkar, A., & Thomas, G. (2009). The legacy of Carville: A history of the last leprosarium in the U.S. *American Journal of Health Studies, 24*(2), 314–325.
21. United States Public Health Service. Office of the Surgeon General and Health Promotion. (1979). *Healthy people: The Surgeon General's report on health promotion and disease prevention*. Washington DC: Author.
22. World Health Organization. (1990). *Facts about WHO*. Geneva, Switzerland: Author.
23. Pan American Health Organization. (1995). Cholera in the Americas. *Epidemiological Bulletin of the Pan American Health Organization, 16*(2). Retrieved February 22, 2010, from http://www.paho.org/english/sha/epibul_95-98/be952choleraam.htm
24. World Health Organization. (2009). *Global epidemics and impact of cholera*. Geneva, Switzerland: World Health Organization. Retrieved February 22, 2010, from http://www.who.int/topics/cholera/impact/en/index.html
25. Knobler, S., Mahmoud, A., Lemon, S, & Pray, L. (Ed.). (2006). The impact of globalization on infectious disease emergence and control: Exploring the consequences and opportunities. *Workshop summary—forum on microbial threats*. Washington, DC: The National Academies Press.
26. Centers for Disease Control and Prevention. (1994). International notes update: Human plague, India, 1994. *Morbidity and Mortality Weekly Report*, 43:761–762. Retrieved March 20, 2010, from http://www.cdc.gov/mmwr/
27. United States Department of Labor, Bureau of Labor Statistics. (2008–2009 ed.). *Occupational outlook handbook, Health educators*. Retrieved February 22, 2010, from http://www.bls.gov/oco/ocos063.htm
28. United States Department of Health and Human Services. Office of Disease Prevention and Health Promotion. (2000). *Healthy people 2010* (2nd ed.). Retrieved February 22, 2010, from http://www.healthypeople.gov/default.htm
29. World Health Organization. (2005). *Global smallpox vaccine reserve: Report by the Secretariat*. Geneva, Switzerland: Author (report to the WHO Executive Board, document EB115/36). Retrieved February 22, 2010, from http://www.who.int/gb/ebwha/pdf_files/EB115/B115_36-en.pdf
30. Howard-Jones, N. (1975). *The scientific background of the International Sanitary Conferences, 1851–1938*. Geneva, Switzerland: World Health Organization.
31. World Health Organization. (2006). *International health regulations, 2005*. Geneva, Switzerland: Author. Retrieved February 22, 2010, from http://www.who.int/csr/ihr/en/
32. World Health Organization. (2002). *Global public health response to natural occurrence, accidental release or deliberate use of biological and chemical agents or radionuclear material that affect health*. Geneva, Switzerland: Author (World Health Assembly resolution WHA55.16). Retrieved March 20, 2010, from http://searo.who.int/meeting/rc/rc55/rc55–6.htm
33. United Nations Economic Commission for Europe. (1992). *Convention on the transboundary effects of industrial accidents*. Geneva, Switzerland: Author. Retrieved February 22, 2010, from http://www.unece.org/env/teia/welcome.htm
34. Centers for Disease Control and Prevention. (2008). The 20th century's ten great public health achievements in the United States. *Morbidity and Mortality Weekly Report, 43*, 761–762.

35. Ottawa Public Health Agency of Canada. (2004). *Information: Global public health intelligence network (GPHIN)*. Ottawa, Canada: Author.

ENHANCED READINGS

World Health Organization. *International classification of disease*. Retrieved March 20, 2010, from http://www.who .int/classifications/icd/ICDrevision.pdf

RELEVANT WEB SITES

United States National Library of Medicine. (1988, April 27). *Images from the history of the public health service*. Bethesda, MD: National Institutes of Health, Department of Health & Human Services. Available at: http:// www.nlm.nih.gov/exhibition/phs_history/contents.html#about

United States Department of Health and Human Services. Office of Disease Prevention and Health Promotion. (2000). *Healthy people 2010* (2nd ed.). Available at: http://www.healthypeople.gov/default.htm

World Health Organization. (2008). The top 10 causes of death, Fact sheet No. 310. Available at: http://www .who.int/mediacentre/factsheets/fs310_2008.pdf

Law, M., Kapur, A. K. & Collishaw, N. (2004, November). Health promotion in Canada 1974–2004 lessons learned. Canadian Medical Association. Retrieved March 20, 2010, from http:www3atelus.net/placer/Kelly/ Health-Promotion-In-Canada-1974-2004.pdf

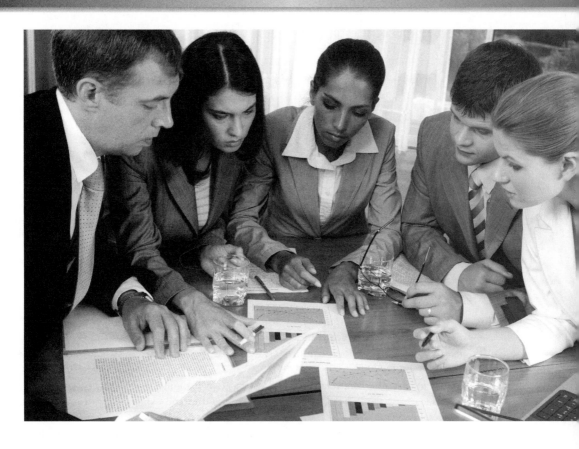

CHAPTER 3

Health Program Planning Models for Change and Prevention

OBJECTIVES AND ASSESSMENTS

This chapter meets the following National Commission for Health Education Credentialing, Inc., Society for Public Health Education, and American Association for Health Education Responsibilities and Competencies for Entry Level and Advanced Level Health Educator competencies.* The learner will:

1. Assess individual and community needs for health education.

This chapter meets the following general learning objectives. The learner will:
1. Compare and contrast health education program models similar to Healthy People 2010.
2. Identify, delineate, and evaluate primary, secondary, and Internet resources on health program planning models.
3. Provide and examine a rationale for health education planning models and programs.
4. Select and assess the basic health needs of communities and explain how to influence healthful behavior.
5. Summarize the components, guidelines, development procedures, and settings of health education programs.
6. Construct examples of basic health education program needs, services, and environmental areas.
7. Examine the content areas for health education programs.
8. Develop at least six basic parts of a program model and evaluate how each is measured.

Sources: Reprinted with permission of NCHEC.

National Commission for Health Education Credentialing, Inc. (NCHEC), Society for Public Health Education (SOPHE), & American Association for Health Education (AAHE). (2006). *A competency-based framework for health educators-2006*. Whitehall, PA: NCHEC.

INTRODUCTION

Health Program Planning Models (HPPMs), along with theories, are essential elements for planning, implementing, and evaluating successful health programs. HPPMs offer a step-by-step process that gives structure to the program, organizes the program, gives specific directions, and provides a framework for planning, implementing, and evaluating health programs. Models are the structure, and the health behavior theory provides the schema for understanding events or situations, explaining and predicting them according to the relationships among the variables.[1] According to Glanz, Rimer, and Viswanath, "Models draw on a number of theories to help understand a specific problem in a particular context or setting."[2(p29)]

Changing the health behaviors and infrastructures of long-entrenched derogatory habits and environments is a difficult task. When committing to a plan of action, planning models offer health educators a road map to follow, helping them achieve the required changes in a systematic and structured format. Unorganized planning for health is chaos, and there is no guarantee that the strategies, interventions, activities, or methods are working toward the goals and objectives. Proper planning is imperative to gaining meaningful results in health programs. Public policy as well as institutional, educational, organizational, and environmental factors are important concepts in planning programs.

There are many models to choose from, and each is unique in its own way. Some work at an individual level, and others work to change whole communities for more healthful living. Research reveals the programs that are most successful, and health educators are advised to adapt these programs to their existing needs. Health educators who want optimal results heed the expression, "Don't reinvent the wheel." They investigate other program models and can use and/or tailor a model to fit their program needs. Investigating previous successful programs and using program replication involves using evidence-based programs that work and adapting them to the current circumstances. Do not try to design a program from scratch unless no other program exists that suits your needs. Aside from wasting energy, the results are not proven through research and you may find yourself mired in details and trying to right a program that has strayed off course. A proper planning model is an essential part of carrying out successful health programs and evidence-based research on programs is essential for success. Find the correct and most productive program model and theory and/or combinations so the path is successful for the health educator leading the program and the participants in the program.

Career Concept

Are you interested in creating innovative programs to help people change harmful health behaviors? You might enjoy being in a medical care setting or a worksite health setting.

FUNCTION OF PLANNING MODELS

A planning model alone is like a puzzle piece that can only be productive if synchronized in conjunction with other pieces of a program plan; in this case, the most important piece would be relative theoretical principles. **Theory** is the glue that completes a successful program, and when utilized correctly,

> **Theory:** A conceptual framework that coordinates with evidence-based health promotion plans and gives credibility to a program.

brings about the desired behavior or social change in most participants and/or groups. If theory is not infused into the HPPM, you have no assurance that changes in any kind of behavior, environment, and/ or society will occur. You are playing "hit or miss" if a plan has no theory. In other words, you do not know if the strategies will accomplish the task if there is no theoretical background to it. The plan and theory should fit the situation and problem.

A model accomplishes the generic planning tasks. It allows for assessing needs, identifying the problem, developing appropriate goals and objectives, selecting and creating strategic plans, educational and environmental and legislative efforts, and specifying the administrative and staff role. It then provides for implementing the model program based on the needs assessment and conducting the process, impact, and outcome evaluations. A planning model provides a step-by-step framework for science-based prevention programming. It is a format for the planning committee, director, and staff. It works only when linked with the goals, objectives, needs assessment, problem identification, theoretical principles, and strategies used for behavior change in individuals, groups, communities, along with social, economic, and educational change, and specific cultural groups.[3]

Models are generalized, hypothetical descriptions of a program plan. They are a systematic way to design a program and administer the program from beginning to end. Parts or combinations of different HPPMs can be used to address problems. Using a variety of models allows for different sequences, emphasis, flexibility, and use of the major components. They must fit the special needs and cultural characteristics of the target group, the community or setting. Adaptation is necessary to adjust to the needs and cultural characteristics of the population or if administrative tasks need improvement. There may not always be a perfect planning model, which again underscores the importance of combining and adapting different models, as well as the theoretical principles used. Models function in several categories. An easy way to remember the basic stages in most models is the acronym PPIE, or the word pie with two P's. The first P task is to perform the needs assessment(s), identify the problem(s), and propose the rationale. The second P, or planning stage, involves the goals, objectives, theory, and strategies. The I is the implementation phase, and the E is the evaluation phase.

CATEGORIES OF HEALTH MODELS

There are three identified categories of health models and theoretical models. These models are individual (**intrapersonal**), **interpersonal**, and **community**, as identified by the National Cancer Institute and the NIH in 2005.[1] Intrapersonal or individual models impact individual knowledge, attitudes, beliefs, and behaviors. Interpersonal models address individual factors as they relate to individual needs, environment, and personal characteristics. Community models cover institutional, community, and

---

Intrapersonal models: Individual models that impact individual knowledge, attitudes, beliefs, and behaviors.
Interpersonal models: Models that address individual factors as they relate to individual needs, environment, and personal characteristics.
Community models: Models that cover institutional, community, and public policy factors.

public policy factors. A fourth model, the **cultural model**, should be added, as it is a necessity today. A cultural model addresses embedded cultural factors and attempts to change those negative ones detrimental to health.

Health educators need to be aware of the major planning models but should always research and understand many different planning models and use integrative, multilevel approaches. These approaches include multiple interventions, strategies, and activities geared to the theory and objectives of the program.

Campbell asserts that a model provides direction and a framework to build with the assumptions formally stated at the beginning.[4] She stated there are "6 generic set of tasks" that are necessary in every HPPM. These six tasks include:

1. Assess the needs of the target population
2. Identify the problem
3. Develop appropriate goals and objectives
4. Create an intervention that is like to achieve desired results
5. Implement the intervention
6. Evaluate the results[4]

The stages for the HABIT model are shown in Table 5–1 in Chapter 5. This model will be discussed in Chapter 5 in conjunction with strategic program planning. It is a new proposed model in a pilot stage, but research shows that its elements are replicated in research based on effective program plans.

Some of the relevant and empirically researched models available are described in this chapter. There is not enough space to delineate every specific part of the health models discussed or to list all models for health. There are many more effective HPPMs. It is recommended that research is necessary when planning programs and deciding on planning models. Health practitioners should realize that these program planning models can be combined and integrated for stronger program plans just as theoretical models can be combined.

HEALTH MODELS

A Systematic Approach to Health Promotion (Healthy People 2010)

A four-part planning model was used to develop *Healthy People 2010*. This model is used for planning at the national, state, or local community levels. The phases include goals, objectives, determinants of health, and health status. The results of this model, *Healthy People 2010*, are delineated in the following discussion. A new planning model is anticipated with the proposed *Healthy People 2020* objectives.[5]

Cultural models: Models that address embedded cultural factors and attempt to change those negative ones detrimental to health.

6 Generic Tasks of Program Models: Assess the needs of the target population, identify the problem, develop appropriate goals and objectives, create an intervention that is like to achieve desired results, implement the intervention, and evaluate the results (Campbell, 2001).

Healthy People 2010 is a comprehensive set of health objectives for the nation to achieve over the first decade of the new century to realize the vision of healthy people living in healthy communities. Created by scientists both inside and outside of government, it identifies a wide range of public health priorities and specific, measurable objectives. Together, these objectives reflect the depth of scientific knowledge as well as the breadth of diversity in the nation's communities. More importantly, they are designed to help the nation achieve *Healthy People 2010*'s two overarching goals—increase quality and years of healthy life and eliminate health disparities.[5]

The nation's progress in achieving the two main goals of *Healthy People 2010* are monitored through 467 objectives in 28 focus areas. Most objectives focus on interventions designed to reduce or eliminate illness, disability, and premature death among individuals and communities. Some focus on broader issues, such as improving access to quality health care, strengthening public health services, and improving the availability and dissemination of health-related information. Each objective had a target date of 2010 for specific improvements to be achieved, and these are being compiled. In addition to the two main goals, three notable goals are promote healthy behavior, prevent and reduce diseases and disorders, and promote healthy communities.[5]

Assessment Protocol for Excellence in Public Health (APEX-PH) (National Association of County and City Health Officials, 1991)

APEX-PH is a planning and assessment process to help county and local health department's respond to "The Future of Public Health." This model states that every public health agency should collect, organize, and analyze information on the health needs of the community. It is a framework for working with community members and organizations to establish the health status and health department's role in the community. It is also integrative and works with other models. It has been replaced by the *MAPP* (i.e., mobilizing for action through planning and partnerships) model, but many agencies like the first phase or organizational assessment that assists in planning efforts. The phases are assessing organizational capacity (internal assessments, *SWOT* [i.e., strengths, weaknesses, opportunities, and threats] analysis), implementing the community process (data collected and analyzed, problems analyzed, and priorities developed), and completing the cycle (develop policies, services, implementation plan, and evaluation plan).[6]

CDCynergy (CDC, 1997)

CDCynergy is an interactive training and decision-supported technological tool designed by the CDC in 1997 and issued in July 1998.[7] An updated version was released in 2001 and became known as the basic edition. The 2003 edition is know as *CDCynergy 3.0, Your Guide to Effective Health Communications*.[8] It is a comprehensive communication plan that allows for a large variety of strategies to address health

---

CDCynergy: An interactive, comprehensive communication plan that allows for planning, implementing, and evaluating program strategies to address the health problems using health communication involvement.

problems. The phases involve health communication in planning, implementing, and evaluating program strategies. Also included are researching the audience, pre-testing, implementation, and evaluation to benefit the participants. *CDCynergy* uses research to help describe the causes of the health problem you plan to address with interventions. It defines the audience segments that are affected by the problem. It is a health communication plan that answers questions in a specific, systematic sequence. There are six phases in this model: define the problem, analyze the problem, plan the intervention, develop the intervention, plan the evaluation, and implement the plan.[8] A breakdown of these phases follows.

Phase 1: Define the Problem

The key element for each phase involves defining the problem, researching the problem, and working with partners. Phase 1 includes conducting relevant research to identify and define the health problem(s) and subgroups to address in interventions. There is a section for assessing the factors and the research variables that affect the direction of the project for applying the SWOT analysis.

Phase 2: Analyze the Problem

This phase designs and develops goals, lists root causes of each problem to be addressed, and considers health ethics. Considerations include engineering, education, policy enforcement, and community service intervention options. The relevant theories, intervention models, and best practice are determined. The interventions selected must address the problem(s). Funding and partnerships are acquired and solidified.

Phase 3: Plan the Intervention

This phase involves deciding the intervention, including determining whether communication is the predominant method or is a support for other interventions. Segmentation of intended audiences is necessary, and communication goals are written for each segment of the audiences. Next, a guide for selecting the appropriate concepts, messages, setting, activities, and materials is designed. Communication goals are rewritten as measurable communication objectives. In addition, plans are confirmed, and time and resources are addressed as needed.

Phase 4: Develop the Intervention

This phase involves developing and testing concepts, messages, materials, and communication channels and settings with the specific audiences. The timetable and budget are drafted. Next, the channel-specific communication activities are selected and tested. The communication implementation plan is constructed using a theoretical focus, and the formative research is conducted. This phase also considers the setting, roles, and responsibilities, and the materials are marketed for dissemination.

Phase 5: Plan the Evaluation

This phase identifies the stakeholders' information needs. The intervention standards are connected with the evaluation type and design. The sources of information, data collection methods used for gathering credible information, data analysis, timetable, budget, and a reporting plan are completed. This phase is when the evaluation implementation plan is shared with stakeholders and staff.

Phase 6: Implement the Plan

The final phase involves executing and managing the communication and evaluation plans. Documenting feedback and lessons learned and modifying the program based on these concerns are accomplished. Then evaluation results are disseminated.[8] There is also a *CDCynergy Lite* version available that is an abbreviated version of *CDCynergy* and includes the same six phases of the communication model.[8]

Community Primary Healthcare Model (CPHC) (WHO, 1978)

The *CPHC* model is based on community need and choice. It developed from the definition of primary health care by the WHO in 1978.[9] It states that health care must be practical, be scientifically based, and use socially acceptable methods and technology that are universally accessible to individuals, families, and communities. Full participation at an affordable price must be maintained at each stage within self-reliance and self-determination principles. It is linked with the country's healthcare system as the central focus and function and with the overall socioeconomic development of the country. It provides for constructing interventions to improve health outcomes and has five principles: equitable distribution, appropriate technology, focus on health promotion and disease prevention, community participation, and a multisectoral approach.[9] The interactive planning process is recommended when implementing this model.[10] This is a process that utilizes systems thinking and design. All the principles of the *CPHC* model linked with the interactive planning process can continuously improve coordinating healthcare services at the local and regional levels if interdisciplinary, intra-organizational, and interorganizational.[11]

Community Wellness Model (CWM) (Jenkins, 1991)

This model helps local resources find solutions for community-based problem solving. The first stage is the single resource level, the second stage involves multiple resources, the third stage is communitywide resources, and the last stage is task force resources.[4] The premise for the *Community Wellness Model* is that wellness is not static but an interrelated, dynamic process that is everchanging and growing. This approach is different from the *Wellness Model* that delineates the illness/wellness continuum from high levels of wellness to premature death.[12] It is also not the same as the Insel and Roth *Dimensions of Wellness*[13] model that consists of physical, emotional, intellectual, spiritual, interpersonal and social, and environmental wellness.

Ecological Model

The *Ecological Model* comprehensively addresses public health problems at multiple levels of influence, combining behavioral and environmental components. Changes and interactions between factors occur over a lifetime and a person's individual and social environmental factors are viewed as targets for affecting positive behaviors. As McLeroy, Bibeau, Steckler, and Glanz explain:

> The model assumes that appropriate changes in the social environment will produce changes in individuals, and that the support of individuals in the population is essential for implementing environmental changes. It addresses interventions aimed at changing the intrapersonal, interpersonal, institutional, community, and public policy factors.[14(p. 351)]

A multilevel interactive approach involves two key concepts. The first is that behavior affects and is affected by these multiple levels of influence. The second is that individual behavior forms and is formed by the social environment. It is a well-known fact that individuals' social environment affects their health. Socially disadvantaged people are more likely to have diseases and injuries. Ecological models use science for prevention and promotion programs that can succeed in populations.[15]

The health determinants are causal in action. They result from a complex interaction of social, economic, environmental, behavioral, and genetic determinants over the course of a person's life. The social environment involves the concept of reciprocal causation or reciprocal determinism, meaning the person, behavior, and social environment affect lifestyle and ultimately health.[1] The dimensions this model identified are the individual, the behavior, the physical environment, the social environment, and cultural factors. **Social determinants** influence behavior and health in positive and negative ways. Early exposure to positive or negative conditions strongly impacts a person's quality and length of life. A safe environment, adequate socioeconomics, important roles in society, adequate housing, higher education levels, and social support within communities are directly related to better health and welfare.[16]

There are different levels of influence for the *Ecological Model*,[1,14] including intrapersonal, interpersonal, institutional or organizational factors, community and public policy levels. The intrapersonal level focuses on a variety of intervention strategies to target individual characteristics that influence behaviors. It is also called the individual level. Individual characteristics that are considered include knowledge, skills, beliefs, experiences, attitudes, behaviors, and personality traits as these individuals interact with the environment and society.

The interpersonal level is based on changing behavior through social influences. It addresses relationships as social identity, support, and role delineation with significant others, including family and friends. It considers the personal influences as well as the influences of other people, the immediate physical environment, and the social networks where people live, work, and play.

Ecological Model: A model that comprehensively addresses public health problems at multiple levels of influence, combining behavioral and environmental components.
Social determinants: Positive or negative conditions in life that influence behavior and health in positive and negative ways.

The **institutional or organizational factors** address rules, regulations, policies, and informal structures that can restrict or support recommended behaviors. Informal rules and policies can become embedded, or **institutionalized**, in communities. This level also involves social institutions and associations that have direct influence over the physical and social environments within an organization. Community factors include standards, norms, and social networks that occur among individuals, groups and organizations, as well as both structural and practical terms of a community.

The **public policy factors** are defined in more global terms, including political boundaries, distribution of resources that manage and direct the lives, and the management, direction, and development of communities. This level is concerned with the local, state, and federal policies and/or laws that regulate and support healthy actions and practices for prevention, early detection, control, and management of disease.[1] As McLeroy et al. state, "The purpose of an ecological model is to focus attention on the environmental causes of behavior and to identify environmental interventions."[14(p366)] Communities are mediating power structures, concerned with the relationships among organizations within a political or geographic area. Health promotion programs where health educators use multiple levels of influence targeted to the specific populations they are serving are more effective in solving health problems. This approach is more likely to maintain prevention efforts over a longer period than any one intervention of the program.[1]

The purpose of the *Ecological Model* is to facilitate interventions within many different levels of influence. The strategies that are most likely to cause change should be used. The program focuses on the different dimensions of the health problems and analyzes the behavioral, epidemiological, social, educational, and ecological factors. The ecological analysis includes organizational, community, administrative, regulatory and policy, intrapersonal, interpersonal, and environmental considerations. A *SORC* analysis is also performed. *SORC* stands for stimuli, organism, responses, and consequences.[17]

In focusing on an individual's behavior and how it is affected by environmental, ecological, and social influences, certain questions need to be asked: Why does the problem exist? What populations need help? What do we need to know about the participant population in order to guide our decision making in regards to the plan, so messages are targeted to the intended audiences and make an impact?

PRECEDE–PROCEED Model (Green & Kreuter, 1975, 1991, 2005)

The *PRECEDE–PROCEED* model by Green and Kreuter is one of the most used and referenced HPPMs.[18] It covers almost every possible situation and causation. If carefully followed, planners can

---

Institutional/organizational factors: The organizational factors that address rules, regulations, policies, and informal structures that can restrict or support the behaviors recommended.
Institutionalized: The state of informal rules and policies that have become embedded in communities.
Public policy factors: Local, state, and federal policies and laws that regulate and support healthy actions, practices, and resource distribution for prevention, early detection, control, and management of diseases.
PRECEDE–PROCEED: A program planning model that covers many different situations and causations. PRECEDE stands for predisposing, reinforcing, and enabling constructs in educational/ecological diagnosis. PROCEED stands for policy, regulatory, and organizational constructs in educational and environmental development.

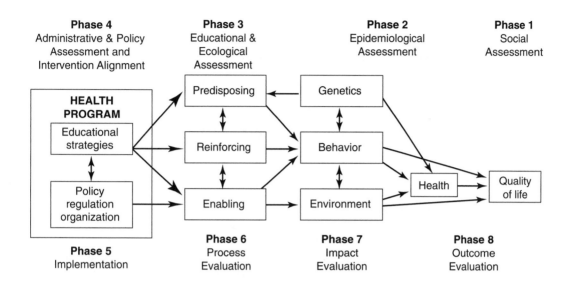

FIGURE 3-1   *PRECEDE-PROCEED* Model

Source: Green, Lawrence and Kreuter, Marshall. *Health Program Planning: An Educational and Ecological Approach, 4e.* 2005. © The McGraw-Hill Companies. Reproduced with permission.

assure they are following an organized and systematic planning model. It has recently been updated, and it seems the authors are continuously updating and revising this wonderful tool for health educators. PRECEDE stands for **p**redisposing, **r**einforcing, and **e**nabling constructs in educational/ecological diagnosis. This phase is crucial for developing effective programs because it focuses on attitudes, values, and beliefs. PROCEED stands for **p**olicy, **r**egulatory, and **o**rganizational constructs in educational and environmental development. The first four phases are the formative evaluation parts involving assessment and the last four phases are the implementation and the summative evaluations.[18] Many of the phases of *PRECEDE-PROCEED* have been replicated and used with many other planning models. It is a very thorough model and covers all aspects affecting a person's health (see **Figure 3–1**).

Areas of the model are described as follows:[18]

- *Phase 1*: Social diagnosis and situational analysis (identify social problem)
- *Phase 2*: Epidemiological diagnosis (genetic factors, behavioral factors, lifestyle, behavioral and environmental factors)
- *Phase 3*: Educational and ecological assessment (predisposing, reinforcing, and enabling factors)
- *Phase 4*: Administrative and policy assessment and intervention alignment implementation (health program including educational strategies and policy; regulation; and organization)
- *Phase 5*: Implementation or beginning the program
- *Phase 6*: Process evaluation determines if program is active and works

- *Phase* 7: Impact evaluation determines if program effects on behavior and environment are adequate
- *Phase* 8: Outcome evaluation determines if quality of life improved

It is important to understand this model can be revised or revisited because of constant analysis and evaluation within the phases.

Expert Methods of Planning and Organization Within Everyone's Reach (EMPOWER) (Green & Kreuter, 1991)

EMPOWER is a wonderful interactive technological tool based on the *PRECEDE–PROCEED* HPPM of Green and Kreuter.[18] *EMPOWER* was developed to support health educators and other professional planners meet the unique needs of a particular local group or community. It enables health promotion professionals to develop expert programs that are effective and responsive to needs. Sequential modules guide the planner through the *PRECEDE–PROCEED* model planning process. The modules include, but are not necessarily limited to, many different assessments. The *EMPOWER* planning and implementation model should produce programs and outcomes that can be evaluated, enabling users to gather and analyze data from different resources. This model is based on cancer prevention and is ideally suited to the new technological world of program planning.[19] It is available on CD-ROM with an instructional booklet. The analyses segments of this model include situational analysis, social analysis, epidemiological analysis, behavioral and environmental analysis, educational and organizational analysis, and administrative and policy analysis.[19]

Generic Health and Fitness Delivery System (GHFDS) (Patton, Cory, Gettman, & Graf, 1986)

This model was not originally developed for health but can be used nonetheless. It is goal oriented and has five processes or stages. It is a dynamic and interactive model that provides an ongoing review and feedback for program delivery to meet the needs of the participants, allowing for modifications and feedback in later steps. The components are needs assessment, goal setting, planning (choosing strategies to meet goals), program implementation or delivery, and evaluation. Each step has two components—education and service. The education component includes cognitive awareness and knowledge experience. The service component provides for experiential learning.[4]

Healthy Plan–*it* (Health Analysis for Planning Prevention Services (CDC, 2000))

The purpose of this model is for planning and managing public health programs using a data-based decision-making process. It is a management system that includes planning, organizing, monitoring,

---

EMPOWER: An interactive technological tool system, based on the *PRECEDE–PROCEED* program planning model, to support professional planners in developing programs to meet the unique needs of a particular local group or community.

and evaluating organizational resources.[20] It was developed by the CDC based on the *Health Analysis for Planning Prevention Services* (HAPPS) and the Sustainable Management Development Program. Public health program management includes preventing or controlling disease, disabilities, and premature mortality. The model has six steps: setting priorities (participatory setting and consensus building), establishing goals (statement of results), setting outcome objectives (measurable outcomes related to goals and the problem), strategizing (methods and interventions), evaluating (measure success of objectives and goals), and budgeting (actual project cost).[20]

Healthy Plan-*it* is a tool for planning and managing public health programs using a data-based decision-making process. It can be ordered as a CD-ROM that contains a participant's manual, a facilitator's manual, and PowerPoint® files with embedded video clips for each of the three modules. Healthy Plan-*it* was developed by the Sustainable Management Development Program, under the CDC's Coordinating Office of Global Health.[20]

Public health program management includes planning, organizing, monitoring, and evaluating the use of organizational resources (including time, personnel, and money) to prevent or control diseases, disabilities, and premature mortality. A description of the modules follows:

- *Module 1*: Problems and Priorities provides a way to rate health priorities through the *Basic Priority Rating System* (BPRS), and a way to determine which priorities make the most sense to address through the *PEARL* assessment system. *PEARL* is an acronym for propriety, economics, acceptability, resources, and legality.
- *Module 2*: Finding Solutions teaches the steps involved in problem solving: identifying determinants and contributing factors to the selected health issue, setting objectives, designing an intervention strategy, and developing a work plan based on a work breakdown structure.
- *Module 3*: Evaluation and Budget provides tools for monitoring and evaluating progress toward achieving the set objectives, creating budgets, and using the budget as a management tool.[20]

Healthy Communities and/or Healthy Cities and/or Healthy People in Healthy Communities (USDHHS, 2001)

The purpose of this model is to assist in planning and organizing community-based health promotion planning programs utilizing the objectives outlined in Healthy People 2010. This planning model includes the following priorities: mobilize key individuals and organizations; assess community needs, strengths, and resources; plan for action; implement the action step; and track progress and outcomes.[21]

Mobilizing Action Through Planning and Partnerships (MAPP) (National Association of County and City Health Officials, 2001)

MAPP is an approach created by the National Association of County and City Health Officials.[22] It was created to assist local public health agencies with local planning. The purpose is to mobilize partnerships and use strategic planning actions to improve health and quality of life. There are six phases of *MAPP* (see **Figure 3–2**). In phase 1, organizing for success and partnership development, planners assess

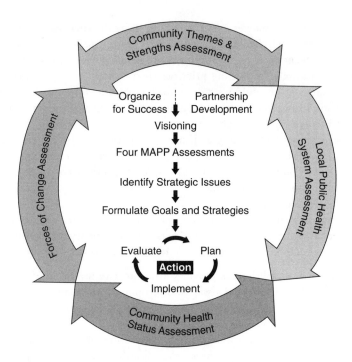

FIGURE 3–2   Mobilizing for Action Through Planning and Partnerships (MAPP) Model

Source: National Association of County and City Health Officials. Available at http://mapp.naccho.MAPP .model.asp. Used with permission.

the process and resources. Phase 2 is a visioning process in which the community is guided through shared vision concepts and common values. Phase 3 includes four *MAPP* assessments that help identify gaps between desired health status and the present status and issues. The four assessments include community themes and strength; local public health assessment and capacity; measurement of the community health status; and change assessment as capacity, including legislation, technology, and social and environmental events. In phase 4, strategic issues are prioritized. In phase 5, goals and strategies are formed to reach the health program's vision. The sixth phase is the action cycle, which includes implementation, evaluation, and dissemination for results.[22]

Multilevel Approach to Community Health (MATCH) (Simons-Morton, Simons-Morton, Parcel, & Bunker, 1988)

This multilevel model establishes connections between health outcomes, intervention objectives, and approaches. It is an ecological model using various levels of framework. It proceeds in a straightforward and direct pattern from the needs assessment and priority setting to the development of effective health programs. It is used when the behavioral and environmental risk as well as the protective disease and/or injury factors are known and action priorities have been previously determined. *MATCH* is comprised of five phases, with steps within the phases.[23] Phase 1, goals selection, includes identifying health status goals, high-priority populations(s), health behavior goals, and environmental factor goals. Phase 2, intervention planning, identifies the targets of intervention action, intervention objectives, and the mediators of the intervention objectives, and selects intervention approaches. Phase 3, program development, involves creating the program units, selecting or developing curricula and intervention guides, developing session plans, and creating or acquiring instructional materials, products and resources. Phase 4, implementation, begins by facilitating adoption, implementation, and maintenance and proceeds to selecting and training the implementers. Phase 5, evaluation, conducts the process, impact, and outcome evaluations.[24]

PEN-3 (Airhihenbuwa, 1989)

Developing culturally appropriate health programs is important in a diverse and changing society. Cultural models are a new way to approach health behavior change. PEN-3 is a highly recognized model that centralizes cultural elements as the most important part of prevention and promotion health behavior programs and adapts preventive health programs to fit specific cultural/community needs. Cultural plans are often overlooked, but should be used or integrated in any health promotion program where culture plays a huge part on the health of the community/group. Most health educators need additional help when working with groups with indigenous cultures.[25]

The *PEN-3* model is a self-empowerment approach or a cultural empowerment application. It is used to develop, implement, and evaluate health programs with three components. Each element has three parts that start with a *P*, an *E* , and an *N*, thus the name *PEN-3*. The original areas of the model that intertwined and/or overlapped included the cultural beliefs (positive, existential, negative), health education program (person, extended family, neighborhood), and educational diagnosis (predisposing, enabling, and nurturing factors).[26]

A revised 2004 model is similar to the original but includes the revised headings of 1) cultural identity, 2) cultural empowerment, and 3) relationships and expectations (see **Figure 3–3**). The cultural identity phase replaces the terms health education program and includes the person, extended family, and neighborhood. The cultural empowerment phase replaces the cultural beliefs phase and includes positive, existential, and negative factors. The relationships and expectations phase replaces the educational diagnosis phase and includes perceptions, enablers, and nurturers.[26] In the cultural identity phase, the focus is on the individual or person who is empowered to make the health decisions. In addressing the extended family, there is a focus not just on the individual person but those who influence his or her life, including the entire family. The neighborhood involves the whole community and its leaders. The relationships and expectations phase of health behavior determines the influences on health actions. There are perceptions or the attitudes, values, and beliefs that can enhance or detract from the motiva-

---

MATCH: A multilevel ecological model that provides a way to establish connections between the health outcomes, intervention objectives, and approaches.

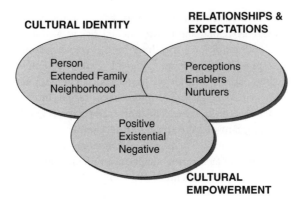

FIGURE 3-3   The *PEN-3 Model*

Source: Courtesy of Dr. Collins Airhihenbuwa, Professor and Head, the Department of Biobehavioral Health, College of Health and Human Development, The Pennsylvania State University.

tion to change behavior. With enablers, cultural, societal, or other forces enhance or detract from the health behavior change. With nurturers, these perceptions are influenced and negotiated by personal friends, family, peers, and the community. The cultural empowerment phase addresses appropriate positive health behaviors or those cultural behaviors known to be beneficial, and they should be kept. The existential behaviors are those cultural behaviors embedded in a group that do not cause any harm. The negative behaviors are the health beliefs and actions known to cause harm; these are the ones to consider changing or eliminating when possible. The E's are the most influential factors in *PEN-3*. For success in behavioral/cultural changes, the extended family, the enablers (sustained positive traditions), and the existential behavior (human and cultural empowerment) are very relevant to this model.[26, 27]

PEN-3 Model framed health-related projects including cancer, hypertension, diabetes, smoking, food choices, and recommendations for national strategies to eliminate health disparities among ethnic minorities for obesity. It uses the cultural context to develop culturally appropriate health promotion programs.[26] This model was used to conduct cultural-based research and develop strategies for combating HIV/AIDS in Africa. It also addresses the stigma and human rights abuses associated with this disease.[27]

Planned Approach to Community Health (PATCH) (CDC, 1984–1985)

The CDC developed *PATCH* in the 1980s in response to a need for a community planning tool. As stated by the CDC, "The goal of *PATCH* is to increase the capacity of communities to plan, implement,

> **PATCH**: A community-based model used by communities to plan, conduct, and evaluate health promotion and disease prevention programs.

and evaluate comprehensive, community-based health promotion programs."[28] *PATCH* is a process that helps establish health promotion and disease prevention programs. It was developed in coordination with state and local health departments and community groups. The team helps collect and use local data to set health priorities to design and evaluate interventions.[29] The theories are organized within the context of the PRECEDE part of the *PRECEDE-PROCEED* model. The philosophy was built on the one developed by the WHO's *Health for All* and the *Ottawa Charter for Health Promotion*.[30] There are five basic phases in the *PATCH* process:[28]

- *Phase I*: Mobilizing the community
- *Phase II*: Collecting and organizing data
- *Phase III*: Choosing health priorities
- *Phase IV*: Developing a comprehensive intervention plan
- *Phase V*: Evaluating *PATCH*

Social Marketing (Kotler & Zaltmane, 1971)

The *Social Marketing Model* was developed for translating marketing strategies into messages. It is also called marketing segmentation. As health educators, we use it to improve health behavior. Just as business marketers brand their products, health educators market good health to consumers. The same plan that markets products for consumers works equally well for marketing health. The model identifies the patterns that show the differences in one target group from another. The benefits for the participants are keyed to the *Social Marketing* strategies and methods. It is consumer driven and works by dividing or segmenting the target audiences into subgroups that are homogenous.

This planning model assesses the needs, analyzes the problems, selects channels and materials, develops materials and pretesting, implements methods, assesses effectiveness, and uses feedback to refine goals. This model identifies the variables used in planning for segmenting the target populations. Selecting channels and materials involves the standard four *p*'s (product, promotion, price, and place), but there is a need to include a fifth *p* for the person (client or participant). Once all of the stages are completed, the evaluation and refinements are used to revise the model. The cycle begins again after the new revisions are in place.[1] The areas of the Social Marketing model are (1) planning and strategy development, (2) developing and pretesting concepts, messages, and materials, (3) implementing the program, and (4) assessing effectiveness and making refinements.[1]

Social Marketing Assessment and Response Tool (SMART) (Neiger, B.L. & Thackery, R., 1998; Walsh et al, 1993)

The *SMART* model is based on social marketing with a formula that merges with health education. It is called a consumer-based planning approach and is a planning protocol where consumers are involved

---

> *Social Marketing Model*: A planning model that assesses the needs, analyzes the problems, selects channels and materials, develops materials and pretesting, implements methods, assesses effectiveness, and uses feedback to segment and improve target populations.

in data collection and program delivery. This model has seven phases: (1) preliminary planning, (2) consumer analysis, (3) market analysis, (4) channel analysis, (5) develop interventions and materials and pre-test these, (6) implementation, and (7) evaluation.[31]

Strategic Prevention Framework (Center for Substance Abuse Prevention)

Most of the models address a current health issue or problem. The paradigm change for the future of health education enhancement, maintenance, and promotion is that efforts depend strategically on prevention, protection, and access to services and address the factors that enhance and hinder health status. The *Strategic Prevention Framework* was developed by the Center for Substance Abuse Prevention (CSAP), which operates under the Substance Abuse and Mental Health Services Administration (SAMHSA) of the USDHHS. Risk factors are elements that predispose a person to specific negative behaviors or conditions individually or within the environment. Protective factors are elements that reduce the influence of negative behaviors or conditions within an individual or the environment. The Strategic Protection Framework addresses risk and protective factors with a five-phase process, including (1) assessment, (2) capacity development, (3) planning, (4) implementation, and (5) evaluation. **Figure 3–4** provides an example of the elements contained in the 5 phases of the *Strategic Protection Framework*. The example in **Figure 3–5** shows the use of the *Strategic Protection Framework* in sustainability and cultural competence as a stimulus and centralized structure for improving health in all people utilizing assessment, capacity building, planning, implementation, and evaluation.[2,10,32]

Strengths, Weaknesses, Opportunities, and Threats Analysis (SWOT) (Johnston, Scholes, & Sexton 1989; Bartol & Martin, 1991)

This model facilitates planning and action in a limited time frame. It includes rapid internal and external assessments, using an organization's strengths, weaknesses, opportunities, and threats. While some proponents argue that too much time is involved in planning, it identifies relevant strengths and addresses weaknesses. Properly coordinating, infusing adequate theory, and establishing a rationale are important element of this model.[21]

The Health Communication Process Model (National Cancer Institute, 2002)

This model provides for assessments of target audience needs at critical points for comprehensive program development and implementation. It is a circular, continuous process of planning and improvement. Although many organizations may not be able to implement the entire process, following the entire model as fully as possible can provide for more productivity, and additional components can be implemented in the future. In this model, stage 1 includes planning and strategy. The assessment of the problem, defining the target audience, goals, and measurable objectives, provides a foundation for this process. Stage 2 is selecting channels and materials. Decisions in this stage guide selection of the correct communication channels, producing effective materials and formats. With

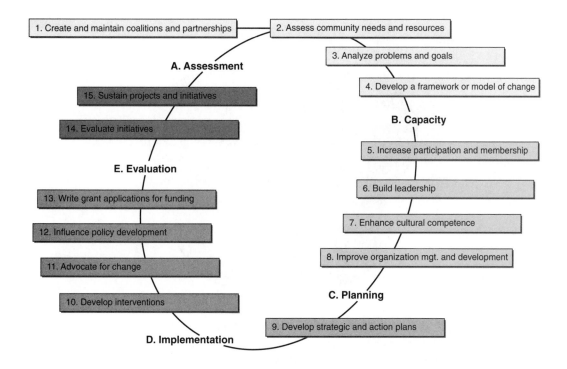

1. Create and maintain coalitions and partnerships — 2. Assess community needs and resources

A. Assessment

3. Analyze problems and goals

4. Develop a framework or model of change

15. Sustain projects and initiatives

14. Evaluate initiatives

B. Capacity

5. Increase participation and membership

E. Evaluation

6. Build leadership

13. Write grant applications for funding

7. Enhance cultural competence

12. Influence policy development

8. Improve organization mgt. and development

11. Advocate for change

10. Develop interventions

C. Planning

9. Develop strategic and action plans

D. Implementation

FIGURE 3–4 Skills Required to Implement the *Strategic Prevention Framework*

Source: Courtesy of the *Community Tool Box*, copyright 2007 by the Work Group for Community Health and Development, University of Kansas. Available online at http://ctb.ku.edu. Used with permission.

program planning completed, stage 3 involves developing materials and pre-testing. Feedback from the intended audience is crucial while testing and developing the messages and materials. Changes should be implemented if the messages and materials need revisions. Stage 4 is the implementation stage. The program begins with the promotion and distribution through all channels to the target audience. Components of the program should be reviewed continuously. These components along with information from audience reactions are tracked so revisions and alterations can occur as needed. The channels and materials having the greatest effect are identified. Stage 5 is assessing effectiveness. The program is evaluated by analyzing the results of measurements used throughout the program. Objectives, planning, implementation, and evaluation are assessed for competence. Stage 6 is feedback to refine the program. Data collection includes the audience, channels, message, and the program effect. The evaluation phase reviews all aspects of the program and identifies strengths to continue and weaknesses to address for the next cycle.[33]

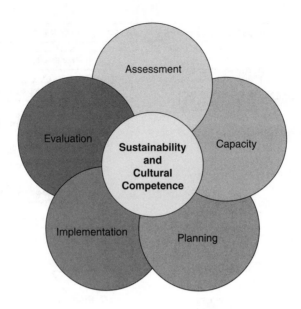

FIGURE 3–5   What is the *Strategic Prevention Framework*?

Source: Courtesy of the *Community Tool Box*, copyright 2007 by the Work Group for Community Health and Development, University of Kansas. Available online at http://ctb.ku.edu. Used with permission.

The Community Tool Box (CTB) (University of Kansas Work Group, 1995–2010)

Building healthier cities and communities involves local people working toward changing health conditions and outcomes. Core competencies, such as community assessment, planning, community mobilization, intervention, advocacy, evaluation, and marketing successful efforts are necessary to support community health promotion efforts. The *CTB* is an effective way to transmit skills through easy access to online information. This information center, maintained by the University of Kansas, began in 1995 and is updated continuously. It is an Internet-based support system for building healthier communities. The *CTB* was officially designated as a WHO Collaborating Center for Community Health and Development in 2004. It was recognized as a model by the CDC. It works in three domains: community and public health, child/youth health and development, and community and capacity development.[32]

There are customized work stations, a curriculum with 16 competencies, and an online documentation and support system (ODSS). The work stations provide support for building community initiatives, including community evaluation, and building capacity for health and development. The curriculum framework outlines an interactive process with six phases and related competencies associated with facilitating community change and improvement. The ODSS provides for online documentation for improvement and evaluation.[32]

The phases of the CTB include (1) understanding community context (for assessing assets and needs), (2) conducting collaborative planning for developing a vision, mission, objectives, strategies, and action plans (VMOSA), (3) developing leadership and enhancing participation (for forming relationships and recruiting participants), (4) initiating community action and intervention (for developing strategies and advocacy), (5) evaluating community initiatives (for program evaluation and community change), and (6) promoting and sustaining the initiative (for grant funding and social marketing). This tool kit is a valuable resource that supports development and evaluation of community health promotion programs.[32]

> **Thought Concept**
>
> *Describe how an HPPM is similar to constructing the framework of a house.*

Developing a Framework Using Logic Models or Intervention Mapping

Logic Models are similar to concept or *Intervention Mapping*. There are HPPMs and theoretical models that use this concept. A theory based on this concept is shown in Chapter 4. Many visual learners physically map out the model framework, theories, and strategies along with the objectives and goals to clarify and arrive at an organized, sequential plan of how the program works. For HPPMs, concept mapping and *Logic Models* are strategic ways to visualize how the elements work in a well-planned and comprehensive program. Many health educators write the elements of a program on paper and then place each item on a bulletin board or chart. That way, each can be moved and manipulated until an acceptable plan of action arises or visual map occurs.[32]

Intervention Mapping provides a framework for effective decision making at each step for health educators planning health programs. The process includes intervention planning, implementation, and evaluation. A health promotion or communication intervention is a planned combination of theoretic methods delivered to target groups. Delivery occurs through a series of strategic planning steps keyed to the goals and objectives and organized into a program. Interventions are designed to change environmental or behavioral factors related to health. Well-defined antecedents or determinants of behavior and environmental conditions are the targets of an intervention. The planning tasks and procedures in Intervention Mapping are not new to health promotion or health communication. However, the specific tasks of each step and the organization of these tasks into a systematic, interrelated approach can accommodate a wide variety of theoretical approaches. This is the innovative approach used in *Intervention Mapping*. The steps of *Intervention Mapping* for HPPMs according to the University of Texas Health Sciences Center at Houston include:[33]

- *Step 1*: Needs assessment or problem analysis
- *Step 2*: Matrices of proximal program objectives
- *Step 3*: Theory-based methods and practical strategies
- *Step 4*: Program
- *Step 5*: Adoption and implementation
- *Step 6*: Evaluation

For more information on these types of models, see the *Community Tool Box*'s detailed resource called the "Outline for Developing a Framework or Model of Change."[32] Also, see Chapter 5 in this book on Health Program Strategic Planning and the National Cancer Institute's reference for more information on VMOSA or vision, mission, objectives, strategies, and assessment.[34]

DOCUMENTING HEALTH INITIATIVES

The Pan American Health Organization's *Guide for Documenting Health Promotion Initiatives* states, "Health promotion is a way of thinking and working that is integrative, intersectoral, population-based, participatory, context-sensitive and acts at many different levels to achieve better health conditions and status in the entire population and especially in those that are most marginalized." According to the PAHO guide, the purpose of health promotion is to provide opportunities for "...critical reflection, capacity building experience, empowerment of your initiative's participants, [and] reflection on health promotion processes, using this as guidance on what information should be collected on health promotion initiatives, and having the potential for helping in advocacy/funding leverage activities."[35(p3)] The guide supports health promotion initiatives that improve and call attention to health programs that promote health and health equity efforts. In response to the need for more data collection and analysis of the effects of health programs, projects, and initiatives, the guide aims to promote and expand evidence-based documentation of efforts taking place in the Americas.

The PAHO guide facilitates ongoing or recent health promotion projects in cities and communities. It can be used in collaboration with many health promotion projects. Research institutions and other partners are encouraged to help with the data collection and analysis process. This guide is meant only as a source of useful questions to guide systematic documentation efforts. Information important to the group in understanding the initiative should also be included. There is a system of templates available for health practitioners to use. Questions are asked to facilitate responses and keep the documentation clear and precise. The outline includes six different areas of templates with questions, charts, and checklists to fill out. These areas are 1) identification of information, 2) description of the context, actors and stakeholders, 3) types and nature of resources and funding, 4) dynamics of the initiative, 5) main achievements, and 6) critical reflections with lessons learned. The guide includes a rating series and a glossary.[35]

The evaluation requires information about the history, context, and accomplishments of the health promotion initiative. It is recommended that multiple stakeholders, especially community members, are interviewed for a complete view of the health promotion program and its effectiveness from a practical viewpoint.[35]

This new initiative provides a sampling of programs for others to replicate and use. It identifies the strengths and weaknesses of ongoing and completed projects and identifies a plethora of programs to guide new and existing health promotion programs. It is a great resource and a learning experience for professionals in the field as well as a learning tool for future practitioners. This project is just beginning, but the future should provide references and a wealth of information for health professionals researching and planning evidence based health promotion initiatives.[35]

MODELS FOR IMPROVED HEALTH

Diverse HPPMs are available for different types of behavior change. Some of the more frequently used and successful models are listed already in this chapter. However, additional models are often used and there are many excellent models in health education. The problem must fit the model and vice versa. Health educators must carefully select a planning model that is well suited to their needs and flexible enough to address the problem from all aspects that affect health in populations.

Different models are appropriate for different situations. Models for intrapersonal, interpersonal, community, and cultural program plans are readily available. Many program plans are available for planning through software analysis and technology, such as *CDCynergy*, *EMPOWER*, *The Community Tool Box*, and the *Health Communication Process Model*. However, there is no perfect model for all situations.

There is a contemporary view of combining models, building a logic model, intervention mapping, and developing a framework. In fact, a visual concept map is a good way to give structure to the processes and assist in finding the proper planning model(s), theory (theories), objectives, and interventions to effect the most change once the root cause of the health problem is identified. Reciprocal causation, or that behavior and change is influenced by many factors, gives rise to multidimensional approaches utilizing all levels of change. Individual behavior change alone is not enough to sustain long-term change that is sustained and institutionalized because support systems, environments, public laws, policies, and regulations all have to change for this to occur. Community programs, rather than individual behavior changes, are ways of effecting large change in a more effective way because of the infrastructure changes to a supportive, healthier environment for the people of those communities. Supporting community organizing and building as well as changing to a supportive environment is a better, more sustainable solution.

A proper knowledge of various planning models is essential in researching the one(s) that fits your needs and includes the appropriate steps for positive changes in health across all dimensions. Many tools for designing appropriate and effective programs for promoting positive behavior change are available to health educators. Ecological approaches can plan sustainable community safety interventions.[36] Combining planning models and developing new intervention mapping models are desirable to cover all possible avenues necessary for healthier communities and a healthier world. Effecting positive change for health cannot occur without a predetermined and structured model and theory to address and prescribe a solution that will hopefully be successful, or that will at least improve conditions as additional programs are applied, improved, and/or replicated. Attacking programs from multiple levels can reap better results than a one-dimensional approach and leave embedded, positive changes or **institutionalization**. Consider all aspects that produce health behavior and environmental and infrastructure changes for sustained health promotion.

SUMMARY

- Community health problems are in essence global threats to our health. One community's problems can threaten the world, so global efforts are imperative to reduce health risks in every country to protect the world.

Institutionalization: The organizational factors that address rules, regulations, policies and informal structures that can restrict or support the behaviors for long term sustainability.

- Health is a prerequisite for economic growth, social systems, and fulfillment of basic human rights. Eliminating health issues and preventing and eradicating diseases are global problems.
- Health educators are a part of the solution to reducing incidence, prevalence, morbidity, mortality, and disability, and to improving quality of life. Proper planning, implementation, and evaluation of health programs give structure, sequence, and empirical research for others to follow.
- There are many health models or program plans that define appropriate steps for successful health programs. Each model is unique and used for different situations, problems, populations, and types of strategies. The goal is to lead a program planner down a successful path or to map for proper evidence-based planning.
- There are six basic parts of a program model: assess the needs of the target population, identify the problem, develop appropriate goals and objectives, create an intervention that is likely to achieve desired results, implement the intervention, and evaluate the results. A planning model must infuse theoretical principles into the total program plan for successful changes in the health of the participants and the community.
- The planning models delineated in this chapter are the more rigorously tested models.
- There are intrapersonal, interpersonal, community, and cultural types of programs.
- Models included are: *Healthy People 2010, APEX-PH, CDCynergy, CPHC, Community Wellness Model, EMPOWER,* Healthy Plan-*it, Healthy Communities and/or Healthy Cities, MAPP, MATCH, PATCH, PRECEDE–PROCEED, Social Marketing, SMART, Strategic Prevention Framework, SWOT Analysis, Ecological Models, GHFDS, Health Communication Process Models, CTB,* and *Intervention/Concept Mapping.*
- A cultural model, *PEN-3,* is included and is recommended in combination with all planning models. In today's diverse and multicultural society, a model should consider all factors that ultimately affect health.
- Multidimensional-level planning models that address all aspects of behavior and environment are recommended.

CONCEPTUAL TERMS

Theory	Public policy factors
Intrapersonal models	*PRECEDE–PROCEED*
Interpersonal models	*EMPOWER*
Community models	*MATCH*
Cultural models	*PATCH*
CDCynergy	*Social Marketing Model*
Ecological Model	Institutionalization
Social determinants	6 Generic Tasks of Program Models
Institutional/organizational factors	
Institutionalized	

REFLECTIVE THINKING

As a professional health educator, you are serving on the board of directors of the mayor's newly formed "Building Youth Initiative". The new initiative is targeting alcohol and drug abuse among young teens. The mayor sent in a proposal for this program to the state attorney general's office, and it was approved for a grant funding the project. The advisory and planning board of directors was formed by the mayor, and this is the first planning meeting. The other board members are suggesting strategies and the director is writing down ideas, but no program planning model or theory is mentioned. You discuss using concept mapping and researching other programs. You recommend using an evidence-based strategic planning model and theory for effecting change using a multilevel and integrative approach. You also suggest involving the community and youth leaders in the planning process. The discussion is called for a vote, and the board decides to implement the strategies listed without using a program planning model or a guiding theory. How can you convince the other board members that evidence-based practice works and that unorganized planning using only strategies may not be successful? How can you advocate for empowering the community and youth by involving them in the planning process? What is your role in trying to change the board's decision? Do you remain on the board or resign in protest?

CONCEPTUAL LEARNING

1. Define and compare intrapersonal, interpersonal, community, and cultural types of program models, and delineate the differences.
2. Classify the different HPPMs listed in the chapter. Compare the differences and similarities for each.
3. List the generic set of tasks present in most HPPMs.
4. Summarize and examine the four stages in *A Systematic Approach to Health Promotion* (*Healthy People 2010*).
5. Develop a justification for the design of the *APEX-PH*.
6. Construct a description of each stage of *CDCynergy*.
7. Explain how the *CPHC* model was developed.
8. Classify and summarize the basic purpose of each of the following models: *Community Wellness Model,* Healthy Plan-*it*, *Healthy Communities and/or Healthy Cities* and/or *Healthy People in Healthy Communities*, *MAPP, and MATCH*.
9. Arrange the following models into like categories of your choosing, and explain why these categories are necessary for different health education programs: *PEN-3, PATCH, PRECEDE–PROCEED, Social Marketing, SMART, Strategic Prevention Framework, SWOT Analysis*, and the *Health Communication Model*.
10. Demonstrate a logic model using concept mapping. Discuss how a logic model was derived.
11. Select one area of the *Ecological Model*, and state what it addresses.
12. List the concepts of a multilevel interactive approach.
13. Differentiate between health determinants and social determinants.
14. Describe the term institutionalized and institutionalization.

15. Demonstrate a public policy factor as well as institutional and/or organizational factors.
16. Evaluate the *EMPOWER* model.

REFERENCES

1. National Cancer Institute. (2005). *Theory at a glance: A guide for health promotion practice* (05–3896). Washington, DC: Author.
2. Glanz, K., Rimer, B. K., & Viswanath, K. (2008). *Health behavior and health education: Theory, research and practice* (4th ed., p. 29). San Francisco: Jossey Bass.
3. Ebi K. L., Gamble J. L. (2005, March). Environmental health perspectives. *PubMed,113*(3), 335–338.
4. Campbell, C. (2009, August 1). Health education planning models: A review of the literature, part II. *MSU Cares: Coordinated access to the research and extension system*. Retrieved February 22, 2010, from Mississippi Cooperative Extension Service at: http://msucares.com/health/health/appa2.htm
5. United States Department of Health and Human Services. Office of Disease Prevention and Health Promotion. (2000). *Healthy people 2010* (2nd ed.). Retrieved February 22, 2010, from http://www.healthypeople.gov/default.htm
6. United States National Association of County Health Officials. (1991). *APEX/PH. Assessment protocol for excellence in public health*. Washington, DC: Author.
7. Centers for Disease Control and Prevention. United States Department of Health and Human Services. (n.d.). *CDCynergy overview*. Atlanta, GA: Author.
8. Centers for Disease Control and Prevention. United States Department of Health and Human Services. (2003). *CDCynergy 3.0: Your guide to effective health communication* (CD ROM). Atlanta, GA: Author.
9. World Health Organization. (1978). *Primary health care: Report of the International Conference on Primary Health Care*. Geneva, Switzerland: Author.
10. Ackoff, R. L. *Management in small doses*. New York: John Wiley & Sons.
11. McBeth, A. J., & Schweer, K. D. (2000). *Building healthy communities: The challenge of health care in the twenty first century*. Boston: Allyn & Bacon.
12. Travis, J. W., & Ryan, R. S. (1988). *The wellness workbook* (2nd ed.). Berkely, CA: Ten Speed Press.
13. Insel, P. M., & Roth, W. T. (2008). *Core concepts in health* (10th ed.). New York: McGraw-Hill.
14. McLeroy, M. W., Bibeau, D., Steckler, A., & Glanz, K. (1988). An ecological perspective on health promotion programs. *Health Education Quarterly*, *15*, 351–377.
15. Gielen, A., Sleet, D. A., & Diclemente, R. (Eds.). (2006). *Ecological models for the prevention of unintentional injury and violence prevention: Behavioral science theories, methods, and applications*. San Francisco: Jossey Bass.
16. Wilkinson R., & Marmot, M. (Eds.). (1998). *Social determinants of health: The solid facts*. Geneva, Switzerland: World Health Organization.
17. Dignan, M. B., & Carr, P. A. (1992). *Program planning for health education and promotion*. Philadelphia, PA: Lea and Febiger.
18. Green, L. W., & Kreuter, M. W. (2005). *Health program planning: An educational and ecological approach* (4th ed.). Boston: McGraw-Hill.
19. Gold, R. S., Green, L. W., & Kreuter, M. W. (1998). *Enabling methods of planning and organizing within everyone's reach (EMPOWER)*. Sudbury, MA: Jones and Bartlett Publishers.
20. Centers for Disease Control and Prevention. (2000). *Healthy Plan-it: A tool for planning and managing public health programs*. Sustainable Management Development Program. Atlanta, GA: Author.
21. McKenzie, J. P., Pinger, R. R., & Lotecki, J. E. (2008). *An introduction to community health* (6th ed.). Sudbury, MA: Jones and Bartlett Publishers.
22. National Association of County and City Health Officials. (2000). *Mobilizing for action through planning and partnerships (MAPP)*. Retrieved March 22, 2010, from http://mapp.naccho.org//topics/infrastructure/MAPP/index.cfm
23. Simmons-Morton, B. G., Green, W. H., & Gottlieb, N. H. (1995). *Introduction to health education and health promotion* (2nd ed.). Prospect Heights, IL: Waveland Press.

24. Hayden, J. (Ed.). (2000). *The health education specialist: A study guide for professional competence* (4th ed.). Whitehall, PA: The National Commission for Health Education Credentialing, Inc.

25. Airhihenbuwa, C. O. (1990). A conceptual model for culturally appropriate health education programs in developing countries. *International Quarterly of Community Health Education, 11*, 53–62.

26. Airhihenbuwa, C. O. (1995). *Health and culture: Beyond the western paradigm.* Thousand Oaks, CA: Sage Publishers.

27. Airhihenbuwa, C. O., & DeWitt W. J. (2004). Culture and African contexts of HIV/AIDs prevention, care and support. *Journal of Social Aspects of HIV/AIDS Research Alliance, 1*(1), 4–13.

28. Centers for Disease Control and Prevention. (1991). Planned approach to community health: Guide for the local coordinator. Washington, DC: United States Department of Health and Human Services.

29. Kreuter, M. W. (1992). PATCH: Its origin, basic concepts, and links to contemporary public health policy. *Journal of Health Education, 23*(3), 135–139.

30. World Health Organization. (1986, November 17–21). Ottawa Charter for health promotion: International conference on health promotion. Ottawa, Ontario, Canada: World Health Organization.

31. Neiger, B., & Thackeray, R. (2002). Application of the SMART model in two successful social marketing projects. *American Journal of Health Education, 33*(5), 301–306.

32. Kansas University Work Group on Health Promotion and Community Development. (2009). *Community Tool Box: Bringing solutions to light.* Lawrence, KS: University of Kansas. Retrieved February 22, 2010, from http://ctb.ku.edu/

33. University of Texas Health Science Center at Houston. *Intervention mapping: An online resource.* Retrieved February 22, 2010, from http://www.sph.uth.tmc.edu/chppr/interventionmapping/

34. National Cancer Institute. (August, 2004). *The Health Communication Process model. Making health communication programs work: A planners guide.* Washington, DC: Department of Health and Human Services, National Cancer Institute, National Institutes of Health.

35. Kansas University Work Group on Health Promotion and Community Development. (2009). *Community Tool Box: Bringing solutions to light. Pan American Health Organization guide for documenting health promotion initiatives* (part A, chap. 2, p. 12). Lawrence, KS: University of Kansas. Retrieved February 22, 2010, from http://ctb.ku.edu/

36. Hanson, J., Vardon, P., McFarlane, K., Lloyd, J., Muller, R., & Durrheim, D. (2005, April). The injury iceberg: An ecological approach to planning sustainable community safety interventions. *Health Promotion Journal of Australia, 16*(1).

ENHANCED READINGS

Kansas University Work Group on Health Promotion and Community Development. (2005). *Community Tool Box: Bringing solutions to light.* Lawrence, KS: University of Kansas. Available at: http://ctb.ku.edu/en/tablecontents/

See:

Part A: Models for Promoting Community Health and Development: Gateways to the Tools (Chapters 1–2)

Part F: Analyzing Community Problems and Designing and Adapting Community Interventions (Chapters 17–19)

Part G: Implementing Promising Community Interventions (Chapters 20–26)

Part H: Cultural Competence, Spirituality, and the Arts and Community Building (Chapters 27–29)

Part J: Evaluating Community Programs and Initiatives (Chapters 36–39)

National Cancer Institute. National Institutes of Health. (2004, August). *Pink Book: Making health communication programs work.* Washington, DC: Department of Health and Human Services, National Cancer Institute and National Institutes of Health. Available at: http://cancer.gov/pinkbook

See:

Introduction
Planning Frameworks, Theories, and Models of Change
How Market Research and Evaluation Fit Into Communication Programs

National Cancer Institute. National Institutes of Health (2005). *Theory at a glance: A guide for health promotion practice* (05–3896). Washington, DC: Department of Health and Human Services, National Cancer Institute. Available at: http://cancer.gov/cancerinformation/theory-at-a-glance
See:

Part 1: Foundations of Theory in Health Promotion and Education
Part 2: Theories and Applications Presents an Ecological Perspective on Health

RELEVANT WEB SITES

American University. (2009). International Institute for Health Promotion. Available at: http://www1.american
.edu/academic.depts/cas/health/iihp/iihpnewsletter.html
Centers for Disease Control and Prevention. (2004). *The burden of chronic diseases and their risk factors: National and state perspectives.* Available at: http://www.cdc.gov/nccdphp/burdenbook2004
Centers for Disease Control and Prevention. (2007). Healthy Plan-*it* Sustainable Management Development Program. Atlanta, GA: Author. Available at: http://www.cdc.gov/globalhealth/SMDP/materials.htm
Centers for Disease Control and Prevention. (2008, October 17). What is public health? The 20th century's ten great public health achievements in the United States. Available at: http://www.whatispublichealth.org/impact/achievements.html
Centers for Disease Control and Prevention. United States Department of Health and Human Services. (n.d.). *CDCynergyLite.* Atlanta, GA: Author. Available at: http://www.cdc.gov/dhdsp/CDCynergy_training/Content/activeinformation/about.htm
Morbidity and Mortality Weekly Report, 43:761–762. Atlanta, GA. Available at: http://www.cdc.gov/mmwr/preview/mmwrhtml/00032992

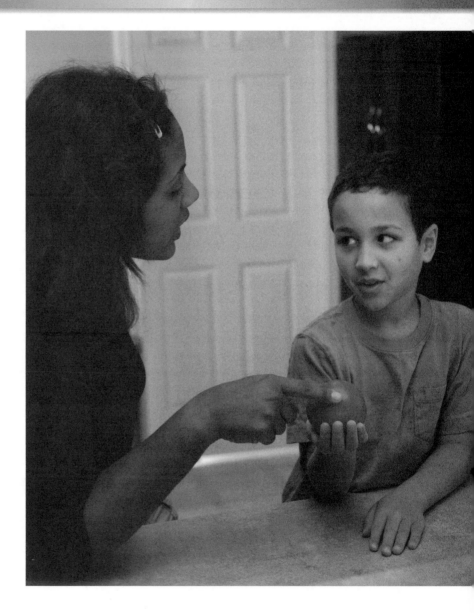

CHAPTER 4

Theoretical Principles and Processes in Health Programs

OBJECTIVES AND ASSESSMENTS

This chapter meets the following National Commission for Health Education Credentialing, Inc., Society for Public Health Education, and American Association for Health Education Responsibilities and Competencies for Entry Level and Advanced Level Health Educator competencies.* The learner will:

1. Assess individual and community needs for health education.
4. Conduct evaluation and research related health education.
7. Apply appropriate research principles and methods in health education.

This chapter meets the following general learning objectives. The learner will:

1. Describe and defend the theories and planning models supporting behavior change.
2. Design an outline for a health promotion program utilizing at least one program planning model and one theory for disease prevention in a community setting.
3. Write, research, and present a health theory project to the class.
4. Demonstrate how health education theory draws from many disciplines and sources.
5. Explain how using evidence-based health promotion plans with empirical research gives credibility to health programs.
6. Construct an example of a cultural strategic planning model and theory using the examples in Chapters 3 and 4.
7. Select an example of a theory from each of the categories, including individual (intrapersonal), interpersonal, community, and cultural.

Sources: Reprinted with permission of NCHEC.

National Commission for Health Education Credentialing, Inc. (NCHEC), Society for Public Health Education (SOPHE), & American Association for Health Education (AAHE). (2006). *A competency-based framework for health educators-2006*. Whitehall, PA: NCHEC.

8. Summarize how multiple theories and plans can be combined within or across multiple levels of influence and practice to solve health problems.

INTRODUCTION

With new therapies, improved communications technology, and coalition efforts to control epidemics, global health has improved. Global action against health risks in one country can help protect all people in all countries. Efforts must go beyond the local level. Human behavior is changing around the world, as is the impact of changes on people's health. Risk factors continue to exist, yet proven theoretical programs can reduce and change some health hazards. Poverty, unsafe water, poor sanitation, lack of access, hygiene, and iron deficiencies are prevalent in underdeveloped countries. In developed countries, we have seen a rise in chronic diseases resulting from lifestyle factors. Unhealthy diets, smoking, obesity, and alcohol abuse are prevalent in the more advanced cultures. Because of globalization, infectious and chronic diseases are spreading to all countries.

Proven health programs based on successful theory and models can assist in global control efforts and possibly eradicate some health risk factors and reduce disease. All countries should work together in advancing global health improvement efforts. Health professionals are an integral part of the solution.[1] Constructing theoretically based and replicable global and community health programs based on empirical research can assist health professional in effecting positive change. Using these proven evidence-based health promotion programs that are replicated is an effective approach. Sharing effective programs among health agencies is a good approach. Planning, implementation, and evaluation of effective health promotion programs are resources that should be shared globally. Health educators are the processors and administrators of successful health programs and are an underrated resource for global health improvements using shared research, data, and successful theoretical models and programs.

THEORY

Health education **theory** draws from many disciplines and sources, including the social sciences, psychology, education, epidemiology, marketing medicine, anthropology, advocacy, the media, the sciences, information technology, and many, many others. Health educators are always trying to find the definitive theory that is effective. Theory is sometimes defined as a set of interrelated "...concepts, definitions, and propositions that explain or predict these events or situations by illustrating the relationships between variables."[2(p4)]

As described by Goldman and Schmalz in 2001,"Theories are summaries of formal or informal observations, presented in a systematic, structured way, that help explain, predict, describe or manage behavior."[3(p278)] A theory is a causal action that brings about behavioral, environmental, and social change. As stated by the National Cancer Institute, "Theory gives planners tools for moving beyond

---

Theory: The conceptual frameworks that coordinate with evidence-based health promotion plans and give credibility to a program.

intuition to design and evaluate health behavior and health promotion interventions based on under-standing of health behavior."[2]

Theories are sometimes called conceptual frameworks or theoretical frameworks. Using empirical and evidence-based research for health promotion plans gives credibility to a program. Theories are valid only if highly developed and rigorously tested. They identify the why, what, and how so investigators can address health problems, create a definitive action plan, and guide the search for targeted health behaviors and environmental changes. Theories define what planners need to know before programs are developed and assist in strategy development. Programs based on theory are predictable and more likely to be successful than those that are not because they apply evidence-based research.[2] Theories related to different levels of causation can help solve multidimensional problems.

> **Career Concept**
>
> *Are you a scientific, hands-on person who enjoys discovering and analyzing information? You may enjoy working in a health-related research setting.*

THEORY AS AN ESSENTIAL PLANNING ELEMENT

The first step when confronted with a health problem is to ask why the problem exists and to try to decipher the answer by identifying the root cause (i.e., behaviors and/or circumstances causing the problems). This investigation goes beyond personal health behaviors and extends to the social, environmental, educational, economic, policy, and legal factors that enable this problem to exist. Individualizing the problem to one of personal responsibility is not a complete cure. A broad, comprehensive, multidimensional and ecological approach is much more effective.[3] In a global sense, this means effecting change not only in one part of the world but using similar approaches worldwide. Investigative approaches are used in a manner similar to the way a private investigator solves a crime. Who, what, when, where, why, and how are questions that may help clarify the nature of the needs and help to target problem(s) and health behaviors.

Theory guides the search for why people do or do not engage in certain health behaviors. It helps define the information that planners need to develop effective programs. It assists in reaching the target audience with the greatest impact with prescriptive strategies. Theory identifies the indicators to monitor and the measurements included for proper program evaluation.[2] What are the root causes of health problems? Some things to consider changing include knowledge, attitudes, and skills of a person(s); actions and beliefs of friends and family; policies and practices within the social, political, civic, religious, and related organizations; community norms and practices; and public health policy, laws, and regulations.[3] Economic situations, cultural practices, deep rooted behaviors and environmental factors peculiar to a particular area or groups of people, and the community and/or country's willingness to change, are all important factors to bear in mind. In a global world without borders, all of these dimensions are important considerations when working with entrenched factors in people's lives.

Planning requires understanding how the parts of the program work together to produce the desired outcome evaluation. Theory enables this understanding. Applying proper theory to planning models helps predict and explain the mechanisms and behaviors for producing change. Theoretical models provide forces that analyze health behavior, apply communication theory in developing educational strategies for behavioral change, and provide guidance for program direction, design, and development of effective strategies for programs targeted to the participants and area (environment). Health education, communications, and health promotion activities are parts of the program. It is important that the participants are involved in planning health education and promotion programs. Program plans are facilitated by many health educators, and this information must be shared through empirical research and publications.[4]

Health program planning is based on a model for the development of education, skills, and environmental changes. The model and theoretical components are necessary for developing structured, theoretically based programs that are aligned with the prioritized health needs and interests of the participants and the community. Any behaviors or other intrinsic elements that affect health adversely need to be targeted in the program plan and theory.

CHARACTERISTICS OF THEORY

According to the National Cancer Institute, "A useful theory helps make assumptions about a behavior, health problem, target population, or environment that are: logical, consistent with everyday observations, similar to those used in previous successful programs, and supported by past research in the same area or related ideas."[2(p7)] It helps explain what influences health behaviors and initiates planning effective interventions, communitywide strategies, services, public policy, and any other changes necessary. The data collection process involves knowing what variables to assess, what interventions to use for participants, how to apply the interventions for the specific populations, and how to predict consequences. Furthermore, it guides the selection of evaluation measures and promotes additional research.[3]

Research has not clearly shown if strategies targeting or tailoring health programs are more effective than generic circumstances. Targeting is creating a single intervention approach for a group by using information about shared characteristics, while tailoring offers change or information strategies for an outcome based on a specific person's unique characteristics.[2] This is an area of concern for health educators and one that definitely deserves more empirical research and evaluation procedures.

COMPONENTS OF THEORY

Concepts are the primary element of the theory. **Constructs** are the key concepts developed for a theory. **Variables** are the "...operational forms of constructs. They define the way a construct is to be measured in a specific situation."[2(p4)] Variables need to be matched to the constructs when the factors identified in the **needs assessment** are evaluated in a theory-driven program (see **Figure 4–1**).

Health problems change with time, technology, and new advances. Some health problems, like biological or chemical hazards and mutations of formerly curable diseases, will demand new approaches.

Concepts: The primary elements of the theory.
Constructs: The key concepts developed for a theory.
Variables: The operational forms of constructs that help delineate the way a construct is measured.
Needs assessments: Research and investigative tools used to determine the root cause or causes of a health problem or problems.

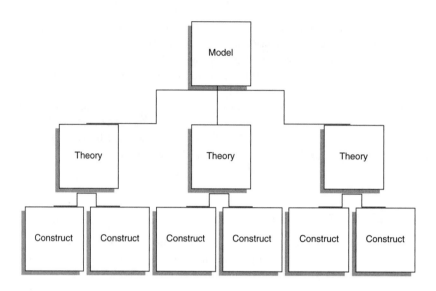

FIGURE 4–1   Constructs, Theories, and a Model

Biology, science, and social disciplines will need to cooperate and invent new strategies and possibly new theories to deal with these emerging health threats. Some theories focus on individuals as the unit of change, while others focus on change in organizations or cultures. Because of these different frames of reference, theories that were very important to public health education a generation ago may be of limited use today.

Theories are explanatory tools that define and describe the relationships among factors and the conditions under which these relationships exist or do not exist. They are evidence based, reflect more certainty than hypotheses or models, are changeable with new evidence or observations, and offer frameworks to understand problems and identify manageable strategies. There is no one right or best theory or combination of theories.[3]

If no theory is involved, however, programmers are stabbing in the dark and cannot be assured of success in their health program or of effecting beneficial change. The health educator plans a program that leads individuals, groups, or communities through the stages of the theory so that behavior change is embedded in the participants' lives and communities; it is institutionalized. Once it is institutionalized the change becomes a part of their daily lives, like brushing their teeth every morning.

What is unique about theory is that sometimes the participants do not realize they are changing their behavior. The effects may seem gradual and accepted, becoming slowly established in that person's life and/or the community. Theory is a systematic way of understanding events or situations that bring about behavior and community change. The theoretical principle(s) explains and predicts the desired behavior change and changes in the environment. Strategic planning models and theory are critical in the success of a behavioral and environmental health program. Theory that produces these outcomes is sometimes called **explanatory theory** or change theory.[2]

CATEGORIES OF THEORY

There are several categories of health theoretical models, including individual (or **intrapersonal**), **interpersonal**, and **community** theories.[2(p45)] Intrapersonal theories deal with individual knowledge, attitudes, beliefs, and behaviors. Interpersonal theories work with individual factors as they relate to environment and personal characteristics. The family and close friends are considered in this theory. Community theories include institutional, community, public policy factors and infrastructure, as well as interpersonal theoretical concepts. It is not unusual to apply theory from all three categories. As well, environmental, policy, and legal changes all contribute to causing a change in individual and group behaviors, environment, and infrastructure. The setting must be a positive one that encourages and leads the participants along the behavior change process. It is not enough to encourage individual behavior change unless the circumstances where the person socializes, lives, and works are conducive to that change.

The author would like to propose a new category—cultural theory. While some researchers feel that a **cultural theory** is the same as a community theory or part of a community theory, there is a distinguishing factor: cultural theory focuses on the factors that are embedded in the population, and these traditions, beliefs, and practices have been in place for years and sometimes centuries. These may or may not be detrimental to the population's health. Such a change is a daunting task and much more difficult than ordinary behavior change. A facet of the cultural theory, which is a challenge for some to accept, is tolerating and working with the positive or least detrimental factors. These types of embedded behavioral, social, environmental, and cultural factors are steeped in history and tradition and must be dealt with deftly. In many cases, rather than relishing the behavioral, social, and environmental structures that are beneficial to health, these cultural factors seem to be somewhat ignored in program theories. Some theories focus on the detrimental cultural factors in health and do not use the positive cultural factors to benefit the program focus—hence the addition of this fourth, cultural category to the three theories normally listed in the literature. With this concept, culture is not in a vacuum, but may be considered along with intrapersonal, interpersonal, and community categories or be viewed as a separate category. Cultural theories should be included in all theories and models to bring about changes within and among cultural systems. With current globalization of business and travel, it is

---

Explanatory theory: Change theory that when combined with strategic planning models is crucial in the success of a health behavior change program.
Intrapersonal theories: Individual theories that deal with individual knowledge, attitudes, beliefs, and behaviors.
Interpersonal theories: Theories that work with individual factors as they relate to environment and personal characteristics.
Community theories: Theories that include institutional, community, and public policy factors that influence health in programs.
Cultural theories: A community theory that addresses the embedded cultural traditions, beliefs, and practices that are detrimental to health in the population.

timely to consider all diverse health influences in planning programs, sharing research, and utilizing multiple theoretical approaches.

The National Cancer Institute in 2005 stated that theory must address health issues in diverse populations.[2] Research findings show that understanding cultural backgrounds and experiences of community members may be more effective. Health practitioners must understand that culture and ethnicity are critical to consider when applying theory to a health problem. This aspect is one that may need revising for different areas of the world.

There are relevant theories that are suited for specific program plans. At the intrapersonal and interpersonal level, theories are broadly called cognitive–behavioral, and key influences on the behavior involves behavioral cognition, knowledge for behavior change, and perceptions, motivations, skills, and the social environment present. Community level models should implement multidimensional approaches to make the social and physical environment conducive to behavior change. Cultural theories address the specific and unique cultural aspects that may need changing, without interfering in the basic cultural grounding of a community. There are some cultural traditions and characteristics that are not as harmful as others, some that planners may not want to change because they are institutionalized and it may cause more harm to change them, and some that could be changed with some minor adjustments. Planners also risk causing too much controversy, and thus the populations may reject all change. The most egregious problems should be addressed first. Sometimes, planners just have to let some traditions and beliefs that do not extremely threaten health remain in order to be successful in other areas. Then, with time and successful programs, health educators can eventually address the least harmful practices if this does not adversely affect the cultural traditions of the group. Don't change the culture; change the circumstances that entrench harmful beliefs and behaviors.

The planner must consider the problem setting, behaviors, the specific site where the program is offered, the specific population (target groups), cultures, family institutions, the behaviors and **environmental changes** required, the type of communication channels and theoretical program that will be most effective, and any other factors identified in the needs assessment that warrant targeting in a health promotion program. The theory and strategic plan must fit the practice setting.[2]

Many different health theories are relevant to health education today. It is important for health educators to be aware of the most relevant and research-based models and theories. Some of the major ones are listed by category in the following discussion. This is not a definitive list but is meant to give a sampling of the relevant, major, evidence-based theories used in health promotion practice.

INDIVIDUAL (INTRAPERSONAL) THEORY

Transtheoretical Model or the Stages of Change (Prochaska & DiClemente, 1979)

The Stages of Change theory involves an individual's readiness to change or attempt to change toward healthy behaviors.[5] The five stages are precontemplation, contemplation, decision/determination, action,

---

Environmental change: The differences in any ecological element during a health promotion program.
Transtheoretical Model or *Stages of Change*: A theory that involves an individual's readiness to change to healthy behaviors.

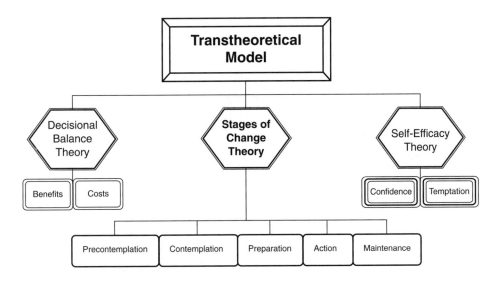

FIGURE 4–2   Transtheoretical Model

and maintenance.[6] This approach helps program planners tailor interventions based on a person's stage of readiness to change. It shows how a person progresses through the stages from not considering change to embracing change in his or her lifestyle. It predicts the potential relapse and repeated change in cycles.[7]

A sixth stage called termination is used by some planners. It indicates when a behavior is embedded in a person and when the person may not normally regress. A classic article written by authors Prochaska, DiClimente, and Norcross in 1992 discusses the use of this theory in changing addictive behavior.[8] Another article discusses the use of this theory in health education for older adults.[5] *The Transtheoretical Model* theory brings the person through the steps necessary for change and is more successful when the environmental circumstances necessary for continuing that change are in place. The model conceptualizes behavior change as a process, not an immediate action in combination with self-efficacy and decisional balance theory (see **Figure** 4–2).

Health Belief Model (Hochbaum, Rosenstock, Leventhal, & Kegeles, 1950; U.S. Public Health Service)

The five phases of this theoretical base are perceived seriousness (severity), perceived susceptibility, perceived **benefits**, perceived **barriers (threats)**, and cues to action (see **Table** 4–1).[9] How these affect the person's healthy behaviors and the cognitive and affective component are paramount.[10] A

Benefits: The positive effects that participants believe a particular behavior or environmental change will bring about.

Barriers: Obstructions that participants believe they may have to overcome to practice beneficial health behaviors or bring about environmental change.

TABLE 4–1 HEALTH BELIEF MODEL	
Behavior is an outcome of ...	
Perceived Susceptibility	The degree to which a person feels at risk for a health problem.
Perceived Severity	The degree to which a person believes the consequences of the health problem will be severe.
Perceived Benefits	The positive outcomes a person believes will result from the action.
Perceived Barriers	The negative outcomes a person believes will result from the action.
Cues to Action	An external event that motivates a person to act.
Self-Efficacy	A person's belief in his or her ability to take action.

second component is how these beliefs are mobilized. The *Health Belief Model (HBM)* has evolved over time and has been effective in identifying factors that affect a person's health behavior. This model has been referred to as a risk perception model. Another phase added later to the *HBM* is self-efficacy, or a person's confidence in his or her ability to perform a certain skill or behavior. It has been successful in prompting people to access preventive services utilizing the self-efficacy addition to the theory.[11]

Since 1950, this model has been used as a reminder to perform preventive services, especially in the medical field.[11] Goldberg, Hapern-Felsher, and Milstein in 2002 published an article that examines a unique aspect of the model—perceived benefits of risky behaviors—which is a paradigm change.[12] Another strategy of this theory is reminders based on health perceptions. When patients receive post-cards or phone calls as reminders for performing normal health services or annual preventive checkups such as mammography, dental checkups, pap smears, prostate checkups, and other preventive exams, this is an example of the *HBM* in action. Health educators must understand the limitations of using perceived seriousness and perceived susceptibility as an intervention strategy and how cues to action should be framed as positive messages. *HBM* is sometimes called a value expectancy model. This theory was used beneficially in a research study by Goldberg, Harpern-Feisher, & Milstein emphasizing the benefits of not drinking alcohol in adolescents.[12]

Consumer Information Processing (NIH, Bettman, 1979)

The *Consumer Information Processing* theory uses the procedure by which consumers acquire and use information for decision making. It was not originally intended to be used in health promotion

Health Belief Model: A medical model that helps establish the factors that affect a person's ability to perform preventive health behaviors.
Consumer Information Processing: A theory that an individual's behavior is determined by the behavioral intention, or the result of attitudes toward the behavior, and subjective perception of norms adjacent to the behavior. This theory uses the process by which consumers acquire and use information for decision making.

programs but for marketing to audiences (consumers) for product promotion. According to the basic concept, people will use health information only when it is available, useful and new, and communicated and presented in a friendly format.[13] The process we go through in interpreting and using health information describes this theory. How it is received is a key factor in how it will be processed and/or adopted.

The components include information processing, information search, decision rules or heuristics, consumption and learning, and information environment.[14] It is especially applicable for health practitioners to understand how information should be given, how consumers use the information targeted to them, and whether that information is rejected or accepted. Also, health communications have changed because of technology, health marketing campaigns, segmentation approaches, tailored messages, the Internet, YouTube, chat lines, blogs, Twitter, streaming videos, online education, Wikis, and other nontraditional sources of information. Consumer tendencies, preferences, and, specifically, needs are considered, and as technology advances, health educators must keep up with the changing times.[15]

Theory of Planned Behavior (TPB) (Fishbein & Ajzen, 1975; Ajzen & Driver, 1986; Ajzen & Madden, 1986)

The *Theory of Planned Behavior (TPB)* is an extension of the original *Theory of Reasoned Action* (TRA) and includes perceived behavioral control. It is concerned with beliefs, attitudes, intent, and behaviors.[16,17] An individual's behavior is determined by the behavioral intention, or the result of attitudes toward the behavior, and subjective perception of norms adjacent to the behavior. Attitudes toward behavior and subjective norms are determined by two constructs.[18] Behavioral outcomes and the subjective importance of those outcomes determine a person's attitude regarding the behavior. Beliefs regarding other people's approval of the behavior and the motivation to comply with those individuals determine a person's subjective norm.[19] This theory examines the factors influencing the relationship between intention and behavior.

TPB focus on intentions to perform a behavior, dependent on attitudes toward the behavior and socially acceptable types of behavior(s) (see **Table 4–2**). How these three processes work together needs to be understood in order to determine whether a change will be accepted and performed. Health practitioners need to examine these three processes when designing programs using *TPB*.

Applications of this theory to programs are varied. Fishbein in 2003 discusses the role of this theory in prevention of HIV.[16] A meta-analysis of the moderation of cognition intension and cognition–behavior relations is examined utilizing *TPB* is discussed by Cook and Sheeran in 2003.[20] Another article uses this theory to examine gender differences in suncreeen usage among young adults.[18]

Theory of Planned Behavior: A theory that helps explain an individual's behavioral intention, the result of attitudes toward the behavior, and perceptions of subjective norms.

TABLE 4–2   THEORY OF PLANNED BEHAVIOR

Theory of Reasoned Action	Theory of Planned Behavior
Attitude • A person's beliefs about what will happen if he or she performs the behavior • A person's judgment of whether the expected outcome is good or bad *Subjective Norms* • A person's beliefs about what other people in his or her social group will think about the behavior • A person's motivation to conform to these perceived norms *Behavioral Intention** • A person's intention to perform a behavior	*Perceived Behavioral Control* • *Control beliefs*: A person's beliefs about factors that will make it easy or difficult to perform the behavior • *Perceived power*: The amount of power a person believes he or she has over performing the behavior

*Influenced by attitude, subjective norms, and perceived behavioral control; behavioral intention is most predictive of actual behavior.

INTERPERSONAL THEORY

Social Cognitive Learning Theory and Social Learning Theory (Bandura, 1977, 1986)

This theory began as *Social Learning Theory*, but was expanded upon by Bandura into *Social Cognitive Learning Theory* or *Social Cognitive Theory*. This theory examines the determinants of behavior. The concept of reciprocal determinism, or the dynamic interactions that occur between a person, the behaviors, and the environment are paramount indicators in this theory.[21] Internal factors include attitudes, values, and beliefs. Behavior is explained as a three-way, dynamic reciprocal theory. It is where the personal factors, environmental influences, and behaviors continually interact. In addition to the major principle of reciprocal determinism, it is important to understand other concepts related to self-efficacy, such as "locus of control" and "learned helplessness" It is important to distinguish these concepts of self-efficacy. Health educators need to become aware of ways to assess self-efficacy and outcome expectations (see **Table 4–3**).

An article by Bandura in 2004 examines health promotion programs by social cognitive means.[22] Bandura's theory is popular for use in many educational settings to improve cognition of new ideas and knowledge. It is a theory that has received a lot of attention in the public school systems to help students process new information.

> *Social Cognitive Learning Theory*: A theory based on reciprocal determinism that helps identify the personal factors, environmental influences, and behaviors that continually intermingle.

TABLE 4-3 SOCIAL COGNITIVE LEARNING THEORY

Individual Characteristics

Self-Efficacy	A person's confidence that he or she can perform a behavior.
Behavioral Capability	A person's level of knowledge and skill in relation to a behavior.
Expectations	What a person thinks will happen if he or she makes a behavior change.
Expectancies	Whether a person thinks the expected outcome is good or likely to be rewarded.
Self-Control	How much control a person has over making a change.
Emotional Coping	A person's ability to deal with emotions involved in a behavior change.

Environmental Factors

Vicarious Learning	A person learns by observing the behavior of others and the consequences of that behavior.
Situation	The social/physical environment in which the behavior takes place, and a person's perception of those factors.
Reinforcement	Positive or negative responses to a person's behavior.
Reciprocal Determinism	The iterative process where a person makes a change based on individual characteristics and social/environmental cues, receives a response, makes adjustments to his or her behavior, and so on.

COMMUNITY THEORY

Community Organization Theory (Ross, Lewin, Rothman, & Tropman, 1987)

This theory emphasizes active participation and development of communities that can better evaluate and solve health and social problems. *Community Organization Theory* involves many different concepts. It is the process by which community groups identify common problems and goals, mobilize resources, and develop and implement strategies. It is a combination of several theories and is not a unified model. This theory also involves participation and involvement of the community in the program process.

Community development opportunities improve and solidify the health of the community. Key concepts are **empowerment**, community competence, participation, and relevance.[23] Other concepts are issues selection and critical consciousness.[13,24] Each competency embodies community participatory

---

Community Organization Theory: A theory that emphasizes active participation and development of communities that can better evaluate and solve health and social problems.
Empowerment: A concept in theory that involves the ability of participants to gain mastery and power over themselves and their community to produce change.

involvement in the process. These processes help the community participants to hold hands and walk along the same path toward a central focus for better health.

The first concept is *empowerment*, or the process of gaining mastery and power over oneself or one's community, to produce change. It gives individuals and communities the tools and responsibility for making decisions that affect them. Empowerment stimulates and activates community members. It is a powerful concept that gives control and performance to the participants and provides ownership of the change. *Community competence* is the ability of a community to engage in effective problem solving. It involves working with the community to identify problems, create consensus, and reach goals. Community competence includes the self-efficacy and behavioral capability to solve problems. *Self-efficacy* is when a person believes he or she can produce a change and understands that knowledge and training must be gained to perform this new change. *Participation and relevance* are when learners become active participants and assist in beginning the program work at the current stage of all participants. This concept can help the community set goals within the context of preexisting goals. These two concepts work together with citizen activation and readiness to change. Reaction to new ideas and the significance and application in daily life give weight to whether this new idea is accepted.

Issue selection is identifying winnable, simple, specific concerns as the focus of action. It helps the community examine how they can communicate the concerns and whether success is likely. This selection helps decide a winnable focus. Some issues are winnable, others take time, and some may not be acceptable at a particular time and in certain circumstances. Choosing issues likely to be accepted or making them more palatable to the audience is an important part of the theoretical and program planning model.[13] *Critical consciousness* is developing an understanding of the root causes of the problems. It should guide consideration of health concerns in a broad perspective of social problems.[24]

Community change affects the greatest numbers of people, environments, and communities. Proper setup and careful consideration of the prominent issues—how it affects people's everyday lives, education, and work—are important when using this theoretical concept.

Social action approaches are used for community organization theory. They are based on social networks and support, the ecological perspective, social systems, and social cognitive learning theory. Focuses include locality or community development, social planning using task and goals, and social action involving problem-solving abilities. Communities coming together for common goals concentrate attention, give power, and help secure funding sources to solve community problems. Such approaches have been used successfully by AIDS activists and advocates for women's health issues. Media advocacy also focuses attention on problems that can be solved when communities work together for a common cause. This theory has contributed to successful community efforts.[13] A powerful 2002 article on the contribution of community organization theory to the Federal Health Start Experience, written by Minkler, Thompson, Bell, and Rose, is worth reading.[25]

Media Advocacy

Media Advocacy refers to the use of the mass media as the resource to advance a social or public policy initiative. Using as many media influences as possible to produce a plethora of messages that are con-

---

Media Advocacy: A theory that uses the mass media as a resource to advance a social or public policy initiative.

sumed and processed by stakeholders works in advertisement. In addition to such commercial activities, this approach is successful in health programs. Advocating health issues through this means is an influential and powerful tool that health educators use to distribute mass messages.

The core competency is framing the issues to maximize impact, rally public support, and advance major policies in a short time period. Public awareness and policy change can be achieved through initiating perception of the health problem, reframing the issue to focus on policy change, presenting media advocacy in a different way, providing support and information through news and feature stories, being available for questions from the media, and reinforcing the newly developed health perception of the original health dilemma. These communications methods define media advocacy and the many different avenues available to health educators by using the media as an avenue for **health behavior change**.[26] Public service announcements are used frequently as a communication tool.

As stated by Glanz, Rimer, and Viswanath, "Media Advocacy activates forces in a social system (that is, media coverage) to help stimulate widespread public concern and action."[27(p393)] Blanketing a health issue through the mass media is a way to effect change in many different people not involved in a health program. It is used for messages of urgency and importance and is a quick and easy way to get the word out. How the message is presented is important. Health practitioners do not like using "scare tactics" to influence the population, but instead prefer positive, meaningful messages that give information and suggestions. Positive messages effect change for a longer time, whereas scare tactics usually cause only temporary change.

Diffusion of Innovations or Adoption and Diffusion (Rogers, Shoemaker, & Preston, 1983)

This theory helps describe the innovation decision process in large organizations.[28] *Diffusion of Innovations* delineates the process whereby new products or messages are introduced and diffused to audiences. The time required for the message to be accepted and/or the behavior to be adopted is called the diffusion process. The audience determines if the message is beneficial (in accordance with their personal needs and wishes), then they understand it, adopt it, and accept it (as a new behavior). The message is reinforced when viewed acceptably by their peers.

People adopt new ideas and changes at different rates. They are categorized as follows by their rate of adoption: innovators, early adopters, early majority, late majority, and late adopters (also called laggards). The theory involves relative advantage, compatibility, complexity, trialability, and observability (see **Table 4–4**). The stages of this communication channel are knowledge, persuasion, decisions, implementation, and confirmation.[28]

A schema to understand this model is to picture a spray can. Where it exits at the spout, the spread of the spray is minimal, but as it diffuses outward, it forms a sort of a reverse funnel effect that continually grows, thus involving more people. The innovators are the first to be reached by the stream of spray, and it dissipates out to eventually envelope the last adopters or the laggards. This theory exem-

---

Health behavior change: A program that uses explanatory theory and the strategic planning model for altering performance or behavior patterns.
Diffusion of Innovations: A theory that delineates the process of how new products and messages are introduced and widely distributed to the audiences.

TABLE 4–4 DIFFUSION OF INNOVATIONS	
Determinants of Diffusion	**Program Considerations**
Relative advantage	Is innovation better than what it will replace?
Compatibility	Does innovation fit with the intended audience?
Complexibility	Is the innovation easy to use?
Trialability	Can the innovation be tried before making the decision to adopt?
Observability	Are the results of the innovation observable and easily measurable?
Impact on social relations	Does the innovation have a disruptive effect on the social environment?
Reversibility	Can the innovation be reversed or discontinued easily?
Communicability	Can the innovation be understood clearly and easily?
Time	Can the innovation be adopted with a minimal investment of time?
Risk and uncertainty level	Can the innovation be adopted with minimal risk and uncertainty?
Commitment	Can the innovation be used effectively with only modest commitment?
Modifiability	Can the innovation be modified and updated over time?

plifies socialization or belonging to a group when audiences recognize that participation in the changes are successful for others and decide they may as well try it and see if they can achieve the same results or they will try it because someone they know is doing it.

Communication channels are an important aspect of this theory. Communication works in two ways: 1) it persuades audiences and mobilizes them to take action, and 2) it emphasizes social network channels for adopting decisions.[13] This theory addresses how new ideas, products, and social practices spread within a society or from one society to another. A randomized control trial was reported by Lowe, Balanda, Stanton, Del Mar, and O'Connor in 2002.[29] This research concerned the dissemination of an Australian prenatal smoking cessation program conducted in hospital settings.

Organizational Development Theory

This theory grew out of the recognition that organizational social processes and structures influence the behavior and motivation of workers. *Organizational Development Theory* identifies problems that impede an organization's functioning. It involves process consultation, the concepts of which are orga-

> *Organizational Development Theory*: A theory that describes the organizational social processes and structures that influence the behavior and motivation of participants and identifies problems that obstruct that function.

nizational development, organizational climate, organizational culture, organizational capacity, action research, and organizational development interventions.[25] It is related to community organization theory in that organizing is important for change in groups.

The key to this theory is that organizations and groups can change when the climate and cultural changes facilitate overall change for all in the organization. The capacity of the organization is important for health practitioners utilizing this theory to consider. The stage must be set so change can occur, and it should be easy to expedite change. The interventions must be in a place that facilitates this change occurring in groups. The suitability of the theory or the fit must be well situated and comfortable for participants. While this theory has a cultural component, it is not the only focus of the theory.

Empowerment Model (Friere, 1970, 1973)

The *Empowerment Model* suggests that a problem-proposing process can help participants feel more powerful, thus freeing them to make healthier behavioral and life choices. It is an educational and prevention theory for health promotion in personal and social arenas. This theory involves the principles of personal decision making, community competence, participation and relevance, issue selection, and critical consciousness-raising principles.[30] It is an ecological approach that considers the importance of the social, economic, and political environment. The theory promotes the participatory approach of group action and specifies that dialogue in communities empowers group beliefs about changes in prevention behavior, health promotion, and health policies.[30] Tai-Seale suggests that the foundation for building community-assumed empowerment has three domains that can intersect, including a shared specific problem, a shared specific interest, and shared residence and general interest.[31] Empowering participants is a way to place the importance of the success on the people involved. Ownership of the program by the ones it is affecting creates a responsibility to continue the programs even if the health educator or the program ceases to exist. Social, political, and psychological empowerment are critical elements that effect the most change for communities.[32]

Sometimes grants are not renewed, programs are transferred to other areas, or agency funding is cut and programs end. With empowerment, the main premise is that by emphasizing ownership, persons are more likely to continue with the changes institutionalized by a health program even after the program is gone. In essence, this is what every health program should accomplish—sustainability.

CULTURAL THEORY

Cultural Transformation Theory (Eisler, 1987)

The *Cultural Transformation Theory* originated from Eisler's research drawing on art, archaeology, religion, social science, history, and other fields.[32] The theory suggests that the earlier human cultures

---

Empowerment Model: A theory that suggests that a problem-proposing process can help participants feel more powerful, thus freeing them to make healthier behavioral and life choices.
Cultural Transformation Theory: A theory that proposes that the diversity of human culture is founded on two basic social models and advocates for the partnership linkage model.

were partnership models, not hierarchial dominator models. This theory proposes that the diversity of human culture is founded on two basic social models. The first is the dominator model, which ranks human members in patriarchies and matriarchies. The other is the partnership model, which links rather than ranks humans.[33]

Thought Concept

Why is changing to a healthier lifestyle so difficult for some people? What barriers exist to preclude behavior change?

These concepts work with cultural traditions and embedded practices. Working with the dominator model currently in place and affecting links with the participants as partners encourages participation. Just doing something because someone (the dominator) says to do it is not enough. Performing a health behavior and environment change as part of a group is a more effective way to increase and embed health promotion in cultures. [33]

SHORT SUMMARY OF ADDITIONAL THEORIES

Behavioral Intention (Fishbein, 1975)

The likelihood that a target audience will adopt a desired behavior is predicted by assessing the attitudes and perceptions of the benefits of the behavior.[19] How the audience members think their peers view the behavior is another factor.[34] The idea is to change or influence these factors so the target audience adopts the desired behavior.[17]

Behaviorism (Skinner, 1974)

This theory centers on observable, external behavioral conditions. The environmental response is behavior change. The positive and negative reinforcers or stimuli used established these patterns of behavior. These patterns are learned responses. Operant conditions manipulate the stimuli to promote the reflex behavior. This process involves learned patterns of behavior, not reinforcement or mental intervention.[27]

Coping Theory (Folkman & Lazarus)

This psychological theory addresses stress, appraisal, coping, and emotions. The parts of the model are cognitive appraisal and coping. Cognitive appraisal consists of primary and secondary appraisal. Coping is the ability to accept constant change that exceeds normal levels. The main methods of coping are problem-focused coping and emotional coping, and the eight approaches include confrontation, distance, self-control, acquiring social support systems, escape and avoidance, accepting responsibility, problem solving, and positive reappraisal. This theory considers situations and personal factors that influence lives. It involves the management of the cognitive and behavioral factors that place increased demands on personal resources.[27]

Each action concludes with a reaction to the situation, so there is a constant state of equilibrium. This theory purports there are stages to change and was a forerunner to the theory of "stages" people go through to bring about change in behavior.[27] Tove and Gjengedal in 2007 discussed the implications of coping theory on patients waiting for testing for possible gastric diseases.[35]

Inoculation Theory (McGuire, 1972)

This theory proposes that an individual will resist persuasive, threatening arguments if they know the content and strategy ahead of time. Media and peer influences can help to provide resistance skills to persuasive communications.[27]

Locus of Control (Rotter, 1954, 1966, 1975)

Locus of Control is a term used to describe expectations held by an individual that a particular event will occur as a result of a specific behavior and is contingent on reinforcement.[36] This concept is divided into internal (self-controlled) or external (outside forces) loci of control.[37] *Locus of Control* describes an individual's expectations concerning an event as a result of specific behavior from internal or external forces. In external *Locus of Control*, an individual believes that the happenings are unrelated to his or her behavior and are beyond personal control. In internal *Locus of Control*, the individual believes that his or her own behavior and/or personal characteristics result in outcomes or events that are controllable by the person. The internal *Locus of Control* factors in self-efficacy and is the desirable state for a person.[38] Mamlin, Harris, and Case in 2001 provided a methodological analysis of research on *Locus of Control* and its application to learning disabilities.[39]

Maslow's Hierarchy of Needs

This theory by Abraham Maslow involves the motivations process that human needs are arranged in a hierarchy according to their relative importance and that each step has to be approached successively. This is a humanistic approach consisting of five tiers, or the **hierarchy of needs**, that all humans must reach to realize their full potential, starting at the bottom (with the most elemental needs) and working upward (see **Figure 4–3**). Maslow's *Theory of Self-Actualization* is based on the resiliency of people. The fist level to be addressed is physiological needs (food, sleep, and sex), then safety needs (survival, security, order, and stability), belongingness and love needs (affection and strong bonding), then self-esteem needs (self-worth), and lastly self-actualization (personal fulfillment and oneness with the universe).[40(pp58–59)]

Organizational Change

This theoretical concept proposes that organizations undertake a series of steps (stages) as they change, including the problem definition step (awareness stage, initiation of action (adoption stage), implemen-

---

Maslow's Hierarchy of Needs: A theory that human needs are arranged in a hierarchy according to their relative importance and that each step needs to be approached successively.

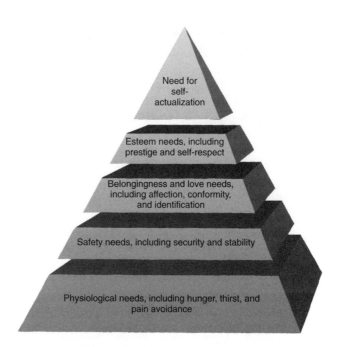

FIGURE 4–3   *Maslow's Hierarchy of Needs*

tation of change step, and institutionalization of change step. It is concerned with the processes and strategies for increasing the chances that healthy policies and programs are adopted and maintained in formal organizations. Four phases to organizational changes have been identified for public health and promotion: organization-wide versus subsystem, transformational versus incremental, remedial versus developmental, and reactive versus proactive.[41] There are many different organizational change theories for public health and promotion. They are more complex to initiate than psychological theories or individual change theories. They give relevant insight into facilitating adoption or institutionalization of change within an organization and help define the barriers to changing behavior.[27]

Persuasions in Communications and/or Communications for Persuasion (McGuire, 1981)

A series of steps causes a person to understand the communications methods and change a behavior. The steps address all of the factors involved in assuring the communication plan's message is successfully disseminated, accepted, staged, and addressed so it is accepted by the intended audience to facilitate behavior change.[13] The communication components all involve a thought process of change.

The steps are exposing the audience to a message; capturing their attention; creating interest; ensuring that they understand the message; personalizing the message; encouraging acceptance; getting the audience to remember, think about, and agree with the message; encouraging the audience to make decisions; influencing their behavior; offering the audience positive reinforcement; and ensuring that they accept the suggested behavior. Through various communication methods, people can become convinced and make positive health decisions. Five communication components are necessary to communicate the message, including credibility of the source, message design, delivery channel, intended audience, and intended behavior.[42]

Self-Efficacy Theory (Bandura, 1986)

Perceived *Self-Efficacy* refers to how capable individuals believe themselves to be in achieving goals. It is defined by individuals' *belief* about their capabilities to execute actions that achieve quality, designated behavior performance, not necessarily the actual skills they possess. This persuasion relies upon short-term achievable goals and credible persuaders. It considers individuals' beliefs about what they will accomplish in the future or outcome expectations.[27] It is a part of *Social Cognitive Theory*, but it is also used in isolation. There are four major ways self-efficacy can be developed, including mastery experience, social modeling, improving physical and emotional states, and verbal persuasion.[22] The role of self-efficacy in facilitating behavior change is discussed by Strecker, Becker, and Rosenstock.[43] An article of particular interest that explores the concept of self-efficacy as a predictor for chronic disease management is provided by Noreen and Dodge.[44]

Learning Theory and Intervention Mapping

While *Concept and Intervention Mapping* and *Logic Models* are used frequently for program planning models, there are theoretical models that expand this concept. Ausubel began the idea of concept mapping in educational psychology in the 1960s and worked with Novak and Hanesian in 1978.[45] This theory was expanded and continues to be extensively researched and developed. The primary idea of Ausubel's theory is that learning new knowledge is based on prior knowledge. The first concept is that knowledge starts with recognition and observation of events with previously learned concepts. We construct concept networks and add to these. The second concept is meaningful learning; this helps the person understand the relationships. Meaningful learning requires recognizing and linking concepts. A third part of the theory is that concepts are of different depth. Concepts can be very general to very specific. General learning concepts include more specific learning concepts. Meaningful learning is placing the new concepts into specific levels in the knowledge structure that are inclusive.[45] William Trochim is well known as a knowledgeable author on *Intervention Mapping*.

As discussed in Chapter 3, plotting ideas is very productive for strategic plans. It provides a structured plan that makes it easy to see patterns and related items because they are displayed visually. This method allows for planning discussion and has been a valuable asset for health agencies, organizations, government entities, and nonprofit organizations. It enhances cooperative planning and facilitation. It offers a visual image of the program plan and incites many creative ideas and formulations, lending structure to the beginning planning stages. The concept identifies the priorities and helps convey the

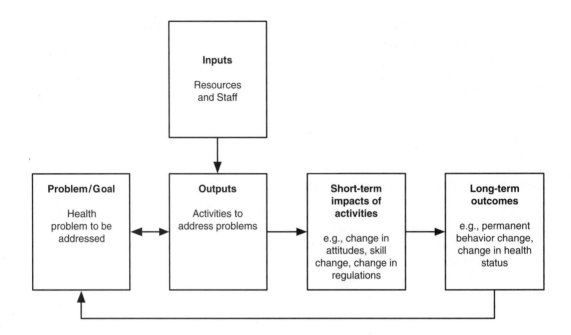

FIGURE 4–4   Example of a Basic *Logic Model*

reality of the project and its purpose for the planning group and the stakeholders. This tool is useful for many health promotion organizations.[46]

It starts with a focus idea and concepts. *Concept Mapping* is the beginning step in defining an organization's mission and vision. The mission and vision focus become established as ideas and connections by individuals form idea clusters. These concepts are visualized or "mapped" as a set of ideas or thoughts from the groups. Cards or computers are used to form piles of these ideas, which are then sorted and categorized. This sorting method encourages ranking and linking of these ideas and prompts discussion, encourages flexibility and allows consensus building, and then facilitates decision making in groups. Consensus decision making is key, as the group itself formulated the ideas or concepts that can facilitate a sharing of the ideas into formulating the mission and vision of the organization. The group's ideas and thoughtful opinions are organized and displayed as it visually paints a picture that all can relate to as their own creation. Thus, ownership is created, and the group empowerment process begins when formulating the mission and vision focus for an organization or program. It is the epitome of a road map to a program planning theoretical model.[46] See **Figure 4–4** for a sample *Logic Model*.

THEORY AND MODELS

Research should be centralized as the input to decide the needs and social conditions of the participants, to assess accessible resources, and to track the progress and effectiveness of the program through the process, impact, and outcome evaluation phases. When applied collectively, theory and planning can generate theoretical concepts that address the specific settings and participants. Using theory and models takes practice, and health practitioners are advised not to reinvent the wheel. They should perform the required research ahead of time to determine if an already established program's theory and model may be replicated or adjusted to suit their particular situation and problem. Knowledge of the theory and comprehensive planning systems is paramount to choosing the correct one(s) to cause the greatest positive effect and success.

Ecological Models—Combinations for Success

Many health educators find that they can achieve the greatest impact by combining theories to address a health problem in programs. Most theories are more robust when they are integrated within a comprehensive planning system. Program planning models are also more intensive and targeted if combined to achieve the maximum effect. Multiple theories, multiple resources, and **integrative plans** can be combined within one level, across levels of practice, and/or combined to address a single problem, and/or combined in planning systems. Pieces of different theories may fit together for a more effective, multiple-theoretical approach. This approach investigates health and behavior at **multiple levels of influence** with multiple theories, thus yielding multiple solutions. Examining health and behavior at multiple levels with multiple theories and multiple planning models increases the chances of successful programs. It attacks the health problems from many different angles with intentional behavior change theory and the correct participatory response for solving the health problems.

There is evidence that multiplicity in theories works. The CDC published articles on injury prevention through the use of multiple theories and integrative plans. There is an overview of programs by the National Center for Injury Prevention and Control[47] showing that ecological models are successful for prevention of unintentional injuries.[48] Also, there is evidence that multilevel and multisource needs assessment data help community interventions when planning programs.[49] Thus, multiple approaches at multiple levels using empirically based programs with integrative approaches can promote safety in health. The process is a kind of program saturation, applying as many theories and strategies as possible to saturate or envelope the group, community, and environment. The results must be sustainable and long-lasting lifestyle and environmental changes. Integrative plans provide recognition on multiple levels of influence. This targeted focus provides a constant reminder of what is essential in planning a program. Changing the environment is a key factor to making the saturation process a part of the daily lives of the participants. Everywhere participants go, they are exposed to the program components and see the changes already taking place. This saturation effect provides the opportunity to change in a conducive and comfortable environment that accepts change and embraces it.

Ecological plans mean that intrapersonal, interpersonal, and community theories can be combined. *Stages of Change*, the *Health Belief Model*, and the *Theory of Planned Behavior* can address individual

---

Integrative plans: Multiple theories and multiple resources combined to address a single problem.
Multiple levels of influence: The use of multiple theories to offer many different experiences and multiple solutions for health programs.

behavior change through strategies such as education, brochures, social marketing campaigns, and interactive technology. Using *Social Cognitive Theory* for interpersonal change can involve advising and mentoring programs. While the environmental changes strategies, including *Media Advocacy* campaigns and policy change can use community theories such as *Diffusion of Innovations* and *Community Organization*.[2] Change is never easy, but it can be made easier through an organized program planning model(s) and theories that help the participants in programs move easily through the tunnel of positive health promotion changes.

THEORETICAL APPLICATIONS

Investing and choosing correct theoretical models and believing in their applicability to health prevention and promotion efforts plays a big part in a program's success. Convincing others to use theory is not always an easy task. They may not be convinced of the theory's application, may not understand it, or may believe that is just a hypothetical concept that may not work. As professionals, it is our duty to acquaint ourselves with current research on theory, stay up to date on current theories used in practice, and research successful programs and theories already in use that can be replicated.

Matching the goals and objectives to a program plan with an appropriate theory and strategies is the first step in attaching the concepts to the program. A well-planned and executed program may only have a small impact in terms of numbers, but all change affects everyone. One tiny effective program, once replicated in other areas and communities, can snowball into many dots on the map of positive health change until all combine to become one highlighted area where change is effected in huge proportions. Effective programs have a ripple effect, and that ripple can reach far and wide—even producing global change.

SMALL PROGRAMS EFFECT GLOBAL CHANGE

As mentioned in Chapter 2, a cure for Hansen's disease was researched and discovered in 1941 at the small Carville leprosarium in Louisiana, run by the U.S. Public Health Service.[50] From 1894 until the 1950s, patients diagnosed with Hansen's disease were quarantined here. Some of these patients at Carville volunteered to participate in an experimental drug therapy program in the 1950s that led to the "Miracle at Carville."[51] This medical treatment was possible through the trial and error of many treatment programs at the facility. At first, Promines the drug discovered here and used for Hansen's disease only helped relieve some symptoms, but it did not eradicate the disease completely because of drug resistance. The multidrug therapy of dapsone, rifampicin, and clofazimine was discovered in 1981 through extensive research programs at Carville. The cure that resulted from years of multiple experimental programs evolved into the multidrug therapy (MDT) currently used throughout the world.[52]

The disease is now controlled due to MDT. Patients and those newly diagnosed in the United States are treated as outpatients, and quarantine is not required. Carville became one of the most sophisticated medical, research, and rehabilitation centers in the world for Hansen's disease treatment.[52] The disease is now curable in all countries where access and resources are available.[53]

The history of Carville, from its humble beginnings to its status as the world-known center for Hansen's disease care, research, rehabilitation, training, and education, is a tribute to effective health

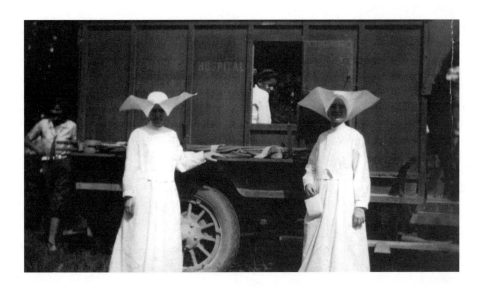

FIGURE 4–5 Two Daughters of Charity Nuns Standing in Front of the Transport Wagon for a Quarantined Hansen's Disease Patient to Carville, LA The Carville leprosarium was the last in the United States (1894–1999).

programs.[54] By the trial and error of many programs, and by sharing results and therapies, one small treatment facility made a difference in the quality of life for patients worldwide. Tenacity, research, and consultation with experts in the field—all accomplished by an organization that was not always highly funded or with sophisticated facilities and equipment—made an enormous contribution to the health of humankind. The Carville physicians, staff, and researchers did not intend to effect change on a global basis. They used the resources available, such as the armadillo, as a research prototype. Their focus was on making the lives of their patients more comfortable and reducing the disease's disabling and painful symptoms. Nonetheless, the dedicated work of people with a vision in a small program produced change on a global track (see **Figure** 4–5).[54]

Sometimes health practitioners become mired in programs that do not seem to be causing the desired effects. Not seeing huge changes or watching participants drop out, revert to unhealthy behaviors, or institute policies and laws not conducive to health progress can lead to what some call "program apathy." It can be difficult to recognize progress in small doses. Continuous progress, though it may not come in large steps, can eventually lead to the definitive answer or health program for that particular need. Small steps in the right direction are just as effective as large steps. Programs must start small sometimes to be replicated. They all lead to the same destination. We cannot give up and must continue working toward a healthier and better world for all citizens.

THEORIES AND MODELS

While theory is the change agent in a program, a planning model is the map to follow when constructing program plans. These two essentially hold hands in the program, keeping the program implementers on task and offering beneficial strategies for the participants.

Health practitioners must understand the procession of criteria for behavior change programs, objectives, and interventions. Interpreting each part of a program model and theory is important to the interventions or strategies. Realizing the importance of the environment or setting and the opportunities for strategies in and out of the setting of the program is crucial. A conceptual framework can facilitate strategies. Exploring health communications and the dissemination of interactive health interventions to the true setting is vital to a program's function. The following basic criteria for dissemination and health interventions are important: reach as many participants as possible, keep the budget costs conservative, and increase efficacy and empowerment for participants by using many diverse theories, strategies, program models, and communications channels. A health educator must determine and measure all factors involving health-related behavior and environmental and infrastructure changes. Interactive communications technologies for health behavior change, decision making, and utilizing many other areas, are where these theories are useful.

Picture the whole process of utilizing **evidence-based program** planning models and theories as a recipe. The main ingredients are assembled in a certain order and used in a certain way, much like the parts of the program planning model. Theory is the spice that compliments and enhances the model and makes it function properly. The correct ingredients are assembled in the program plan. They are measured very carefully. The ingredients are then mixed in a certain order and baked so that the end result is a perfectly cooked culinary delight that is consumed by the participants. Choosing models and theories that have proven their worth through empirical research is like following a tried and true recipe handed down for generations. A program planning model and theory are going to be more successful, affect more participants, and yield higher results when using and/or replicating evidence based programs with theories and models used successfully by other health educators through empirical research. Doing comprehensive research ahead of time is key to choosing theories and models that meet the program needs. Using proven approaches will save you the time and trouble of experimenting with a plan and theory that may not be as successful. Use the resources available to you, and include the participants in the planning process. Using scientifically based programs, innovative methodology and strategies, cutting-edge initiatives, adequate funding sources, validated public health practices, capacity building, quality improvement processes, and continuous evaluation of all possible health and socio-environmental determinants leads to effective health promotion and disease prevention programs. Such an approach is a tried and true recipe for producing a successful multilevel health education program, one that critics will compliment and cynics will applaud—the greatest compliment to the "chef," or health educator administrator. While following these recipes, though, do not be afraid to try and investigate other innovative models, strategies, and theories along with the evidence-based practices, and evaluate their results. This is how you may discover some other relevant program parts that work.

Evidence-based Programs and Practice: These are programs that are research based with proven empirical verification of effectiveness.

Environmental factors and behavior change predict a range of health-related behaviors. Using theoretical models and concepts to develop a conceptual framework of health behavior change is smart and keeps the focus on achieving the program goals and objectives. Public health communications play a huge role in changing environmental and behavioral factors and performing effective, theoretical-based health programs and research for health promotion, disease prevention, and disease management. This knowledge is considered critical to the development of effective public health behavior and education programs. Infrastructure is always an important consideration. Economic and living conditions, availability of food, water, shelter, and access to health care services are huge health considerations, especially in underdeveloped and poverty stricken areas.

Marketing professionals change people's behavior on a daily basis with advertising and convince them to try certain products. *Media Advocacy*, *Consumer Marketing*, *Social Marketing Theory*, and many other theories are used in business, industry, and commercial messages. As health practitioners, we can use the same approaches to change improper health behavior patterns and environments to improved health behavior patterns for health literacy, prevention, promotion, protection, access, enhancement, and maintenance.

SUMMARY

- Health education theory draws from many disciplines and sources.
- Health educators are always trying to find the definitive theory that is successful with specific types of behavioral/environmental change for evidence-based programs/practices.
- Theory and practice in health education is based on behavioral, sociological, biological, psychological, and scientific disciplines.
- Using evidence-based health promotion plans with empirical research gives credibility to a program.
- Strategic planning models and theory are critical in the success of a health behavior change program. Such theory is sometimes called explanatory theory or change theory.
- Concepts are the primary element of the theory. Constructs are the key concepts developed for a theory. Variables are the set forms of constructs.
- The categories of theories include individual (intrapersonal), interpersonal, community, and cultural.
- Individual theories are intrapersonal change theories and include *Stages of Change*, *Health Belief Model*, *Consumer Information Processing*, and *Theory of Planned Behavior*.
- Interpersonal theory involves the individual and significant others and includes *Social Cognitive Learning Theory*.
- Community theories involve all individual and environmental factors affecting change. Types included are *Community Organization*, *Media Advocacy*, *Diffusion of Innovations*, *Organizational Development Theory*, *Community Organization Theories*, and the *Empowerment Model*.
- Cultural theory includes the *Cultural Transformation Theory*.
- Additional prominent theories include *Behavioral Intention*, *Behaviorism*, *Coping Theory*, *Field Theory*, *Inoculation Theory*, *Locus of Control*, *Maslow's Hierarchy of Needs*, *Organizational Change*, *Persuasions in Communications*, and *Self-Efficacy Theory*.

- Multiple theories and plans can be combined within or across levels of practice and combined in planning systems.
- Theory investigates health and behavior at multiple levels of influence, using multiple theories and, hopefully, solving health problems with multiple solutions.

CONCEPTUAL TERMS

Theory	*Consumer Information Processing*
Concepts	*Theory of Planned Behavior*
Constructs	*Social Cognitive Learning Theory*
Variables	*Community Organization Theory*
Needs assessments	Empowerment
Explanatory theory	*Media Advocacy*
Intrapersonal theories	Health behavior change
Interpersonal theories	*Diffusion of Innovations*
Community theories	*Organizational Development Theory*
Cultural theories	*Empowerment Model*
Environmental change	*Cultural Transformation Theory*
Transtheoretical Model or *Stages of Change*	*Maslow's Hierarchy of Needs*
Benefits	Integrative plans
Barriers	Multiple levels of influence
Health Belief Model	Evidence-based Programs and Practice

REFLECTIVE THINKING

Health educators frequently discuss why people do not want to change to become healthier. As purists, we cannot always understand the reasoning behind resisting such a change. Some of it is human nature itself; change is difficult and continuance is more difficult. Some of it has to do with lifestyle choices. There is always the factor that the person is content and does not want to embrace change.

Here is a true story. Harold was 79 years of age. He had high blood pressure and was in for his annual checkup. Harold's regular physician had retired, and he had a new physician without a lot of experience working with older adults. The physician aggressively attacked Harold's lifestyle. He told him he needed to change his diet, exercise more, and lose some weight. The physician said he needed to cut out certain foods, including bacon and fried eggs as his staple breakfast fare. The physician gave him a diet to follow, recommended walking every day, and asked him to start recording his diet, activity patterns, and weight daily, and to return in a month. Harold laughed. He told the physician that he had a very good life, loved to eat, hated to exercise, and wasn't interested in losing weight at his age. He said he had taken high blood pressure medication for many years, and it had served him well. Harold said that he was happy and was not willing to change at this point in his life. The physician, in response, told Harold he could no longer serve as his primary care doctor and referred him to another physician. Harold left and continued with his present lifestyle. He lived to be 90 years of age.

What factors enabled Harold to live so long with an unhealthy lifestyle? Would you have tried to change Harold's mind after hearing his response? What theory would you have used to try to convince Harold to change his lifestyle? Just how far can you go without forcing a lifestyle change? Was Harold justified in his way of thinking? Would his quality of life have been better if he had changed?

CONCEPTUAL LEARNING

1. Summarize the following terms, and select an example of each from the theories listed in the chapter: theory, explanatory or change theory, concepts, constructs, and variables.
2. Cite an example of each of the following four types of theory, and compare the concepts: individual or intrapersonal theory, interpersonal theory, community theory, and cultural theory.
3. Discuss the different stages of the *Transtheoretical Model* or *Stages of Change Theory*. Demonstrate what can happen when someone regresses in this theory and how they may recover.
4. Compare the perceived seriousness, perceived susceptibility, benefits, and barriers aspects of the *Health Belief Model*, and provide an example of each.
5. Compose a communications message for a patient demonstrating the cues to action part of the *Health Belief Model*.
6. Propose a scenario demonstrating that multiple theories and plans can be combined for multiple levels of influence, and describe how doing so leads to multiple solutions.
7. Assemble peer-reviewed research journal articles for health programs using intrapersonal theory, interpersonal theory, community theory, and cultural theory. Identify the main health problems and the strategies used for each program, and discuss the similarities and differences.
8. Compare and contrast the strategies used for two health programs that you located from peer-reviewed professional journals. Identify the effectiveness for the different levels of theory.

REFERENCES

1. Pfizer Global Pharmaceuticals. (2009). *Milestones in public health: Accomplishments in health over the last 100 years.* New York: Author.
2. National Cancer Institute. (2005). *Theory at a glance: A guide for health promotion practice* (05–3896). Washington, DC: Department of Health and Human Services.
3. Goldman, K. D., & Schmalz, K. J. (2001). Tools of the trade theoretically speaking: Overview and summary of key health education theories. *Health Promotion Practice, 2*(4), 277–281.
4. Dignan, M. B., & Carr, P. A. (1992). *Program planning for health education and promotion.* Philadelphia: Lea and Febiger.
5. Lach, H. W., Everard, K. M., Highstein, G., & Brownson, C. A. (2004). Application of the transtheoretical model to health education for older adults. *Health Promotion Practice, 5*(1), 88–93.
6. Prochaska, J. O., & Velicer, W. F. (1997). The transtheoretical model of health behavior change. *American Journal of Health Promotion, 12*, 38–48.
7. Doyle, E., & Ward, S. (2001). *The process of community health education and promotion.* Mountain View, CA: Mayfield Publishing.
8. Prochaska, J. O., DiClimente, C. C., & Norcross, J. C. (1992). In search of how people change: Applications to addictive behaviors. *American Psychologist, 47*(9), 1102–1114.
9. Becker, M. (Ed.). (1974). *The health belief model and personal health behavior.* Thorofare, NJ: Slack.
10. Rosenstock, I. M. (1974). Historical origins of the health belief model. *Health Education Monographs, 2*, 328–335.

11. Janz, N. K., & Becker, M. A. (1984). The health belief model: A decade later. *Health Education Quarterly, 11,* 1–47.
12. Goldberg, J. H, Hapern-Felsher, B. L., & Milstein, S. G. (2002). Beyond invulnerability: The importance of benefits in adolescents' decision to drink alcohol. *Health psychology, 21*(5), 477–484.
13. National Cancer Institute. (2004, August). *Making health communications programs work: A planner's guide.* Washington, DC: Department of Health and Human Services.
14. Bettman, J. R. (1979). *An information processing theory of consumer choice.* Reading, MA: Addison-Wesley.
15. McKenzie, J. F, Neiger, B. L., & Thackery, R. (2009). *Planning, implementing, and evaluating health promotion programs: A primer* (5th ed.). New York: Pearson Benjamin Cummings.
16. Fishbein, M. (2003). The role of theory in HIV prevention. *AIDS Care, 12*(3), 273–278.
17. Ajzen, I., & Fishbein, M. (1980). *Understanding attitudes and predicting social behavior.* Englewood Cliffs, NJ: Prentice Hall.
18. Abroms, L., Jorgensen, C. M., Southwell, B. G., Geller, A. C., & Emmons, K. M. (2003). Gender differences in young adults' beliefs about sunscreen use. *Health Education & Behavior, 30*(1), 29–43.
19. Ajzen, I. (1988). *Attitudes, personality, and behavior.* Belmont, CA: Dorsey.
20. Cook, R., & Sheeran, P. (2004). Moderation of cognition-intention and cognition-behavior relations: A meta-analysis of properties of variables from the theory of planned behavior. *British Journal of Social Psychology, 43,* 159–186.
21. Bandura, A. (1977). *Social learning theory.* Englewood Cliffs, NJ: Prentice Hall.
22. Bandura, A. (2004). Health promotion by social cognitive means. *Health Education and Behavior, 31,* 143–164.
23. Minkler, M., & Wallerstein, N. (1999). Improving health through community organization and community building: A health education perspective. In K. Minkler (Ed.), *Community organizing and community building for health* (pp. 30–52). New Brunswick, NJ: Rutgers University Press.
24. Rothman, J., & Tropman, J. E. (1987). Models of community organization and macro practice perspectives: Their mixing and phasing. In F. M. Cox, J. L. Erlich, J. Rothman, & J. E. Tropman (Eds.), *Strategies of community organization: Macro practice* (pp. 3–26). Itasca, IL: F. E. Peacock.
25. Minkler, M., Thompson, M., Bell, J., & Rose, K. (2002). Contributions of community involvement to organizational level empowerment. The Federal Health Start Experience. *Health Education & Behavior, 28*(6), 783–807.
26. Wallack, L. (1990). Media advocacy: Promoting health through mass communication. In K. Glanz, F. M. Lewis, & B. K. Rimer (Eds.). *Health behavior and health education: Theory, research, and practice.* San Francisco: Jossey Bass.
27. Glanz, K., Rimer, B. K, & Viswanath, K. (2008). *Health behavior and health education: Theory, research and practice* (4th ed.). San Francisco: Jossey Bass.
28. Rogers, E. M. (1994). *Diffusion of innovation* (4th ed.). New York: Free Press.
29. Lowe, J. B., Balanda, K. P., Stanton, W. R., Del Mar, C., & O'Connor, V. (2002). Dissemination of an efficacious antenatal smoking cessation program in public hospitals in Australia: A randomized control trial. *Health Education and Behavior, 29*(5), 608–619.
30. Wallerstein, N., & Bernstein, E. (1988). Empowerment education: Freire's ideas adapted to health education. *Health Education Quarterly, 15,* 379–394.
31. Tai-Seale, T. (2001). Understanding health empowerment. *The Health Educator, 33*(1), 23–29.
32. McKenzie, J., M., Pinger, R. R, & Kotecki, J. E. (2008). *An introduction to community health* (6th ed.). Sudbury, MA: Jones and Bartlett Publishers.
33. McBeth, A. J., & Schweer, K. D. (2000). *Building healthy communities: The challenge of health care in the twenty first century.* Boston: Allyn & Bacon.
34. Fishbein, M., Bandura, A., Triandis, H. C., Kanfer, F. H., Becker, M. H., & Middlestadt, S. E. (1991, October 3–5). *Factors influencing behavior and behavior change* (Final Report, Theories Workshop). Bethesda, MD: National Institute of Mental Health.
35. Tove, G., & Gjengedal, E. (2007). Preparative waiting and coping theory with patients going through gastric diagnosis. *Journal of Advanced Nursing, 57*(1), 87–94.

36. Rotter, J. (1954). *Social learning and clinical psychology*. Englewood Cliffs, NJ: Prentice Hall.

37. Rotter, J. (1966). Generalized expectancies for internal versus external control of reinforcement. *Psychological Monographs, 1*(609).

38. Rotter, J. (1975). Some problems and misconceptions related to the construct of internal versus external control of reinforcement. *Journal of Consulting and Clinical Psychology, 43*, 56–67.

39. Mamlin, N., Harris, K. R., & Case, L. P. (2001). A methodological analysis of research on locus of control and learning disabilities: Rethinking a common assumption. *The Journal of Special Education, 34*(4), 214–225.

40. Seaward, B. L. (2001). *Health of the human spirit*. Needham Heights, MA: Allyn & Bacon.

41. McNamara, C. (2006). Clearing up the language about organization change and development. In *Field guide to consulting and organizational development: A collaborative and systems approach to performance, change, and learning*. Minneapolis, MN: Authenticity Consulting.

42. McGuire, W. J. (1984). Public communication as a strategy for introducing health-promoting behavioral change. *Preventive Medicine, 13*(3), 299–313.

43. Strecker, V. J., DeVellis, B. M., Becker, M. H., & Rosenstock, I. M. (1986). The role of self-efficacy in achieving health behavior change. *Health Education and Behavior, 13*(1), 73–91.

44. Noreen, M., & Dodge, J. A. (1999). Exploring self-efficacy as a predictor of disease management. *Health Education and Behavior, 26*(1), 72–78.

45. Ausubel, D., Novak, J., & Hanesian, H. (1978). *Educational psychology: A cognitive view* (2nd ed.). New York: Holt, Rinehart & Winston.

46. Trochim, W. K. (1998). *An introduction to concept mapping for planning and evaluation*. Retrieved March 22, 2010, from http://www.socialresearchmethods.net/research/epp1.htm

47. Sleet, D. A., Bonzo, S., & Branche, C. (1998). An overview of the National Center for Injury Prevention and Control at the Centers for Disease Control and Prevention. *Injury Prevention, 4*(4), 308–312.

48. Allegrante, J. P., Marks, R., & Hanson, D. W. (2006). Ecological models for the prevention of unintentional injury. In A. Gielen, D. A. Sleet, & R. Diclemente (Eds.), *Injury and violence prevention: Behavioral science theories, Methods, and applications*. San Francisco: Jossey Bass.

49. Levy, S. R., Anderson, E. E., Issel, L. M., Willis, M. A., Dancy, B. L., Jacobson, K. M., et al. (2004). Using multilevel, multisource needs assessment data for planning community interventions. *Health Promotion Practice, 5*(1), 59–68.

50. Parascandola, J. (1994). The Gillis W. Long Hansen's Disease Center at Carville. *Public Health Reports, 109*(6), 728–730.

51. Martin, B. (1950). *Miracle at Carville*. Garden City, NY: Doubleday Press.

52. World Health Organization. (1994). *Chemotherapy of leprosy: Report of a WHO study group*. Geneva, Switzerland: Author.

53. World Health Organization. (2008). *Leprosy*. Retrieved May 15, 2008, from http://www.who.int/lep/en

54. Hernandez, B. L. M., Vengurlekar, R., Kelkar, A., & Thomas, G. (2009). The legacy of Carville: A history of the last leprosarium in the U.S. *American Journal of Health Studies, 24*(2), 314–325.

ENHANCED READINGS

Kansas University Work Group on Health Promotion and Community Development. (2005). *Community Tool Box: Bringing solutions to light*. Lawrence, KS: University of Kansas. Available at: http://ctb.ku.edu/en/tablecontents/
See:

Part M: Social Marketing and Institutionalization of the Initiative (Chapters 45–46)

National Cancer Institute and National Institutes of Health. (2004, August). *Pink Book: Making health communication programs work: A planner's guide*. Washington, DC: Department of Health and Human Services. Available at: http://cancer.gov/pinkbook

See:

Introduction
Planning Frameworks, Theories, and Models of Change
How Market Research and Evaluation Fit into Communication Programs
Chapters 4 and 5
Appendix B: Selected Planning Frameworks, Social Science Theories, and Models of Change

National Cancer Institute and National Institutes of Health. (2005). *Theory at a glance: A guide for health promotion practice.* Washington, DC: Department of Health and Human Services. Available at: http://cancer.gov/cancerinformation/theory-at-a-glance
See:

Parts I–III

RELEVANT WEB SITES

United States Department of Health and Human Services, Health Resources and Services Administration. (2007). *National Hansen's disease (leprosy) program: History.* Available at: http://www.hrsa.gov/hansens/default.htm

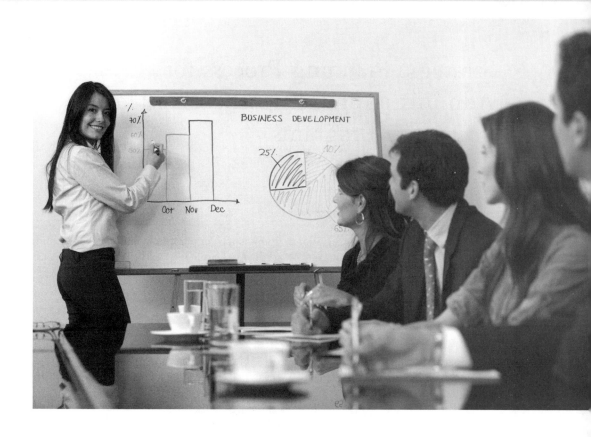

Strategic Planning Process for Administering Comprehensive Health Education Programs

OBJECTIVES AND ASSESSMENTS

This chapter meets the following National Commission for Health Education Credentialing, Inc., Society for Public Health Education, and American Association for Health Education Responsibilities and Competencies for Entry Level and Advanced Level Health Educator competencies.* The learner will:

2. Plan strategies, interventions and health education programs.
4. Conduct evaluation and research related to health education.

This chapter meets the following general learning objectives. The learner will:

1. Define and discuss the terms health literacy, prevention, promotion, protection, enhancement, maintenance, and access.
2. Write, research, and orally present a health project to the class.
3. Identify national, state, and local laws, policies, and regulations affecting community health.
4. List and define the content areas for health education programs.
5. Compose five reasons why strategic plans are necessary to measure success in health programs.
6. Defend the ideas of evidence-based planning for best health practices.
7. Distinguish between each step in the HABIT model strategic framework.

Sources: Reprinted with permission of NCHEC.

   National Commission for Health Education Credentialing, Inc. (NCHEC), Society for Public Health Education (SOPHE), & American Association for Health Education (AAHE). (2006). *A competency-based framework for health educators-2006*. Whitehall, PA: NCHEC.

INTRODUCTION

The Millennium Development Goals Report of 2008 has as its theme to "End Poverty by 2015." Conceived by the United Nations, the report presents a lofty goal. The goals are to end poverty and hunger; provide universal education, gender equality, child health, maternal health; combat HIV/AIDS; achieve environmental sustainability; and engender global partnership. Progress has been made in the world, but the global economic shortfall and higher prices for food have impeded the progress. A midway assessment by the United Nations Secretary, General Ban Ki-moon, said that despite some success, the progress has declined and the target goal to end poverty may not be met by 2015.[1]

This initiative offers a useful example of health programs on a global effort. Even if the intended results and progress may not occur as quickly as anticipated, health educators must persevere until the problem is solved. Can we ever solve all of these problems? We may not entirely succeed, but not trying has even more far-reaching detrimental consequences. We may take large steps toward progress, backward steps sometimes, and even go in the back door to make changes so we can eventually enter through the front door. But regardless of the approach, continuing efforts are paramount to improving and making our world a healthier and safer place to live. We owe this to the next generation and we owe it to ourselves to leave an indelible mark of health improvement for future populations. We must make a difference for all mankind, and this is where most health educators practice and where the profession leads them. Most community health promotion programs are not on a large scale and do not affect large groups. These smaller efforts give impetus to other communities and global health networks and coalitions around the world. Small steps are necessary to move toward the path of better health for a global tomorrow. Knowing how to administer programs is a skill that can be learned, and there are tools available to help health educators become successful.

Career Concept

Do you enjoy traveling to different countries and interacting with people from different cultures and diverse backgrounds? You may enjoy working in a health private voluntary organization, a nonprofit organization, or a private industrial company.

BACKGROUND ON THE NATURE OF HEALTH PROGRAM PLANS

Planning involves examining all aspects that influence health in populations. There are many determinants for health in humans. Historic and environmental influences, population movement, political change, war, technologic advances, famine, poverty, and many other variables affect health. For example, an effect of war is that many grandparents become caregivers for children of deployed military personnel. One effect usually causes a multiplicity of other effects. Thus, many factors, other than physical health, influence health in humans. To determine health status, certain facts need to be known and specific related data need to be collected. This information is used by many countries to make health-related decisions concerning legislation and actions.[2] As global situations change, these changes produce a ripple effect—one health influence may affect another one—sometimes making data collection difficult and requiring immediate programs and program focus changes.

The data that needs to be examined include information on the population, vital statistics, health statistics, and health services statistics. Data on the population include the number of people and demographic information such as gender, age, ethnic origin, geographic distribution, and other characteristics. Vital statistics include live births; deaths by gender, age, and cause; marriage; divorce; and related information. Health statistics include morbidity by type, severity, and outcome (illness or accident); reportable diseases; disabilities; prevalence; epidemics; and other specific statistics unique to a region. Health services involve the type and quantity of facilities and services, personnel qualifications, payment information, health insurance information, cost information, and hospital, health centers, and clinic operations—as well as other diverse aspects that may be divided into subcategories.[2]

Once data collection is complete, a picture begins to emerge that defines certain deficiencies and areas that need improving such as methods for prevention, promotion, protection, literacy, access, maintenance, and enhancement. A *program* in health education and promotion, according to Dignan and Carr, is "a package of services or information that is intended to produce a particular result. Successful programs require specific and clear goals and objectives, combined with reasonable and appropriate methods for satisfying the objectives and thereby reaching the goals."[3(p5)] **Program plans** are statements that are documented and describe the services package that works toward achieving a specific purpose. They specify what is maintained or changed for focusing and determining outcomes. The model provides the basics for developing a structured program of instruction and theory as the driving force to produce the intended outcome.[3] Multistrategy health communication programs are preferable for multiple types of change.[4]

A sample title for a program proposal includes the basic elements to thoroughly describe what will be done. The who, what, when, where, why, and how need to be included. The *what* explains the specific type of program and program topics such as prevention, promotion, education, access, environmental changes, etc., or combinations of these. Planners can add any other characteristics to describe the type of program or extenuating circumstances (including limitations and delimitations). The *why* should describe the type of program or problem that needs to be solved and the disease (or problem and issues) or behaviors contributing to the problem. The *who* identifies the number of participants and the specific demographics of the participants. The *where* indicates the specific practice setting and the social, cultural, policy, regulatory, and environmental climate that influences participants. The *how* explains the process for conducting the program: How will the goals and objectives be achieved? How will interventions address the issues/problems for the participants? How will specific measurements be used to evaluate if the goals and objectives were achieved? The how also includes the program budget and what can be done with the money allocated. The *when* is the length of time for the program and specific starting and ending dates.

Here is an example of a simple program proposal title: A Four-Year Sexually Transmitted Infections Education and Prevention Program (STIEPP): A Comparison of Pretest and Posttest SEXED Survey Scores in 400 Randomly Selected Male and Female University Students (18–24 Years). This title describes what type of program will be used (prevention and education); why the program is needed [to address a disease or problem (sexually transmitted infections)]; how it will be conducted (random selection of participants); data collection or measurement used (to compare pre- and posttest SEXED survey results); who will participate (400 male and female students, ages 18–24 years); when it will be

---

Program plan: Structured outlines that are documented and describe what works to achieve a specific purpose and produce the intended outcome.

conducted (the length of time is 4 years); and where it will be conducted (at a university). While the title may seem long, it delineates exactly the program purpose, the research data that needs collecting, and the participants.

A STRATEGIC PLAN

Strategic written plans, sometimes called action plans, are always smart ways to measure success.[5] Proper planning is important to determine a health program focus.[3] It also assists in understanding the health issue, determining communication roles, identifying strategies for the preferred behavior change, establishing a development process, creating a plan that supports measurable objectives, setting program priorities, assigning all responsibilities, and continuously evaluating progress.[4] Health education programs need to function efficiently and effectively to bring about the desired changes in participants and communities and to promote prevention, promotion, protection, access, enhancement, and maintenance. **Multiple interventions** at **multiple levels** using evidence-based practice are essential for proper planning.[6] An **empirical review** of relevant literature is helpful in identifying similar programs, replicable programs, and multiple interventions and levels. Proven programs are recommended. The **HABIT model** draws from many diverse models to deliver a comprehensive program plan addressing the needs, interests, and problems of a community program or a school health education program.

Planning goes from a larger conceptual model to a very detailed and lengthy strategically planned concept model supported by a specific written plan. Breckon, Harvey, and Lancaster in 1998 stated that planners should plan the process, with the people, with the data, with permanence, with priorities, with measurable outcomes, and with evaluation.[7] In their words, "In the context of population health program planning,...the notion of **best practices** should be viewed as a process of careful, **evidence-based planning** that enables planners to tailor strategies and methods to the unique circumstances of a given place or population."[8(p21)]

In a strategically planned program model with relevant theory embedded, there are two types of research in developing effective programs. Formative research is a process that develops, defines, and refines the concepts before fully implementing them. Summative research is a process of monitoring to compare impact and outcomes against the specifically defined program objectives and strategies. A

Multiple interventions: The use of many different types of strategies across all levels of influence for more effective program planning.

Multiple levels: The use of many levels of influence drawing from evidence-based practice for more effective and proper planning.

Empirical review: A review of relevant research literature for identifying similar programs, replicable programs, and multiple interventions and levels.

HABIT model: A model that takes the health educator through the stages of a health administrative program using strategic planning; the acronym HABIT stands for hiring, assessing, building, implementing, and testing.

Best practices: The ideal approach to help planners manage strategies and methods for particular circumstances for a program.

Evidence-based planning: Detailed program plans that are based on research with proven empirical verification.

strategic plan not only gives structure to a program, it is a road map for the executive director or school administrator, program staff, and the planning/advisory/steering committee to follow to ensure success. It is important to use evidence-based recommendations and findings for what works to promote health in communities. For school-based initiatives, the planning process is similar; however, a health supervisor or principal may be the person in charge of the program instead of an executive director. The staff would be the certified teachers, and the advisory committee would be the school health advisory committee.

HIRE, ASSESS, BUILD, IMPLEMENT, TEST (HABIT) MODEL (MICHIELS-HERNANDEZ, 2009)

A new model developed by the author takes the health educator through the stages of a health program administration model using strategic planning (see **Figure 5–1**). The acronym HABIT describes the end result of the program and stands for hire, assess, build, implement, and test. This model implies that the behavior and other environmental and policy changes become habit forming and conclude in habits that are embedded in individuals, groups, and communities. The stages listed take into consideration that a program administrator (e.g., director, executive director, CEO, school administrator) is already in place at the site. For the purposes of this chapter, the executive director (ED) title and school

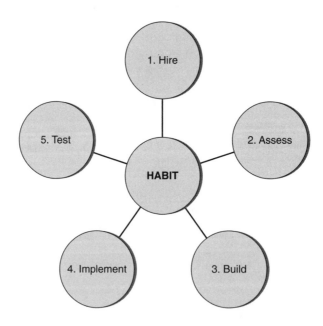

FIGURE 5–1   HABIT Model

administrator (SA) titles are used. However, school-based initiatives should be planned in the same manner whether in conjunction with a community program or a school-based curriculum. Also, the planning/advisory/steering committee will be referred to as the planning committee. In a school-based situation, this could be the school health advisory committee or a committee could be formed. The employed staff along with the ED will be referred to as the program team, and meetings will be called staff committee meetings. These terms could include school-based initiatives where the staff would be the certified teachers and the SA would be school-based personnel such as supervisors or other administrators.

The HABIT program planning model is a sequential and coordinated process to guide health educators in administering and planning programs (see **Table 5–1**). It includes the basics identified in many other planning models, along with an administrative order that gives a program administrator or school administrator a very specific structure to follow. An ecological model focuses on individual and social environmental factors for health prevention and promotion efforts. Using this approach, these changes should produce individual behavior change, community or group change, and support for the changes. These concepts are infused within the model.[9] The basic steps for strategic planning using the stages for the HABIT model are:

Hire the program staff and team.
Assess and identify the needs and problems of participants/community.
Build the strategic program plan model, theories, and strategies.
Implement the program.
Test the program.

The following discussion provides a detailed view of each of the steps.

1. Hire the Program Staff and Team

The first task before a program even begins is to secure a **human subjects review board** approval as required by the agency, organization, or university and meet these requirements. The human subjects review board approval and the research procedures are delineated. Once a new program is funded or facilitated, a strategic planning model is used to facilitate the planning process. Even if a needs assessment was performed (to apply for the funding for a grant or program), if enough time elapsed between writing the program and funding, a new assessment and refined rationale may be necessary. The problem or issue was identified in the grant or need assessment and needs to be addressed as well as the issue that contributed to the problem. Sometimes, the parameters of the program may change and the human subjects review board must approve changes before the program can proceed.

Human subjects review boards: Governmental, agency, university, medical center, and other review boards that monitor all programs and research involving human subjects.

TABLE 5-1   STEPS OF THE HABIT MODEL

1. Hire the Program Staff and Team
  a. Director assembles, interviews, and hires program staff as needed
  b. Define job descriptions
  c. Develop staff budget
  c. Hire program manager(s) and staff (invite community leaders and program participants to assist)

2. Assess and Identify the Needs and Problems of Participants or the Community
  a. Assess or redefine needs assessment and build rationale
    (1) Primary and secondary data collection
    (2) Quantitative and qualitative data diagnosis
        (a) Epidemiological data
        (b) Ecological and environmental data
        (c) Educational data
        (d) Health status data
        (e) Behavioral and cultural data
            (i)   Predisposing
            (ii) Reinforcing
            (iii) Enabling factors
  b. Define administrative tasks, organizational plan, policy development
  c. Identify and define problem
    (1) Global
    (2) Local
  d. Define participant population
    (1) Age
    (2) Gender
    (3) Linguistics
    (4) Minorities
    (5) Specially challenged populations
    (6) Literacy levels
    (7) Cultural traits
  e. Redefine rationale
  f. Define benefits and values
  g. Form advisory/steering council or committees, and define tasks
    (1) Participants population
    (2) Doers
    (3) Influencers
    (4) Sponsoring agency representative(s)
    (5) Community leaders
    (6) Stakeholders

3. Build the Strategic Program Plan Model, Theories, Strategies, and Evaluation Plan
  a. Program team and advisory committee develops strategic plan with scope and sequence charts
  b. Define vision and mission
  c. Write goals and objectives based on needs assessment, problem, and rationale
  d. Develop model, theory, and strategies, and evaluation design (process, impact, and outcome)

TABLE 5–1   *(Continued)*

　　　(1) Match to vision and mission
　　　(2) Match to needs assessment, problems identified, and rationale
　　　(3) Match to goals and objectives
　　　(4) Specificity to participant population, culture, and determinants of health
　　　(5) Specificity to environment, ecological, policies, laws, legislation, and education changes needed
　e. Develop budget
　f. Define timetable
　g. Develop resources
　h. Define proposed solution and results
　i. Develop evaluation plan and specify data collection techniques (process, impact, outcome)
　j. Pilot program or perform pretest of program
　　　(1) Process evaluation
　　　(2) Impact and outcome evaluation
　　　(3) Change and improve program
　　　(4) Refine budget and timetable

4. Implement the Program
　a. Develop tasks and resources
　b. Go over strategic plan, management plan, and administrative/staff tasks
　c. Introduce program to participants
　d. Conduct program
　e. Perform process and impact evaluations
　　　(1) Make minor changes (improve program strategic plan as needed)
　　　(2) Make minor revisions (improve budget and timetable as needed)
　f. Collect data continuously

5. Test the Program
　a. Perform program outcome evaluation (internal and external)
　　　(1) Reexamine strategic plan
　　　(2) Final data collection
　　　(3) Analyze data
　　　(4) Report results to manager and staff
　　　(5) Apply findings
　b. Evaluate program managers and staff
　c. Make recommendations for change
　d. Improve program for replication
　e. Complete the evaluation report and disseminate results

The problem must be identified and then justified in the final rationale. In the case of grant funding or university programs, this board approval must be secured and its approval received before the program or any planning begins. Community or public health or governmental programs will need to submit information to other human subjects board. Agencies without these forms, may want to consider adopting a model to use (see Table 7–1 for a sample).

Once hired, the ED or SA has a formidable task ahead. Assembling the program team is the beginning. The needs assessment helps determine the type of employee skills and experiences needed for the program team. Experience with the issue, with the specific participants, and with the necessary technology is considered along with the proper degree, education, and training in working with these specific participants and/or students.

For step 1 of the HABIT model, the ED or SA assembles, interviews, and hires the program team or staff committee. The program staff is hired unless the staff already exists. Salaries are defined for the employees and staff, if not previously done. These salaries are included if a grant is received, for specific or new employees, or if a new agency was created; if a grant is renewed, salaries of existing employees are included. The budget for the program staff, if a community agency or school is already in existence, may or may not be separated from the program budget, except in grant funding. Sometimes, only certain jobs may be included in a grant if an agency or school district was already established and desires a new program or a supplement to the existing programs offered.

Job descriptions and the staff budget must be established. The job descriptions should be clearly outlined. Job descriptions include the responsibilities of the director, programmer, evaluator, advisory committee, and contractors in terms of staffing, managing facilities, obtaining informed consent, and ensuring the security of data collected. For school health purposes, the term staff will be used synonymously with a community program. If there is a large data collection process and a lot of statistical information to be entered, you may want to consider a statistician and/or data processor, even if only on a part-time basis.

During the interview process, it is essential to invite community leaders and program participants to assist in the job selection process, if possible. Doing so could encourage partnerships, and researching appropriate community leaders is important. You only need two people along with the director for interviews and staff selection. If more are required, an uneven number is needed for a vote to preclude a tie vote, but if there is a tie, the director needs the final say in the hiring if there is not a consensus. Needless to say, the job descriptions are formulated to meet the program needs and include degreed and certified health educators for the program manager(s) and staff. If medical staff members are hired, such as nurses or physicians, their job descriptions and degrees should be appropriate for the role they play in the program. Staff persons, if included, should have appropriate job requirements to carry out the tasks required.

Before hiring, the ED or SA must complete an employee manual and have it approved by the planning committee. This manual should be given to each new employee and is required reading. Also, a written contract specifying job requirements and stipulating that the manual be read and understood is recommended. An attorney needs to be consulted for the manual and the contract to make sure all legal ramifications are controlled.

Hiring is only the first step with employees. Just like the program, they need to be evaluated regularly to make sure the planning and program activities are being carried out in a professional and efficient manner. The ED or SA meets with the staff every week from the beginning until the end of the program, ensuring that the whole team is on task and that assigned tasks are completed on time. The ED or SA also plans a general agenda to follow for each meeting and asks for input from the advisory/steering/planning committee or school health advisory committee and the program team (employees). Ethical practices, which are discussed in Chapter 7, are paramount for a professional health education program and must be enforced. Cultural sensitivity training for the program team is a good recommendation, especially when minority groups are involved in the participant population.

2. Assess and Identify the Needs and Problems of Participants or the Community

Once the staff is hired, the second step involves assessing the needs and assembling the advisory/steering committee or school health advisory committee. As explained in step 1, a needs assessment may need to be done again, even if it was in the initial step in funding or grant procurement. Any needs assessment more than six months old needs to be repeated. Also, a needs assessment for resources and identifying the resources necessary and available in the area is done. Plans to recruit additional resources or purchase needs to be decided as well as funding necessary for purchased items. These budgetary items are considered in conjunction with the other planning factors.

It is imperative that the ED or SA clearly delineate the job descriptions for the program team and the responsible person(s) for data collection for the needs assessment and the evaluation data collection.. Quantitative and qualitative data to collect on the participants and the community and/or school includes but is not limited to demographic, epidemiological, economical, and environmental data, as well as data related to education level, health, culture, and behaviors. You want to assess the knowledge, attitudes, skills, behavior, beliefs, health status, culture, religion, skills, policies, stakeholders, organizational structure, health risks, standard of living, literacy levels, access to health services, and any other mitigating factors affecting the participants and the community.[10]

For culture and behaviors, look at **predisposing**, **reinforcing**, and **enabling factors**.[8] List the positive and negative aspects of each of these three factors for the participants. Predisposing factors provide a reason or motivation to perform a behavior, including knowledge, attitudes, readiness, and beliefs. Reinforcing factors continually encourage certain behaviors due to social support, rewards, and praise. Enabling factors allow people to act on their own inclinations due to support, resources, assistance, and services. Tolerance and respect are definitive factors when working with specific cultures. Diagnosing the size of the health problem and the risk factors are basic to planning. Global and local health, political factors, and economic issues need to be defined along with preventive and protective factors already in place.

Define the administrative tasks, the organizational plan, and any policy development necessary for the program. Recognize the **global problems**, and relate them to the local problem. Identify characteristics of the participant population, including age, gender, linguistics, minority profile, specially challenged populations, literacy levels, linguistics, cultural traits, and any other factors. These steps

---

Predisposing factors: Factors that provide a reason or motivation to perform a behavior, including knowledge, attitudes, readiness, and beliefs.
Reinforcing factors: Factors that continually encourage certain behaviors due to social support, rewards, and praise.
Enabling factors: Factors that allow people to act on their own inclinations due to support, resources, assistance, and services.
Global problems: All influences affect the global structure. Environments, politics, infrastructures, and social/cultural patterns vary in many different countries and parts of the world. Recognizing these differences and working with supportive laws, policies, regulations, and norms can support environmental changes and communities.

help the program planners to build a **rationale**, or if it was initially developed in a grant proposal, to refine the rationale. Next, define or redefine the rationale (why), benefits, and values of the program for participants and the community. The rationale may have been established if this was grant funded, but taking a second look or defining it clearly is imperative; it may need more specific development or expansion depending on the recent data collected. It must reasonably explain why the program is necessary with support from relevant data. If a rationale or focus changes in a grant, the funding agency must approve significant changes according to the grant criteria.

Data collection instruments need to be determined for the needs assessment. Also, the same types of data or additional data collection techniques available are selected for use during the evaluation phases later on in the planning process. The reliability and validity of any instruments used need to be determined and are important for accurate data collection. There are different types of assessment techniques. **Primary data collection techniques** are those in which the program team collects the evidence; information comes from the "horse's mouth," or firsthand information sources, including the participants or other community leaders. **Secondary data collection techniques** involve data collected by someone else (e.g., city health departments, U.S. Census Bureau, county agencies, epidemiological reports).[10] Primary data are recognized as the most accurate for the community at a given time, but secondary data are readily available and can offer a snapshot of the community. Both are necessary to get a clear image of the health of the community.

Different data collection techniques are used for primary and secondary sources. **Quantitative assessment techniques** include primary data such as needs assessment surveys, other surveys, health risk assessments, nominal group process reports, self-reports, community assets and resource findings, baseline measures of behavior, public records, archival data, and many more sources.[4,11] The secondary sources, such as public records and archival data, are available from existing data, records, or resource inventories from agencies (city, government, and state), existing records, literature, vital statistics, hospital and healthcare records, incidents reports, demographic reports, etc.[10]

Self-assessments or self-reports are written questionnaires submitted via mail, e-mail, or fax and could include personal diaries or program records.[10] Respondents report on themselves. The health educator needs to overcome bias, and wording is important. The questionnaire should be valid and reliable, using preexisting measures when possible.[11] Indirect observations can be done using proxy measures; for example, the program coordinator could measure weight or blood pressure to confirm if self-reports on these measures by the participants were correct. Self-directed assessments are surveys that act as screening tests for determining propensity to conditions or diseases (such as heredity or lifestyle) and are commonly called health risk assessments.

Rationale: The reason a program is necessary, supported by relevant data.
Primary data collection techniques: Techniques in which evidence is collected by the program team; it is firsthand information.
Secondary data collection techniques: Techniques in which evidence is collected by someone else or accessed from another source.
Quantitative assessment techniques: Data collections using numbers.

Qualitative assessment techniques include focus groups, community forums, nominal group processes, interviews, SWOT analyses (strengths, weaknesses, opportunities, and threats), and ethnographic techniques such as observation. Interviews include telephone interviews (random digit dialing), face-to-face or in-depth interviews, e-mail interviews, Internet chat sessions, and group interviews. Observation techniques include direct observation and meetings.[5,10,11]

There are individual data collection techniques and multistep techniques. Individual data collection techniques include a single step. Single-step survey techniques utilize the participant population and significant others using written questionnaires, telephone, or face-to-face interviews. Key informants include individuals with knowledge and ability to report the need. They are respected in the community but sometimes give biased information. A multistep survey includes the Delphi technique, which is a series of questionnaires (distributed by mail or e-mail). This technique begins with a set of broad questions being sent out to participants. The responses to the questions are analyzed and a series of new questions evolve from the results that narrow the topic and these newly constructed questions are sent out again for review. These responses are analyzed and even more specific questions are compiled according to these analyzed results. This process continues and new questionnaires may continually request additional information until finally a consensus from all participants is reached from the analyzed results.[5,11]

A community forum is when a large group of people from the target population meet and discuss needs. A moderator shares the purpose, and recorders take notes. With focus groups, a skilled moderator, drawing from prepared questions, leads a small group of 8–12 people in discussion of an issue. Several focus groups may be invited to gather information. Nominal group process includes a few knowledgeable representatives of the target population (usually 5–7 people). These experts are invited to qualify and quantify needs. Self-directed assessments are a screening test of health assessments; they include health risk assessments.[4,5]

Health assessment tools can be found in *The Seventeenth Mental Measurements Yearbook*, by the Buros Institute.[12] It is a good resource for psychological tests and measurements along with validity and reliability data information. Author information is included with most instruments listed. The *SPM Handbook of Health Assessment Tools* is another resource used by many health educators.[13] These data collection methods, used for needs assessments, and the information listed here are also considered for the evaluation design and plan.

The ED or SA administrator consults with community leaders and the program team for possible members for the planning committee. Then, the ED or SA starts recruiting the committee and includes some of the community participants, population, doers, influencers, sponsoring agency representatives, community leaders, key persons, and stakeholders. This step may need to precede the needs assessment and job descriptions so the community is involved in this step or so community leaders can be recruited to assist in the process. Besides the ED or SA, key staff members (2–3) may be included on the planning committee. The ED or school administrator also plans with the staff on a weekly basis, but having key staff on the planning committee allows for a smooth transition to what the planning committee dictates and what the staff carries out. The ED or SA heads the committee, key program managers, and the community participants who make up the planning team. Keep the total number of participants

---

Qualitative assessment techniques: Data collections acquired from conversations, direct observations, and interviews.

at an odd number for voting purposes—otherwise you may end up with a tie vote quite often. Robert's rules of order should be used for all meetings.[14]

3. Build the Program Model, Theories, and Strategies

A model facilitates the planning or building process. Even if a needs assessment was performed (to apply for the funding for a grant or program), if enough time elapsed between writing the program and funding, a new assessment and rationale are necessary. Included in this plan are the policy, legislative, and educational changes. Internal and external changes are necessary for a program. Internally, the changes occur within the individuals and the society where they live. Externally, the changes are peripheral, such as environment, policies, education, and legislative efforts. School-based efforts may be more internalized, but external changes are necessary to support a climate for change for the students within that community and outside the school setting. For effective change, internal and external elements can help ensure institutionalized change.

The needs assessment, vision, mission, goals, and objectives are written, in coordination with the building and implementation of the planning model, theory, and strategies. Each component is matched to the strategic planning model and to one another in a coordinated effort that is specific to the participant population/community and most effective to accomplish the behavior change. The rationale is the reason for the program, and these issues are addressed in the strategic plan.

The needs assessment is analyzed, and any problems encountered in the needs assessments are targeted in the program that is built or designed. The third step is to build this targeted program plan—a **health program strategic plan** with an identified scope and sequence of the program's focus to target the identified problems.[3,5] Thus, the scope and sequence of the program is delineated. The program team and the advisory committee define the vision and mission statements appropriate for the program based on the analyses of data collected and other information in step 1.

The needs assessment, mission, goals, and objectives are written in coordination with the strategic planning model, data collection methods, and strategies. The theoretical principle(s) appropriate to the situation is chosen along with the other elements. Then, each is matched to one another in a coordinated effort that is specific to the participant population/community and most likely to accomplish the changes in the community, education, environment, and other changes necessary to accomplish the goals.

A **vision statement** expresses where you hope the community will be in the future. A shared vision is one that promotes ownership by all parties involved. It is a commitment to work together for a better community and/or school and a better health future for all. It is truly the dream or utopia. It states what things will look like if the issue is addressed perfectly and positive results are achieved. It articulates the beliefs and governing principles of the organization to the community or school (or both) and staff.[5] Of course, the vision statement may or may not be reached in the first year of a program; indeed it may take many years to achieve it. A **mission statement** is what the organization represents at the

---

Health program strategic plan: A targeted program plan with an identified scope and sequence of the program's focus to target the identified problems.
Vision statement: A forecast of where you hope the community/group will be in the future; a predictive statement for a program.
Mission statement: A statement of what you will achieve and a reason for applying your program to this objective.

present time. It states what you are going to do and why, and it broadly defines how the community can achieve it. It is a concrete statement, concise and inclusive, that is oriented on action and outcome.[5] It is grounded and states what is feasible in a short period of time. The vision and mission statements should be reevaluated every year in a program. While they are not as measurable as specific objectives, the reality is that they do have a chance of success. The difference between a vision and a mission statement is that a vision statement predicts what you hope the agency, school, or organization will be in the future when the program is successfully implemented, and the mission statement states what the program represents at the present time.

The goals and objectives are the next basics to define and build. The goals, objectives, theory, strategies and other program components address the health problem through prevention, promotion, access to services, literacy, enhancement, and maintenance factors. A **goal** is a broad statement about where you want to go.[14] It is the aim or target for the community and participants to achieve.[11] It is different from a vision statement in that it precipitates action and serves as a guide for the specific objectives. According to *Healthy People 2010*:[15(p1)]

> The goals provide a general focus and direction. Once the goals are in place, they serve as topical headings for the objectives. The objectives are formulated that relate to the goals. The goals, in turn, serve as a guide for developing these...set or sets of...objectives that will measure actual progress within a specified amount of time.

There is no set number of goals for a program; rather, goals are the broad headings under which the specific measurable objectives align. It is important that the ED or SA clarify the program goals continuously throughout the planning and implementation process.[3] Underneath each goal, the specific objectives are listed. All **objectives** must be measurable, and this information, once collected, ensures accurate testing or evaluation during and after the health program. The objectives focus on the determinants of health. These determinants cover the combined effects of the whole program. The physical and social environments of the individual and community, the policies, and the interventions are included. The ultimate result is to promote health, prevent disease, ensure access to quality health care, afford protection, increase literacy, and maintain and enhance the improvement of health as a result of the plan.[16]

The types of health objectives include administrative, **learning**, **behavioral**, **program or community**, cultural, **environmental**, and public law and/or policy. Administrative objectives are the **process objectives** or tasks involved in planning an implementing the program. Learning objectives are changes in the participant's knowledge (cognitive), attitudes (affective), and behaviors (psychomotor), or KAB. Behavioral objectives are changes in the individual participant's health behavior and may

---

Goal: A broad statement of the program's aim; the objective for the community and participants to achieve.
Objectives: The specific, measurable written statements of achievements for the program and/or participants; this collected information ensures accurate testing or evaluation during and after the health program.
Learning objectives: Changes in the participant's knowledge, attitudes, and behaviors in a program.
Behavioral objectives: Changes in the individual participant's health behavior(s) in a program.
Program or community objectives: Changes in the overall health statistics (quality of life) of the participants/community/group in a program.
Environmental objectives: Changes in a program such as prevention and promotion factors and removing barriers in a program.
Process objectives: The administrative tasks for a program.

relate to cultural behavior patterns that need changing. Cultural objectives are those that change or reinvent harmful cultural attitudes and skills. Program or community objectives are changes in the overall health statistics (quality of life) (see **Table 5–2**). Environmental objectives are changes such as removing barriers and adding prevention and promotion factors.[5,10,11] Public policy, laws, and regulations are political and infrastructure changes. While some believe these factors are not necessarily objectives, they are vital to a program in which regulation changes are paramount to success and should be delineated in the objectives section.

The theoretical principle appropriate to the situation is chosen and linked with the goals and objectives and strategies or methods. Theory is the conceptual structure for well-defined research and informed practice. Theories explain behavior and then recommend methods to achieve a particular behavior change.[6] Theories about behavior help explain the "why" of people's action. As stated by Doyle and Ward, "Theory based educational methods may well prove to be the most effective in helping people change health related behaviors."[17(p159)]

Different types of theories best fit different health programs, but multiple theories are used for multiple solutions and are highly recommended. There are also theories best suited to individual, interpersonal, community, and cultural changes in behavior. Rigorously tested theories and factual empirical evidence are needed to continuously test the usefulness of theories.[6] Building on marketing principles, theory is used in advertising, business, public relations, and even industry to help bring about the desired behavior change in people. In marketing, it may well be how to get someone to buy a product, and in business or industry, it may help employees become more efficient and effective. As health educators, we want people in a program to "buy in" to the product of changing to healthier lives, and theoretical principles used appropriately help achieve that goal. See Chapter 4 for specific theoretical program models.

Once the theory is chosen, the strategies need to be developed. Strategies are the methods, instructional techniques, interventions, and/or activities that produce the changes needed through the theoretical behavior change process. As changes in the participants and the social/environmental occur, strategies are formed with the planning committee and program team. As usual, the theory or theories are matched to the vision and mission statements, goals, objectives, needs assessment data, strategies, participant population characteristics, problem, solution, budget, resources and evaluation (process, impact, and outcome).

Intervention strategies assess specific targeted issues. The cause of the problem is determined and addressed. The intervention goals are addressed. For strategies, they should be acceptable to the program population, culturally sensitive, and appropriate for the participants' demographic profile and other characteristics of their lifestyle. Identify the methods and activities for education. Also, consider the correct literacy levels and how the materials will be used.[4] The communication methods should suit the participants and the skills and information they need.[3] Many different methods need to be explored to appeal to all types of learners. Technological methods can be used to reach both auditory learners and visual learners. Auditory learners comprehend better through listening skills while visual learners need materials as visual aids to aid comprehension. Many interactive learning methods that appeal to a wide range of people are used. However, participants may need technology skills to access technological strategies. A summary of different methods and strategies is available in different sources.[3–5,11] Program staff must understand and carry out the pivotal activities that give participants the skills necessary to proceed through the activities for a successful program.[3]

TABLE 5–2   **COMMUNITY ANTISMOKING CAMPAIGN OBJECTIVES**

Program Objectives	Examples	Evaluation	Targeted Results
Administrative/ Process	Tasks by administration staff such as designing brochures and media campaign	Formative (Process) Examples: brochures printed and distributed targeting different community age groups; media advocacy on reducing risk of second hand smoke in the community and reducing smoking behaviors	Dissemination
Learning	Change in knowledge, attitudes, and/or skills of participants	Summative (Impact) Examples: skills developed and acquired; awareness and consciousness raising in community organizations; public service announcements and media proliferation; antismoking programs implemented through local churches and education programs in local schools	Health literacy, health education, and access to services
Behavioral	Behavior change to nonsmoking behavior	Modified, discontinued, or adapted new behavior Examples: patrons adhering to nonsmoking in restaurants, bars, and workplaces; large percentage of program participants quit smoking; education program prevents smoking behaviors adopted by youth	Health prevention
Environmental	Environmental changes or adaptations in restaurants and bars	Barriers removed and protective measures in place Example: secondhand smoke eliminated from city and state governments buildings, restaurants, workplaces, and bars. Secondhand smoke eliminated in homes where smokers quit	Health protection

(Continues)

TABLE 5–2   (Continued)

Program Objectives	Examples	Evaluation	Targeted Results
Cultural	Adaptation, change, or removal in cultural knowledge, attitudes, and/or skills of participants	Remove, change, or adaptation of cultural practices that harm health Examples: many program participants adopt nonsmoking behaviors and/or quit smoking; smoking sociability practices discontinued in restaurants, workplaces, and bars; nonsmoking accepted by program participants; city and state buildings adopt nonsmoking policy	Health promotion
Program	Change in health status or quality of life	Measurement data shows reduced risk and benefits Examples: number of restaurants and bars adhering to nonsmoking mandates and reduced risk of secondhand smoke for customers and other businesses adopting practice; city and state buildings have reduced risk of secondhand smoke; large percentage of homes adhering to non-smoking practices and reduced risk of second hand smoke.	Health enhancement
Public Law, Policies	Mandated change in behaviors and environment	Change instituted Example: nonsmoking city ordinance passed for city and state buildings, restaurants, bars, and businesses (workplaces) resulting in reduced risk of secondhand smoke and nonsmoking behaviors adopted by community participants	Health maintenance

Source: Adapted from McKenzie, J. F., Pinger, R. R., & Koteck, J. E. (2008). *An introduction to community health.* Sudbury, MA: Jones and Bartlett Publishers; Deeds, S. F. (1992). *The health education specialist: Self-study for professional competence.* Los Alamitos, CA: Loose Canon; Cleary, J. J., & Neiger, B. L. (1998). *The certified health education specialist: A self-study guide for professional competence* (3rd ed). Allentown, PA: National Commission for Health Education Credentialing; McKenzie, J. F., Neiger, B. L., & Thackeray, R. (2009). *Planning, implementing, and evaluating health promotion programs: A primer* (5th ed.). San Francisco, CA: Benjamin Cummings.

The evaluation design is decided and the process, income, and outcome data collection techniques are defined. These techniques are the same ones listed previously for the needs assessment. Next, the budget is defined or redefined depending on the parameters. The resources, budget, and timetable need to be planned in conjunction with the strategies in a strategic plan. Again, the vision, missions, goals, objectives, needs assessments, participant population characteristics, budget, and resources are matched to these strategies and to each other. The resources need to be identified. Any in-kind contributions are factored in, as long as there is not an agenda tied to them. The budget and accrued resources will dictate what interventions or strategies are feasible for the number of participants and/or the length of time for the program. Always allow for those unexpected extras in the budget. Do not forget anything, even the small items. If not budgeted, and if a necessary part of the program, you may find that they have to be sponsored or that a fundraiser may be necessary. This means anything needed to keep the program going and to accommodate people in the program—even toilet paper—must be accounted for. Then, the budget is defined or redefined depending on the parameters. Understand the difference between cost-benefit and cost-effectiveness.[11]

A timetable is developed (scope and sequence chart), and resources are developed and sought. The **timetable plan** is then matched to all of the considerations thus far described, and job descriptions may need to be refined or reassigned. Next, the ED or SA needs to inform the participants and use communication strategies to gain support for the program. The interrelationships among activities need to be illustrated.[3,18] McBeth and Schweer suggest using an interactive planning process to show how the activities relate to the other program components and to define the scope and sequencing of the program.[18]

Charting activities is a way to visually show the interrelationships between the vision, missions, goals, objectives, needs assessments, participant population characteristics, budget, timetable, resources, solution, and intended results for a true strategic plan. These are all matched to one another so all program components relate and make sense. Charting helps the ED or SA to administrate and manage and the staff to effectively carry out the program with a clear direction and purpose. McKenzie, Neiger, and Thackeray recommend the simplest chart, called a Key Activity Chart.[11] It involves three steps: key activities (tasks), estimate of dates to be accomplished, and time allocation for each. Dignan and Carr recommend PERT (Program Evaluation and Review Techniques). Although this method is one of the most complex to use, it helps give specificity to a program.[3(p130)] A GANT chart[19] is another time line and task development chart that is user friendly and recommended by McKenzie et al. as well as the Critical Path Method.[11,20] The ED or SA administrator and planning team need to decide what type of visual mapping best fits the program. Each day of the program is specifically planned ahead of time so everything is in place and all participants, materials, equipment, and responsible staff are available for each strategic stage of the program. This must include the vision, mission, goals, objectives, responsible staff person(s), and theoretical principles addressed; the planning stage of the model, strategies, deadlines, evaluations; the budget and materials and equipment needed; the follow-up tasks, and contingency plans in the tasks.

Timetable plan: A description of how the activities relate to the other program components and the scope and sequencing of the program.

A proposed solution and manner of recording results is developed along with the evaluation plan. An evaluation determines if the goals were achieved. An evaluation plan (process, impact, and outcome) is developed based on the needs assessment, vision, mission, goals, objectives, strategies, and theory. Measurements developed in the planning process are evaluated along the way, during the program, and after the program. An evaluation is an ongoing evolving process that can be flexible when the objectives are not being accomplished because of something that can be easily changed.

A pilot program is recommended. If not used, then a preliminary review, minipilot, or field study is recommended. A process evaluation takes place during the pilot program and pretests the program plan and budget. Evaluation, changes, and improvements are done. Anything that needs further refinement is changed, including minor refinements to any of the program elements—the vision, mission, goals, budget, timetable, model, objectives, resources, strategies, theory, etc. During this portion, review the existing materials, develop and test messages (concepts), plan what materials to develop, develop the messages and materials, and pretest messages and materials for communications.[4] Plan for the production process and distribute communications. Select materials that fit the strategy, appeal to the audience, and convey the correct message. In addition, the budget needs to be reconsidered after purchasing for the pilot program, and an impact evaluation is done. Expected changes and improvements, and the timetable may need adjusting. The process evaluation that takes place during the pilot program pretests the plan. Problems defined in the needs assessment are targeted. Evaluation, changes, and improvements are done all while collecting data. Anything that needs further refinement is changed, including minor refinements to the budget, timetable, model, objectives, strategies, etc.

The policies, legislation, and communications plan must be compiled and aligned with the mission and vision statements, goals, and objectives. A program in and of itself is not a sufficient way to effect lasting change. Alignment with the mass media, policy makers, social change agents, and community leaders for the needed changes in the community is essential to avoid a one-dimensional program change that may not succeed because it has not affected the infrastructure. Essentially, the outcome should work on environmental, ecological, and public policy levels to secure the changing health environment for longevity.

4. Implement the Program

The fourth step is to implement the program. The program participants are notified, and the program is conducted by the team. Dignan and Carr (1992) recommend five phases for implementation: (1) preparing the targets for change, (2) specifying tasks and estimating resource needs, (3) developing a plan for introducing the program, (4) establishing a management system, and (5) putting the program plan into action.[5] The fifth phase depends on the first four phases. It also includes implementing and facilitating the environmental, ecological, and public policy changes. Prevention, promotion, protection, access to services, literacy maintenance, and enhancement are all factors included in this implementation phase.

The ED or SA and planning team need to develop or use prepared materials before implementation. Implementation means beginning the program. It is in this stage that the staff administers the outlined program and involves the participants. Make sure all legal concerns have been addressed, including liability, informed consent, and negligence. Addressing medical concerns, program safety, emergency care, and notification system procedures can decrease the risk of liability. Registration and record keeping, reporting, and documenting procedures need to be established ahead of time. A procedural and/or participants manual may need to be developed and distributed. Procedures for dealing with problems need to be disseminated to the program team by the ED or SA. The moral and ethical concerns and confidentiality with the program team need to be established ahead of time.[11]

Make sure the advisory committee and program team are on board with the implementation and meet regularly to discuss progress and concerns as well as the evaluation data collected. The planning timetable should be addressed daily, with progress noted. Again, job descriptions are clearly outlined ahead of time so everyone understands their responsibilities in carrying out the program. The ED or SA needs to constantly assess whether the program is being carried out ethically, efficiently, and responsibly.

The ED or SA is responsible for administering the program and solving any problems. The program is conducted by the team. To begin implementation, the program participants are notified to begin the program or for a school-based program, the students are available to begin the program instruction. The advisory committee meets on a weekly basis with the director and key staff persons for the first month and this tapers off to every two weeks and/or every month as needed. The ED or SA and staff meet daily the first few weeks and may meet weekly once the program becomes more established. The data collected and progress on the timetable plan should be available at each planning committee and staff meeting. Find a day and time in advance that the planning committee or staff committee is available to meet quickly in case of major problems.

The impact evaluation is performed during implementation. As the results are compiled, minor program changes are made based on the evaluation. Any minor revisions are done, including to the budget and timetable, as necessary. Data collection is continuous and recorded daily. Adjustments that are immediately necessary should be tackled and problems need to be solved immediately. The ED or SA ensures that the daily program is carried out, troubleshooting any problems and making any minor program refinements. As well, the program team meets weekly as needed. The ED or SA oversees the staff in recording progress and data during the implementation phase. Remember that any substantive changes need to go before the planning committee.

Implementation is the most critical part of the program. The focus of the program guides this whole process. Poorly administered and unorganized programs are usually doomed. The ED or SA needs to be on "red alert" at all times to solve problems and make sure the program runs smoothly, effectively, and efficiently. Changes necessary must be made and program glitches solved quickly.

5. Test the Program

The fifth step is to test the strengths and weaknesses of the health promotions program or program efficacy. From beginning to end, the team goes back and assesses the administration of the program (**process evaluation**) and the behavior changes of participants (**impact evaluation**). They also conduct

---

Process evaluation: An assessment of the administration of the program.
Impact evaluation: An assessment of the behavioral and other positive changes of the participants of a program.

the last test—the evaluation of the final program (**outcome evaluation**) on health-related quality of life. Indicators of success and the type and design of the evaluation are determined ahead of time. All objectives are considered, and data are collected on administrative, learning, behavioral, cultural, program, and public policy and law components.

The data collection and analyses of the program provide the facts that determine how effective the program was in achieving the goals and objectives. Look at the evaluation purpose and examine the questions that need to be answered. Examine the methodology, instrumentation, data collection process, and analysis and reporting methods.[10]

Many planners budget for data entry persons and data analyzers to assist with the huge task of recording items on a daily basis. If outside evaluators are used, their cost should be budgeted. Cleaning staff, utilities, phone service, office supplies, and other items are included in the budgetary evaluation. For schools, the coordinated school health program needs to be evaluated.

The formative and summative evaluations are necessary. These include the process, impact, and outcome evaluations. **Formative evaluation** includes information collected from the administrative or process evaluation and from the pilot program's evaluation. **Summative evaluation** includes information collected from the impact and outcome evaluations and enables conclusions and benefits of the program based on the collected information.[9] Evaluations can seem threatening, especially to employees; however, they are necessary and measure the effectiveness of the program and of the planners and implementers. The evaluation offers information about the functionality, effectiveness, and efficiency of the program and the implementers and helps make future decisions for the program. The outcome evaluation tests the feasibility of the goals and objectives and the effectiveness of the strategies in accomplishing the focus and improving quality of life for the participants. The evaluation process begins with program planning; each of the following program components should be considered: planning (the whole process), data collection, data analysis, reporting, and application.[11(pp296–297)]

The outcome evaluation not only evaluates the program, but should decide if the program staff should be rehired and if any changes not identified in the pilot program or other evaluations are needed.[3] The ED or SA is evaluated by the planning team and an outside evaluator. All employees and the planning committee are also evaluated by the outside evaluator. Program results or evaluations are the essential elements and determinations of relationships and differences. They essentially are why the program was conducted.

The outcome or final evaluation of the program should also use an inside and outside evaluator for clarity. This gives the program an unbiased view (outside evaluator) and also helps the program managers, staff, and planning committee take a good look at their own accomplishments and problems (inside evaluation). The program, managers, and staff should be evaluated along with the planning committee members by inside and outside evaluators. Changes are recommended to improve the program once it continues or is replicated.

Outcome evaluation: The final evaluation conducted; it assesses the total program results on health-related quality of life.

Formative evaluation: Evaluation that includes information collected during the process evaluation and pilot program evaluation of a program.

Summative evaluation: Evaluation that includes information collected from the impact and outcome evaluations. This collected information determines the conclusions and benefits of the program.

The planning committee assesses the committee members, ED or SA and employees. The committee is involved in employee decisions. If the committee, based on unfavorable evaluations, has decided to terminate someone, the ED or SA, assuming their evaluations were complimentary, carries out the job. Firing is never an easy task, but purging the weak spots is paramount to achieving a good program. New administrators usually have a hard time firing someone, especially if the person is the family breadwinner. Although a painful task, and one that causes an administrator to question his or her own decision making, it is a necessary part of the job. Most people who have been fired for established reasons find other employment. If they were sufficiently warned, and rules established by the governing office (such as the Office of Equal Opportunity in the United States, a school district, or other similar entities in other countries) were followed, it is not a problem. Replacing the person may take time and that also has to be considered in the decision-making process. Again, an employee manual with strict policies is important, and an employee contract is necessary so there are no legal ramifications.

A thorough program evaluation considers absolutely everything internally and externally. And yes, that even means whether there was enough toilet paper (cost, amount, etc.). The vision, missions, goals, objectives, needs assessments, budget, strategies, employees, resources, planning timetable, planning committee, and all outcomes are assessed. Resources also include where the program was conducted and all facilities. Other targets of the plan such as environmental, educational, community, and cultural factors are evaluated. The evaluation report is disseminated through the proper channels. Decisions are made, the program refined, and the whole process started again after one year if the program funding continues based on the program's feasibility and potential for replication.

Again, the main goal of evaluation is to see if the focus was achieved and the quality of life (health status) of the participants improved. According to *Healthy People 2010*, "The ultimate measure of success in any health improvement effort is the health status of the target population."[15(p1)] The quality of life must be positively affected. If the program continues the next year, goals and objectives achieved and maintained are deleted, those not achieved are carried over, and new goals and objectives are added.

If the program is continued, then program revisions take place after the program evaluation. The program team determines if the goals and objectives are appropriate or require changes or revisions or if new ones are needed. If there were objectives or strategies that did not work, determine what can be changed or what additional efforts are needed. Identify the effective program strategies. Continued and/or strengthen the successful strategies, add new ones as necessary, and decide whether to extend the participants population. Factor the cost effectiveness of the activities, and determine what continues and what might need changing or revising. Program support needs to be reestablished, and all results must be shared with the participants, stakeholders, and others involved. Evidence needs to be communicated. The last suggestion is to know when to terminate a program. This is always a difficult decision, but sometimes it is necessary if the program was not effective. Effective programs need to be continued, and a new commitment to the program is necessary by all the stakeholders and the program team.[10]

An excellent resource for using evidence-based programs for public health decision making is the CDC's *Guide to Community Preventive Services*.[21(p1)] It can assist health decision making and includes basic principles and methods of the overall process. Included are evidence-based recommendations and findings for promoting health programs in communities. It includes a broad scope of health topics, systematic reviews, methods, and assistance to identify effective strategies. There are over 200 resources to assist in program choices and policies to improve health and prevent disease in a community. Systematic reviews are used to answer questions about community health programs.[21]

School-based resources include the National Health Education Standards,[22] *Characteristics of Effective Health Education Curriculum* from the Division of Adolescent and School Health program,[23] and CDC's Health Education Curriculum Analysis Tool.[24] There are excellent resources and information on evaluation for community programs available from McDermott and Sarvela,[25] *Healthy People 2010* and *2020*,[15] *Community Tool Box: Bringing Solutions to Light*,[5] and *Making Health Communication Programs Work*.[4]

Thought Concept

Why are community health programs relevant to global health?

TOLERANCE, RESPECT, AND RESPONSIBILITY TOWARD ALL PARTICIPANTS

As always, there are three principles of human interactions that should be promoted through the program by all planners. These principles involve the treatment of the program participants and using culturally appropriate techniques in health programs. When working with diverse groups and cultures, it is imperative that participants do not feel isolated, different, or discriminated against. These three rules must guide program values and behaviors for administrators and staff. They are tolerance, respect, and responsibility.

Tolerance is an important underlying element in a health program. Even if you do not agree with individuals' lifestyles or approve of their habits, beliefs, values, or even the way they dress or look, complete tolerance for all participants must be practiced regardless of behaviors, gender, race, religions, cultural practices, or other characteristics considered different than the norm. "Victim blaming," or the attitude that participants brought a problem on themselves, is not compatible with health ethics or program goals and has no place in a program. Prejudices of any kind are not acceptable in health programs run by professional health educators. Tolerance is an important concept. We may not like or condone the way individuals behave, but we should not judge their circumstances against our own standards and expect them to act as we might in the same situation. Gender equity also falls in this spectrum. Gender inequality is pervasive and sometimes subtle. Sometimes it is not even blatantly expressed but is enmeshed in cultural, religious, and traditional beliefs. It is something that needs to be addressed very carefully with nonbiased efforts. Embedded gender inequality is difficult to overcome and can pose problems for females in supervisory and managerial positions or for participants in a program. Some programs may not be as successful because participants do not believe the person in charge is capable of conducting the program. Overcoming such prejudice requires sensitivity training and a paradigm change in the participants. If it is cultural, it needs to be addressed in the program plan. There may be a lack of tolerance for females or gender discrimination, which is unethical.

The second premise is respect. All humans deserve respect, regardless of their lifestyle, whether or not they follow the dictates of the program, whether or not they drop out, or if they simply do not want to change. Respect each person as a human being with rights and privileges and, yes, the ability to make his or her own decisions in life...whether good or bad. In other words, do not condemn anyone. Choices are personal and often based on many factors including society, family, environment, access to services, special circumstances, or other mitigating factors. These factors may or may not be controllable at points in time.

As in any other circumstance, tolerance and respect are also important when a participant decides to drop out of a program or otherwise not adhere rigidly to the program components. In school-based programs, the good news is that the student will be back for the next school year and perhaps may still change at a later date. Some people, however, may not truly wish to change their behavior, and employees need to realize that free will is important. Some people do not want to change and may never change. Additional efforts should be involved, including environmental, educational, policy, regulatory, and any other efforts that affect health. Respect is giving the proper courtesy and consideration to all program participants and recognizing that each person and circumstance is different. Change may come more easily for some than for others, but health educators must respect everyone's right to choose to participate or not. Also, sometimes extenuating circumstances may cause some not to be as successful. Individual human rights and dignity must be respected, even if a person chooses to drop out of a program or to not adhere strictly to the outlined guidelines and procedures. Efforts should continue with someone with this attitude, and tolerance and respect for different opinions must be upheld. Again, this also relates to respect for gender, religious views, lifestyle, and all other human characteristics.

The third premise is responsibility. A health educator and staff have a responsibility to carry out the program to the best of their ability, to treat participants with tolerance and respect, and to accomplish the end result. Anyone who does not buy in to and completely support the program and the participants does not belong. Employees have ownership in the program and ultimately possess the power to help the program be effective or not. Employees are accountable to the integrity of the program, and this demands they must be willing to accept 100% commitment to the goals and objectives of the program and to the program participants. Working toward those program goals and ultimately achieving the goals is dependent on the program implementers. The program depends on the employees to carry it out ethically, responsibly, and with commitment. Ultimately, the carrying out of the program and the outcome results rest in their hands. Although some program participants may not buy in to the program, the implementers are bound by ethics to continually try to engage the participants in beneficial behavior change by using the ecological approach of all possible health influences and resources, and utilizing as many health determinants as possible. A planner has a responsibility to carry out a program with efficiency, fairness, and adherence to the guidelines and objectives of the program. As such, a planner has a responsibility to the program and the profession to carry out the responsibilities and competencies for Entry, Advanced 1 and Advanced 2 health educators. These guidelines are given in **A Competency-Based Framework for Health Educators-2006**.[26,27] As well, all health educators must uphold the "Code of Ethics" for health professionals as shown in Chapter 7.[28]

A Competency-Based Framework for Health Educators-2006: The undergraduate and graduate standards of the health profession adopted by many universities and associations/organizations that outline the basic responsibilities and competencies for health educators.

A Competency-Based Framework for Graduate-Level Health Educators: The ten unique roles and services of graduate-prepared health educators adopted by many universities and associations/organizations and outline the basic responsibilities and competencies for graduate level health educators in 1999. It was replaced by the Competencies Update Project (CUP) of 2006.

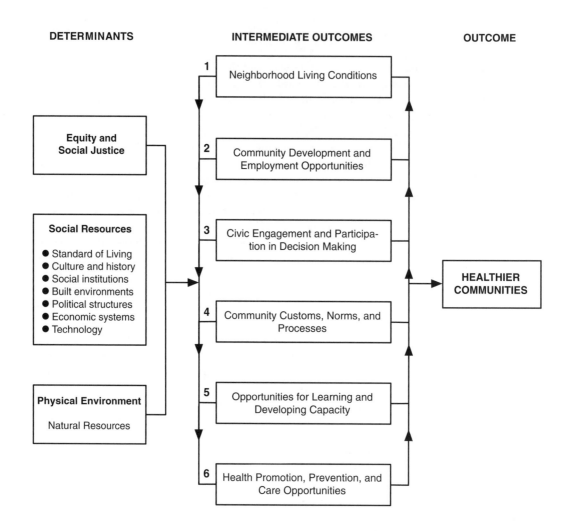

FIGURE 5–2   CDC Sociocultural Framework for Addressing Health Disparities

The CDC sociocultural framework for addressing health disparities provides an outline that embodies the tolerance, respect, and responsibility principles that health educators should embrace. It discusses the determinants including equity and social justice, social resources, and the physical environment or natural resources. Social resources include standards of living, culture (history), social institutions, built environments, politics, economy, and technology. It includes the intermediate outcomes as living conditions, development and employment, civic engagement and decision making, customs and norms, learning and capacity development, and health promotion, prevention, and care opportunities. See the CDC sociocultural framework in **Figure** 5–2.

HEALTH EDUCATORS IN GLOBAL PROGRAMS

The ultimate aim of the program is always to improve the health status of the participants, provide a higher quality of life for them and the community using all strategies and theories possible to engage the stakeholders, and institutionalize change using multiple resources and approaches across many levels of influence. Personal, social, environmental, and educational change as well as laws and policies ensure adherence. There are different types of programs available, including prevention, promotion, protection, access, literacy, and enhancement and maintenance, all of which should draw from different strategies and empirically researched theories. Programs using all types are more successful. Using a strategic planning model, with proper research and evaluation methods, increases effectiveness and utility. Thus, the end result is always better health for a higher quality of life on a local and global level.

The Coalition for National Health Organizations published "Marketing the Health Education Profession: Knowledge, Attitudes and Hiring Practices of Employers."[29] This publication defined health education and included a survey of employers. The results show that we still have a long way to go to promote the profession. The report defined what a health educator does and includes the many skills involved in carrying out global programs. This summarized many of the same skills listed in the HABIT model as performed by the health educators. The skills are:[29]

1. A health education specialist is skilled in promoting behaviors that help individuals, families, and their communities maximize and maintain the quality of their life and health.
2. A health education specialist facilitates collaboration between the individual and health service organization to address the growing demand for comprehensive public health education.
3. A health education specialist is an expert in designing and delivering evidence-based, cost-effective health education programs that really work.
4. A health education specialist incorporates the teaching–learning process to make a positive impact on individual and community health.
5. Health education specialists are best prepared to assess health education needs and the impact of health service organizations in the community.
6. Programs designed by a health education specialist effectively incorporate the teaching–learning process to change behavior and improve patient outcomes.
7. A health education specialist applies teaching techniques and behavior modification strategies to help the organization advance its public health goals.
8. A health education specialist evaluates the effectiveness of health education program, products, and services.
9. A health education specialist advocates for and implements changes in policies, procedures, rules, and regulation to advance the public's health.
10. A health education specialist partners with the clinical provider to plan, conduct, and evaluate programs designed to improve patient outcomes.

CONCLUSION

Global achievements in reducing HIV/AIDS, increasing enrollment in primary education, and reducing deaths in children under 5 years have been seen prior to 2008. While progress has been made and

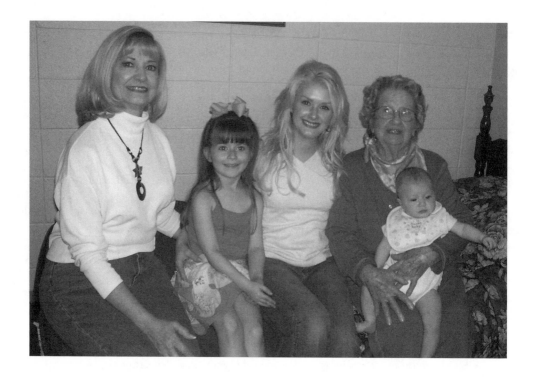

FIGURE 5–3   Family Photo   This photo of a four-generation family shows that people in developed countries are living longer, presenting new healthcare challenges for society.

poverty has been reduced in the world, a pervasive global economic slowdown and rise in prices, especially food and oil resources, is occurring as we embark toward the year 2015. The United Nations Millennium Development Goals for 2015 have a slowdown in their progression. The advances in the fight against poverty and hunger may not be realized. Government and stakeholder efforts need to be revitalized for creating productive and decent employment, eliminating disparities, reducing maternal mortality, and improving sanitation.[1] In developed nations, older adults are living longer, and this presents challenges for basic human needs, appropriate care facilities, and managed health care that promotes a high quality of life. Living longer does not always mean living better, and our older adults may need specialized care in their later years (see **Figure 5–3**).

There is still work to do and many programs to plan. Step-by-step achievements, improved results of health promotion plans, and adequate research improve health in incremental stages. This is the work of programs and the people administrating them. Success in one program is beneficial for replication and continued improvement. Little by little, effective health promotion plans carried out improve our world. We have a lot of work to do, and there will always be new challenges and new improvements in health. To that end, health educators are a vital piece of the global health puzzle. Improving, continuing, and advancing research and programs continues and emerges as the primary reason that health educators practice.

Global programs are where health educators need to revitalize their efforts. Sharing information, programs, and effective health promotion efforts is needed. We live in a society in which gradually diminishing borders, rampant technology advances, informative mass media sources, and Internet access worldwide have all changed the way that health educators practice. We need to embrace the new technologies and access and use them as tools in educating and promoting health. Community programs and school-based programs with successful strategic plans need to share and replicate with others across the globe. Programs that begin in school settings have the potential of affecting lives for many years to come as long as the student is enrolled. Changing to healthier communities can have a diffusion effect on other communities. Working together and supportive efforts can achieve more than single health programs on their own. Global access to effective programs, global sharing, and global coalitions are necessary. Global efforts exist, but many more are needed.

SUMMARY

- Strategic written plans are always smart ways to function in a society and measure success; these are sometimes called action plans.
- Proper planning is important to determine a program focus, understand the health issue, determine communication roles, identify strategies for the preferred changes, establish a development process, create a plan that supports measurable objectives, determine a budget, set program priorities, assign all responsibilities, and continuously evaluate progress.
- Best practices are viewed as a process of careful, evidence-based planning that enables planners to tailor strategies and methods to the unique circumstances of a given place or population. The HABIT model provides a strategic framework for program development.
  - Step 1 is to hire the program team, including the program manager(s) and staff. The director assembles, interviews, and hires program staff as needed. Job descriptions are defined, staff budget is developed, and community leaders and program participants are assembled.
  - Step 2 is to perform a needs assessment to determine the program needs using quantitative and qualitative data diagnoses. Epidemiological, ecological, environmental, educational, health, and cultural data are assessed. The predisposing, reinforcing, and enabling cultural and behavioral factors are identified. The administrative tasks, organizational plan, and policies are developed. The major problem(s) is identified, and the participant population is defined. The rationale is redefined, the benefits and values are listed, and the advisory/steering committee is chosen.
  - Step 3 includes planning the program. The vision and mission statements, goals, objectives, theory, and strategies are all identified and matched to each other as specified by the participant population. The budget, timetable, resources, proposed solutions, and anticipated results are outlined. The process, impact, and outcome evaluation plans are designed. The pilot program pretests the program, and changes are implemented.
  - Step 4 is program implementation. Program participants are notified and the program is conducted. Data collection begins and the impact evaluation determines modification.

○ Step 5 is the final evaluation. The outcome evaluation evaluates the program and the program team. Improvements are recommended for program replication or continuation. All program staff members are also evaluated.

CONCEPTUAL TERMS

Program plan
Multiple interventions
Multiple levels
Empirical review
HABIT model
Best practices
Evidence-based planning
Human subjects review boards
Predisposing factors
Reinforcing factors
Enabling factors
Global problems
Rationale
Primary data collection techniques
Secondary data collection techniques
Quantitative assessment techniques
Qualitative assessment techniques

Health program strategic plan
Vision statement
Mission statement
Goal
Objectives
Types of objectives: process, learning, behavioral, program or community, and environmental
Timetable plan
Process evaluation
Impact evaluation
Outcome evaluation
Formative evaluation
Summative evaluation
A Competency-Based Framework for Health Educators
A Competency-Based Framework for Graduate-Level Health Educators

REFLECTIVE THINKING

You are a program director working in a community agency with a focus on improving parenting skills of single parents. Your job when you were hired was to work on improving nutrition levels in the children and parents with a food plan utilizing a prepared program with all of the components supplied. The agency recently acquired a grant for promoting physical activity for the preschool children enrolled in the program. Your executive director just told you that you are in charge of the new program and someone else will take over the nutrition program. Your responsibilities are to train the teachers working with the groups of children and parents to promote activities at the program site and to train the parents in physical activities to perform at home with their children. You have limited experience working with preschool children and even less experience working with physical activity programs. What do you tell your supervisor? Do you ask to be removed from the program? Do you decide to do the best job you can? What other options do you have? Should you resign? What is your best option if you decide to stay?

CONCEPTUAL LEARNING

1. Summarize the basic components of a strategic written plan.
2. Define and contrast a health program and a program planning model.

3. Construct a concept map showing the areas of the HABIT model.

4. Identify and examine the skills needed for an executive director or coordinator of a health promotion program.

5. Compare each phase of the HABIT model. List all of the processes involved in each step, and summarize the purpose of each step.

6. Research a journal article using a health program planning model and theory. Determine the model, theories, and strategies used, and compare the differences and similarities to the HABIT model.

REFERENCES

1. United Nations. (2008). *The Millennium Development Goals Report 2008*. Retrieved July 25, 2009, from http://www.un.org/millenniumgoals/

2. Basch, P. F. (1990). *Textbook of international health*. New York: Oxford University Press.

3. Dignan, M. B., & Carr, P. A. (1992). *Program planning for health education and promotion*. Philadelphia: Lea and Febiger.

4. National Cancer Institute. (2001). *Making health communication programs work* (revised ed.). Washington, DC: U.S. Department of Health and Human Services.

5. Kansas University Work Group on Health Promotion and Community Development. (2005). *Community Tool Box: Bringing solutions to light*. Lawrence, KS: University of Kansas. Retrieved February 26, 2010, from http://ctb.ku.edu/

6. Glanz, K., Rimer, B. K., & Viswanath, K. (2008). *Health behavior and health education: Theory, research, and practice* (4th ed.). San Francisco: Jossey Bass.

7. Breckon, D. J., Harvey, J. R., & Lancaster, R. B. (1998). *Community health education: Settings, roles, and skills for the 21st Century* (4th ed.). Gaithersburg, MD: Aspen.

8. Green, L. W., & Kreuter, M. W. (2005). *Health program planning: An educational and ecological approach* (4th ed.). Boston: McGraw-Hill.

9. McLeroy, M. W., Bibeau, D., Steckler, A., & Glanz, K. (1988). An ecological perspective on health promotion programs. *Health Education Quarterly*, *15*, 351–377.

10. Hayden, J. (Ed.) (2000). *The health education specialist: A study guide for professional competence* (4th ed., revised from S. Deeds, 1999). Whitehall, PA: The National Commission for Health Education Credentialing, Inc.

11. McKenzie, J. F., Neiger, B. L., & Thackeray, R. (2008). *Planning, implementing, and evaluating health promotion programs* (5th ed.). San Francisco: Pearson Benjamin Cummings.

12. Geisinger, K. F., Spies, R. A., Carlson, J. F., & Plake, B. S. (Eds.) (2007). *The seventeenth mental measurements yearbook*. Lincoln, NE: Buros Institute at the University of Nebraska Press.

13. Hyner, G. C., Peterson, K. W., Travis, J. W., Dewey, J. E., Forester, J. J., & Framer, E. M. (1999). *SPM handbook of health assessment tools*. Pittsburgh, PA: The Society of Prospective Medicine, The Institute for Health and Productivity Management.

14. Robert, H. M., Evans, W. J., Honemann, D. H., & Belch, T. (2000). *Robert's rules of order, newly revised* (10th ed.). Cambridge, MA: Da Capo Press (Perseus Publishing).

15. United States Department of Health and Human Services. Office of Disease Prevention and Health Promotion. (2000). *Healthy people 2010* (2nd ed.). Retrieved February 26, 2010, from http://www.healthypeople.gov/default.htm

16. Simons-Morton, B. G., Greene, W. H., & Gottlieb, N. H. (1995). *Introduction to health education and health promotion*. Prospect Heights, IL: Waveland.

17. Doyle, E., & Ward, S. (2001). *The process of community health education and promotion*. Mountain View, CA: Mayfield Publishing.

18. McBeth, A. J., & Schweer, K. D. (2000). *Building healthy communities: The challenge of health care in the twenty first century*. Boston: Allyn & Bacon.

19. Timmreck, T. C. (2003). *Planning, program development, and evaluation*. Sudbury, MA: Jones and Bartlett Publishers.
20. Modell, M. E. (1996). *A professional's guide to system analysis* (2nd ed.). Boston: McGraw-Hill.
21. Centers for Disease Control and Prevention. (2009). *Community preventive services. The community guide: What works to promote health*. Atlanta, GA: National Center for Health Marketing.
22. The Joint Committee on National Health Education Standards. (2007). *National health education standards: Achieving excellence* (2nd ed.). Atlanta, GA: American Cancer Society.
23. Centers for Disease Control and Prevention. (2007). *Healthy youth and characteristics of effective health education curricula*. Retrieved February 26, 2010, from http://www.cdc.gov/HealthyYouth/index.htm
24. Centers for Disease Control and Prevention. (2009). *Health education curriculum analysis tool (HECAT) index*. Retrieved February 26, 2010, from http://www.cdc.gov/HealthyYouth/HECAT/index.htm
25. McDermott, R. J., & Sarvela, P. D. (1999). *Health education, evaluation, and measurement, a practitioner's perspective* (2nd ed.). Boston: McGraw-Hill.
26. National Commission for Health Education Credentialing (NCHEC), Society for Public Health Educators (SOPHE), American Association for Health Education (AAHE). (2006). *A competency-based framework for health educators-2006*. Whitehall, PA: National Commission for Health Education Credentialing, Inc.
27. American Association for Health Education, National Commission for Health Education Credentialing, Inc., & the Society for Public Health Educators. (1999). *A competency-based framework for graduate-level health educators*. Reston, VA: Authors.
28. Coalition of National Health Education Organizations. (1999). *Code of ethics for the health education profession*. Retrieved February 26, 2010, from http://www.cnheo.org/
29. Hezel Associates. (2007, July). *Marketing the health education profession: Knowledge, attitudes and hiring practices of employers*. A study commissioned by the Coalition of National Health Education Organizations, American Association for Health Education, National Commission for Health Education Credentialing, Society for Public Health Education, American College Health Association, Eta Sigma Gamma. Retrieved February 26, 2010, from http://www.cnheo.org

ENHANCED READINGS

Kansas University Work Group on Health Promotion and Community Development. (2005). *Community Tool Box: Bringing solutions to light*. Lawrence, KS: University of Kansas. Available at: http://ctb.ku.edu/en/tablecontents/
See:

Part D: Developing a Strategic Plan, Organizational Structure, and Training System (Chapters 8–12)

National Cancer Institute and National Institutes of Health. (2004, August). *Pink Book: Making health communication programs work: A planner's guide*. Washington, DC: Department of Health and Human Services. Available at: http://cancer.gov/pinkbook
See:

The Stages of the Health Communication Process (Stages 1–4)

Sciaccca, J., Dennis, D. L., & Black, D. R. (2004). Are interventions for informed, efficacious, precontemplators unethical? *American Journal of Health Education*, 35(6), 322–327.

RELEVANT WEB SITES

National Center for Chronic Disease Prevention and Health Promotion. (2009). *School Health Index*. Healthy Youth. Available at: http://www.cdc.gov/nccdphp/dash/SHI/

The University of Texas, Health Science Center at Houston. (2010). *Intervention mapping.* Available at: http://www
.sph.uth.tmc.edu/chppr/interventionmapping/

World Health Organization. (2010). *Global campaign for violence prevention.* Available at: http://www.who.int/
violence_injury_prevention/violence/global_campaign/en/index.html

World Health Organization. (2010). *Health topics.* Available at: http://www.who.int/topics/en/ (This page offers
links to projects, initiatives, activities, information, and contacts, organized by health and development
topics.)

CHAPTER 6

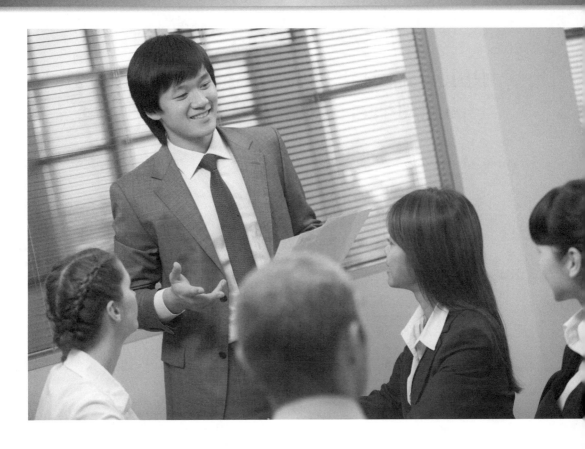

Philosophical Reflections on Health and Health Practices

OBJECTIVES AND ASSESSMENTS

This chapter meets the following National Commission for Health Education Credentialing, Inc., Society for Public Health Education, and American Association for Health Education Competency-Based Framework for Entry Level and Advanced Level Health Educator Competencies.* The learner will:

6. Serve as a health education resource person.
7. Communicate and advocate for health and health education.

This chapter meets the following learning objectives. The learner will:

1. Identify and comprehend basic health education philosophies.
2. Explain how philosophy is conceptual rather than factual.
3. Construct a definition of philosophy using the information in the book.
4. Examine John Dewey's struggles with morality and ethical philosophies.
5. Summarize philosophers contemplating moral issues of goodness and truth.
6. Compare and contrast the four types of philosophies.
7. Describe each philosophy examined in the chapter for deriving a personal health philosophy.
8. Discuss why students of health and health educators need to determine a personal health philosophy but must back it up with reputable sources.
9. Relate and analyze three examples of how health philosophies can change through the years.

Source: Reprinted with permission of NCHEC.

    National Commission for Health Education Credentialing, Inc. (NCHEC), Society for Public Health Education (SOPHE), & American Association for Health Education (AAHE). (2006). *A competency-based framework for health educators-2006*. Whitehall, PA: NCHEC.

INTRODUCTION

Philosophy comes from the Greek words *philein*, meaning to love, and *sophia*, meaning love of wisdom.[1(p1)] *The New Concise Webster's Dictionary* defines it as "the study of life and what it means, how we should live, etc."[2(p214)] *Webster's Online Dictionary* states that the work of philosophers is to "generally frame problems in a logical manner then work towards a solution based on logical processes and reasoning, based on a critical reading and response to previous work in this area."[1(p1)]

FORMULATING A PHILOSOPHY

A health education philosophy needs to be formulated (see **Figure 6–1**). To begin a health philosophy, examine health problems carefully based on all known facts, and proceed logically to solve them. The next step is to defend the solution(s) and engage in literal processes to ascertain the truth. The scientific method involves all of these processes and does not depend on just physical experimentation. The scientific method progresses from observation, formulation of a hypothesis, and further experimentation. Philosophy proceeds logically from formulating, reasoning, and arguing the solutions and then counter-arguing. This process continues until a final solution is found.[1] If the problem is solved, a new philosophy or an update, alterion, or addition to a philosophy may be necessary.

Philosophy determines health problems and includes cultural problems. It concerns human relationships and the patterns established by these relationships. Deciphering the relationships and patterns and finding ways to focus on healthful changes that are reasonable are required to formulate the philosophy. The task of a philosophy is to get beyond the status quo and construct a paradigm change. All factors that affect health and all patterns that need changing should be considered. Look at the global health problems, including lack of access to basic health services and basic human needs such as food, clothing, and shelter. Humankind has tried to change these problems for many years, and some efforts have been successful. It is with forethought, observation, experiences, and contemplative thinking that health philosophies are born. Not all philosophies come to fruition, but as professionals, we must continually contemplate philosophical advances and pursue the improved health of society. Philosophy examines practical problems from a broader domain.

MaGill and McGreal state that a philosophy is a "broadening of the base of understanding of those truths by which men ought to live" and specifically acts as a key to understanding all people. Philosophers attempt to provide adequate reasons and justifications for their beliefs or clarify and examine the basis for the beliefs.[3(pxiii)] Archie and Archie write, "Philosophy is an investigation of the fundamental questions of human existence. Such questions include wondering about such things as the meaning of life, what kinds of things the universe is made of, whether there can be a theory of everything, how we can know what's the right thing to do, and what is the beautiful in life and art."[4(p5)]

Philosophy is an examination that a person undertakes to arrive at the true meaning of life as he or she sees it. The study of philosophy works with concepts and can include facts, while the activity of

---

Philosophy: A logical reasoning and solution about the meaning and importance of life and actions to promote it.

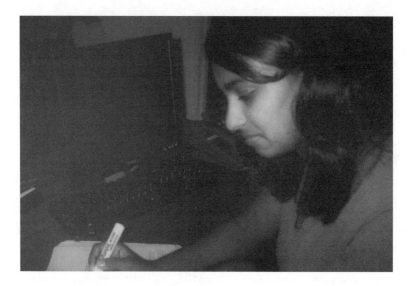

Figure 6–1   Student Studying   Health students should begin formulating a health philosophy and update it periodically.

philosophy seeks understanding rather than knowledge. The reasoning process is important in the study of philosophy.[4] Axioms are general principles of philosophy. They help to reason from general statements to logical, specific conclusions and propositions; this process is referred to as deduction. In contrast, observation and examination of the facts may lead to a general conclusion in a process known as induction.[3] The goal is realizing what the right thing to do is for the health of all persons. According to the *Stanford Encyclopedia of Philosophy*, a **constructivist** view of philosophy is thinking in terms of health, disease, and normality.[5(p1)]

Philosophers of science have largely relied on the knowledge of their field of study to draw hypothetical conclusions. These conclusions are based on the state of scientific concepts and the nature of conceptual change in science. The new philosophy of inquiry is a prevalent one used by scientists and philosophers. Quantitative evidence is necessary for this philosophy, but it has benefits. Experimental philosophy includes tools and encourages two-way interactions between the scientists and philosophers.[6]

Constructivist: A philosophy that concerns the formulation of knowledge; a learning premise used mainly in the educational setting.

This concept of hypothetical conclusions based on fact is definitely related to health. The health field is still finding new ways to improve the health of populations based on factual, empirically-based research.

Reflective thinking is necessary for formulating a philosophy of any kind. It also requires the scrutiny of knowledge from various perspectives.[7] An idea, once formulated, needs to be expanded, picked apart, dissected, and evaluated by any and every means possible. Then, discussion and questions about the true part or parts of the philosophy need to be initiated. Rethinking the solutions and reexamining the meaning of the philosophy is performed. Finally, a consensus can be reached.

Many different types of philosophies embrace health education. Altruism is volunteerism and acting for the good of all concerned. It involves analytical statements that something must be true because of the meaning of the terms used.[3] A concept is an idea or thought process. Humanism embraces the centrality of man. Inference is the process of reasoning from one idea or ideas—termed the premise—to a logical relationship or conclusion.

Stoicism endorses a life of virtue. It includes action and endurance in arduous times. This philosophy seems to embody the life of Mother Teresa. She administered to the sick and needy her entire life and lived a modest, unselfish, and difficult life. Her life was devoted to ministering to the less fortunate. Her philosophy was that every life is important and deserves care. Active devotion, caring, empathy, and nonjudgmental and nonprejudicial actions cause effective change. It is not enough to empathize with a group; action truly does speak louder than words in the case of the less fortunate. She embodied an unselfish and dedicated lifestyle and truly saw a lot of suffering and many deaths, but she never gave up[8] (see **Figure 6–2**).

Philosophies are formed, causal action ensues, and the result is, hopefully, change for the better. So, what happens once the change has taken place? The philosopher must always be open to change, new ideas, and new technologies and discoveries that may produce debate and reconciliation. If a problem is solved, new issues or problems emerge. In some cases, the greater problems are attacked first. If they are solved, then the lesser problems can be the new focus.

A philosophy is never a blanket statement for all times. It is a statement that can be modified, transformed, amended, and even revolutionized through time. Though some philosophies seem timeless, even they may someday become irrelevant or need new adjustments and alterations. The profession of health education is ever-changing, and health educators must be ready to adjust their stance and embrace new philosophies, technologies, theories, strategies, and ways of practice.

Career Concept

Do you enjoy writing and being a detective looking for clues? You may want to consider becoming a health journalist.

PROMINENT PHILOSOPHERS THROUGH THE AGES

Early Philosophies

The following philosophies were selected from many different types because their principles align with some existing health philosophies. This is not an exhaustive effort, but an effort to present major philosophies whose concepts could possibly relate to and/or influence health philosophies. An examination

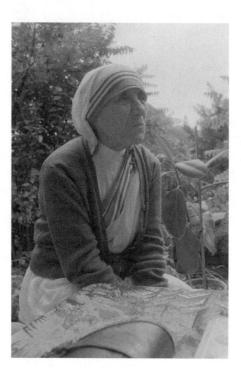

Figure 6–2   Mother Teresa

of other philosophies can help spark a realization for you and can influence how you decide to formulate your own health philosophy.

Aristotle's philosophy of change was based on four kinds of causes: material cause, formal cause, final cause, and efficient cause. The material cause is that out of which something is created. Formal cause is the plan or idea out of which that something is created. Final cause is the purpose for which something is made. Efficient cause is the event producing the result. This philosophy, in the literal sense, is not unlike what happens in a health program. The cause is determined, a plan or idea is created, the plan becomes implemented as a program, and hopefully the result is what was originally conceived.[3]

Confucius (see **Figure 6–3**), in the late 6th or early 5th century BC, proposed *jên* as the ideal relationship among humans; thus it is the perfect virtue of persons. A person's actions are controlled by the propriety rules. The ideal person practices *jên* and seeks the right way in life according to this philosophy.[3(p5)] Heraclitus rationalized that all things are one, but the profound statement was that a person's character determines, inevitably, his or her destiny.[3(pp12,15)]

René Descartes in 1637 stated that the philosophical method is not to accept an idea clearly beyond doubt as truth. The process is to divide complex questions into simpler basic questions, to proceed from simple to complex, and to review all steps to make sure there are no inconsistencies.[3(p380)]

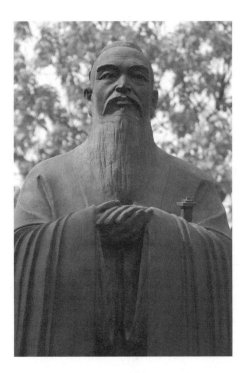

Figure 6–3   Confucius   Confucius said that *jên* is the ideal relationship among humans.

John Stuart Mill's essay on liberty in the 1800s declared that individual liberty should be constrained only when a person commits harm to others. He would probably be called a "liberal" today. The philosophy he advanced is referred to as **utilitarianism**.[3(p664)]

Later Philosophies

John Dewey in 1922 published a philosophy of human nature and conflict on morality and ethics. He proposed that good and bad virtues developed during interactions of humans and the social environment.[3(p835)] **Pragmatism**, based on Dewey's philosophy, is concerned with humanity, social adjustment, and improving the goals of life.[9] **Existentialism** is an extension of pragmatism and addresses psychology and human conditions, including human emotions. Ernst Cassirer (1874–1945)

Utilitarianism: A philosophy advanced by John Stuart Mill concerning individual civil liberties that should not be impeded unless the individual causes extreme harm to another person.
Pragmatism: A philosophy about humanity and social justice.
Existentialism: An extension of the pragmatist philosophy; it is about emotions and humanism.

affirmed that the mind interprets experience through symbols. The cognitive forms are affected by language and myth. These, in cooperation with science, are forms of human expression. As humans respond with their needs, items in that experience then become symbolic to them.[9]

William David Ross a **formalist**, in 1930, insisted that right, duty, and obligations are concepts that are not explained in terms of "goodness" but use intellectual intuition. He further explained that conflicts of moral principles are explained only under particular circumstances.[3(p929)] Jacques Maritain in 1932 proposed that man has several kinds of knowledge, including sensation, reasons, revelation, and mystical union.[3(p964)]

Knowledge, morality, righteousness, character, truth, liberty, humanity, ethics, and cognition are common philosophical threads that weave through health philosophies espoused today. A study of philosophy through the ages reveals that many early philosophers were seeking righteousness and truth. These concepts still exist today. Some are still valid and bear understanding. Others need adjustment, a different twist, or they need to be combined with other philosophies instead of being viewed as a single, narrowly focused philosophy.

TYPES OF PHILOSOPHIES

Scientific methods in philosophy concern the ability to know and use science, logic, and math. Today, the philosophers tend to turn away from traditional philosophies, looking more toward practical principles and views of humankind and adjusting to the changing world. Major philosophers addressed many of the central problems in the history of human thought.[7] Health philosophers used and developed basic strategies to reflect their philosophical tenets.[10(p11)]

Most disciplines are represented by the many different types of philosophies, since there are major philosophies about science, education, religion, and government. There are different philosophies within each of these disciplines. Philosophers study each philosophy based on four basic criteria: **logic, epistemology, metaphysics,** and **axiology**.[3]

Logic involves using scientific methods. This embodies the health program using science and research as the programmatic focus. Epistemology is the study of knowledge and is based on observing what we know. Evidence-based practice using goals, objectives, strategies, and evaluation helps determine the most effective program solutions for the different types of problems. Epistemology and logic include literacy, prevention, and promotion, which involve the realities of disease, disease transmission,

---

Formalist: A philosophy of concepts that are explained in terms of intellectual intuition concerning rights, duties, and obligations.

Logic: One of the four criteria of philosophies; it involves the use of scientific methods and research as the programmatic focus.

Epistemology: One of the four criteria of philosophies; known as the study of knowledge, it is based on observation of the known and uses evidence-based practice for determining the most effective solutions to problems.

Metaphysics: One of the four criteria of philosophy; called ontology, it includes the study of reality and change.

Axiology: One of the four criteria of philosophy; it works with goodness and studies values, ethics, and aesthetics.

treatment, and recovery. Metaphysics, or ontology, is the study of reality and how change occurs in the world. Metaphysics includes health access to resources and health maintenance. Measurement and evaluation document the change occurring in programs. Axiology deals with the nature of good and is the study of value, including ethics and aesthetics.[3,4] The pursuit of ethics and aesthetics as in axiology is paramount to the health philosophies of protection and enhancement. A higher quality of life is the goal of any health program and should always be used as the focal pursuit.

The constructivist philosophy according to von Glasersfeld is basically a theory of knowledge.[11] The roots are in philosophy and psychology. It is sometimes called a theory from knowledge to practice. A constructivist concept might be operationalized in an instructional setting. The basic meaning of the constructivist philosophy is to construct knowledge. It is a learning theory used by educators. Some concepts of constructivism are student-directed goals, problem solving, conceptual interrelatedness, authentic assessment, teachers as facilitators, and metacognition. How people, especially students, learn is a concept that most educators embrace. Rather than providing a specific methodology or pedagogy, constructivism offers a way of constructing learning strategies that impact cognition and understanding.[11]

The pragmatist/existentialist philosophy does not rely on exact sciences but rather on perceptions, feelings, and human kindness.[3] Today's philosophers, including health philosophers, seem to have moved beyond scientific-based facts to include humanism with emotions. While we still need science and proven facts, valuing and respecting humans are essential to health education practice.

GLOBAL PHILOSOPHIES OF UNIVERSITY DEPARTMENTS OF HEALTH

Many universities have a philosophy of training and study within the departments of health promotion, public health, or community health, or other similar titles. Students may not realize there is a philosophy regarding their training and education as health professionals. Universities involved in training health educators and professionals ground their efforts in research and experiences within the departments. The courses should follow the undergraduate and graduate competencies provided by the profession (see Chapter 7).

Commonalities in course content among different departments in different countries emerged from a recent investigation. A global Internet survey by WHO examined the philosophies of the nature and extent of health promotion education and training. The 43 responses were mainly from within the European region.[12]

Common themes emerged from the respondents. The principles used in the Ottawa Charter[13] and interdisciplinary learning were prevalent in the research results. Colleagues from around the world responded to questions regarding their course content and delivery. The European models described a philosophy of imparting relevant basic skills, critical evaluation techniques, and an appreciation of factors affecting health, healthcare delivery, and health policy formulation. The University of Toronto graduate department emphasized the social determinants of health. This university stated it held a strong social science philosophy in health and health promotion. Texas Woman's University's philosophy is to prepare health education specialists with the knowledge, skills, and confidence to assist achievement of self-elected health goals. San Diego State University's philosophy is grounded in behavior modification applications to community health promotion and a strong research base.[12]

The meanings of the survey and interpretation of the results are dependent on a short response time and small response rate. Although level of training, such as undergraduate or graduate work, had different meanings, there were patterns. Five different approaches emerged: medical, social, behavioral, environmental, and educational. There was an agreement regarding the philosophical roots of training programs for health promotion. The themes were "a commitment to interdisciplinary teaching and learning, development of skills and knowledges associated with the new public health, and the principles of the Ottawa Charter."[12(p306)] Despite differences in organization and training levels, some continuity in the approach and **philosophy** to the educational programs across the globe were found. The future for the 21st century for health promotion training seems to be in consensus across borders of the globe. So, the educational background of students is based on philosophical premises determined by their university department.

OTTAWA CHARTER

The Ottawa Charter was an international initiative to achieve health for all by the year 2000. The concept is important to mention in developing a philosophy because it was built on a global concept and global efforts that transcend countries, communities, and municipalities. The conference was facilitated by a new movement to improve public health around the globe. It began with defining health promotion as a way for people to increase, improve, and control their own health. It advocated for mental, physical, and social well-being by identifying aspirations, fulfilling needs, and changing or coping with environments. It emphasized personal and social resources and went from a concept of healthy lifestyle to one of well-being.[12]

The Ottawa Charter asserted that improvements in health require a firm foundation, with the prerequisites of peace, shelter, education, food, income, stable ecosystem, sustainable resources, social justice, and equity. It promoted the global premise that health educators need to advocate, enable, mediate, and endorse health promotion action means; secure a commitment to health promotion; and call for international action.[12]

The objectives behind health promotion action means included (1) building healthy public health policy, (2) creating supportive environments, (3) strengthening community action, (4) developing personal skills, (5) reorienting health services, and (6) moving into the future. Moving into the future involved holism, caring, and ecology strategies as guiding principles in health promotion. The charter ended with a call for international action to join forces in supporting health-promoting strategies in line with the moral and social values advocated in the charter. This document is worth reading because it was a global effort by WHO and international health agencies to improve the health of the globe and support strategies and programs within and across the world.[12]

SAMPLE PHILOSOPHY ON AGING

C. Everett Koop, former U.S. Surgeon General, presented a philosophy of aging in 1982 that many health educators still embrace today. This was a classic article on spirituality and the connection to

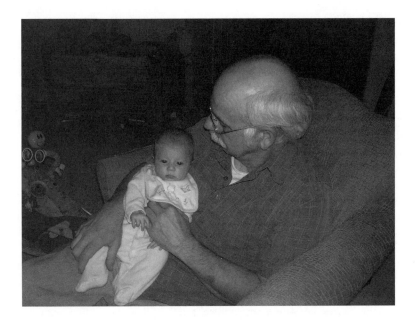

Figure 6–4   Older Man and Baby   A spiritual philosophy is endorsed for older adults.

health. His philosophy included physical, mental, and spiritual health. This philosophy included the basic necessities in life as well as the esoteric philosophy of spirituality, less endorsed by the medical profession at the time. This approach is also endorsed by hospice care, stress management specialists, and many medical associations today. Health educators can promote this philosophy to help people cope with and endure everyday health afflictions and diseases. Difficult decisions about aging, overcoming the barriers to aging, and the terminal nature of the aging process have to be considered. A new way of looking at this is through spiritual health. Spirituality is a concept in health that has produced results not only in the area of aging, but in holistic health areas too (see **Figure 6–4**).[14]

HEALTH PHILOSOPHICAL ROOTS

The *Stanford Encyclopedia of Philosophy* states, "Health and disease are critical concepts in bioethics with far-reaching social and political implications." It further elaborates that, "the concepts of health and disease connect with philosophical issues about function and explanation of the biomedical sciences, and theories of ethical well-being." These two must work together in harmony.[5(p1)]

Thinking clearly and rationally and looking to the future are necessary to develop a philosophy of health. A forward-thinking philosophy is a foundation and involves attitudes, values, behaviors, and true perceptions. It is a framework with goals and truth seeking. A basic philosophy of health should involve a unified view and help make a person a more critical thinker. This effort requires understanding the processes of health and what works, what might be initiated and successful, and what is valued, important, and prized. While individual opinion is valued in a philosophy of health, it should be backed up by empirical research. In most cases, several philosophical concepts will be included.

Smith in 2006 described several health philosophical tenets, including the **holistic** approach, empowerment, **behavior change/modification**, and lifestyle changes.[10] O'Rourke listed five tenets, including the micro-perspective (behavior change), trilogy (behavior change and health improvement through individual responsibility and personal behaviors), macro-perspective, the **functional/utilitarian philosophy**, and the **egalitarian philosophy**. O'Rourke, however, does not endorse the first two approaches listed.[15]

Cottrell, Girvan, and McKenzie cited five predominant health philosophies, including behavior change, cognitive-based philosophy, decision-making philosophy, freeing/functioning philosophy, and the social change philosophy.[16(pp86-87)] The authors based their opinions on a 1995 study by Welle, Russell, and Kittleson.

Organizing these lists of philosophies by professionals into similar categories produced the following health education philosophies to examine for this chapter: holistic, empowerment, behavior change/modification, **cognitive-based and healthy decision making**, changing attitudes, macro-perspective, universal philosophy, functional/utilitarian, and egalitarian philosophy. While many of these philosophies overlap, they are presented as evidence of different viewpoints among health professionals. No judgments are given; each is presented as a different type promoted by different health educators. Also, no philosophy is self-inclusive. Like theory and program models, you can integrate and merge philosophies to develop your own. Multilevel, integrative philosophies are recommended.

Holistic Philosophy

This philosophy asserts that the physical, mental, spiritual, emotional, and social components all influence our well-being. It was in defining these concepts that measurements were enacted to compress the

---

Holistic: Relating to the physical, mental, spiritual, emotional, and social components that influence human well-being.

Empowerment philosophy: This is a philosophy of enablement or shared power where groups/communities are given the skills and knowledge to continue positive change on their own.

Behavior change/modification: A philosophy that concerns individual modification of habits, but can include group/community changes.

Functional/utilitarian philosophy: A philosophy concerned with the change to a productive infrastructure in communities that leads to better and healthier lives.

Egalitarian philosophy: A philosophy that involves cooperation and support to change society's infrastructure for the betterment of all.

Cognitive-based and healthy decision making: A philosophy that espouses increasing the knowledge base and skills of individuals so they can make wise choices and decisions in life.

language used to define the various functioning of humans.[10] Greenberg felt that an all-encompassing definition with all outside influences on health included was a more universal expression of the daily aspects in our lives that affect our health.[17]

Empowerment Philosophy

Empowerment is a community theory, but it is also a community philosophy, thus empowerment works in both realms. Wallenstein and Bernstein in 1988 suggested that Frere's empowerment education theory could be adapted to health education.[18] Hinkler, Thompson, Bell, and Rose in 2002 used community involvement to bring about organizational-level empowerment in "The Federal Healthy Start Experience."[19]

Tai-Seale in 2001 stated that health educators should use the premise of assumed empowerment. The author advocates that health educators should enable or assist others to empower themselves. The basic foundation for building community-assumed empowerment includes shared residence and general interest, shared specific interest, and shared specific problem. According to Tai-Seale:

> This can be facilitated by (1) assembling those with a shared problem, (2) establishing the goal of assumed empowerment, (3) making clear how the health promoter may assist those assembled, and (4) facilitating (not dominating) collective discussion, decision making, and group action by promoting internal leadership, affinity, and skill building.[20(p28)]

Community/organizational empowerment is a way of reaching more changes through community efforts, rather than just individual behavior change, according to Hinkler and Wallerstein.[19]

Behavior Change/Modification Philosophy

The behavior change method has included everything from reward and punishment, or behavior modification, to aversion therapy.[10] It involves using contracts, goals setting, and self-monitoring to modify or change an unhealthy habit. Many theoretical concepts, such as those of McGuire in 1984, espouse individual and interpersonal behavior change/modification.[21] Prochaska and Velicer in 1997 supported behavior change using public communication and the transtheoretical model.[22] O'Rourke in 2006 advocated a microbehavioral change philosophy focused on individual responsibility.[15] Healthy behavior and lifestyle coupled with individual responsibility and collective responsibility created what he called the trilogy. The author felt the focus on health improvement through individual responsibility and personal behavior focusing on the leading causes of death could possibly lead to victim blaming.[15(p8)]

Change Individual Attitudes in About Lifestyle Factors Philosophy

Ajzen and Fishbein in 1980 promoted the idea of behavioral intention.[23] While behavior change and modification are similar to this idea, they can be precipitated by illness, and a person may feel they have to change to live longer. The target audience's decision to adopt a desired behavior is predicted by assessing the attitudes and perceptions of the benefits of the behavior. How audience members think their peers view the behavior is another factor. The idea is to change or influence these factors so the audience adopts the desired behavior.

Cognitive-Based and Healthy Decision Making Philosophy

This philosophy relies on the acquisition of credible content and the attainment of skills. The idea is to increase the knowledge base of individuals, as in health education in the public schools, so persons have the necessary information to make decisions. As an American Association of Health Education position statement, "Philosophy of Health Education," asserted, "The ultimate goal of health education is to enable individuals to use knowledge in ways that transform unhealthy habits into healthy habits."[24(p1)] It further stated that health education helps the learner utilize knowledge in making wise decisions and choices that encourage experimentation and evaluation throughout life. This gives the learner the skills to decipher messages in terms of their potential benefit to self and society as well.

Macro-perspective Philosophy

O'Rourke in 2006 defined the macro-perspective as encompassing collective responsibility and community involvement through participation and process and service on board.[15] Collective "leverage" indicated how the goal can be achieved, promoting healthy people and healthy communities by collective action. This can influence health in entire communities,[25] which is what most people feel was accomplished by the Healthy People initiative of 2000.[26] O'Rourke, however, suggested that this initiative did not really accomplish collective efforts, calling it the "trilogy."[15]

Functional/Utilitarian Philosophy

According to O'Rourke in 2006, the functional/utilitarian philosophy "views health education/ promotion as a means to an end (a healthier more productive society) and not the end in terms of healthier people."[15(p9)] The purpose is to improve the health of all citizens, which is achieved by promoting a healthy workforce or a healthy public school population for enhancing learning. Thus, a productive workforce, community, and society are the end result.

Egalitarian Philosophy

O'Rourke in 2006 cited Berzucha with the philosophy of improving health through the egalitarian philosophy.[15] Berzucha in 2001 stated that a hierarchal structure in society determines people's life span and is reflected by the gap between poor and rich. When there is a large gap, sometimes the upper echelon wields power and domination over the less fortunate. According to this philosophy, feelings of support, friendship, cooperation, and sociability predominate. It allows that individual behavior change is not as effective as changing the structure within societies.[15]

Universal Philosophy

O'Rourke proposed that the Siegrist philosophy should be brought to the forefront again.[15(p9)] Promoted in 1946, this philosophy as summarized by O'Rourke said that health education and promotion are the result of adequate economics, safe environments, high-quality education, meaningful employment, valuing collective responsibility, promoting solidarity, rejecting social Darwinism, and encouraging all citizens to care for each other and value individual contributions.

This philosophy involves everything relevant to a person's health. It encompasses all social demographics, health literacy, education, access, prevention, promotion, and protection efforts as well as public policies, law, environment, and culture. It is more or less a collective view of all influences in a person's life. Some have called this an eclectic philosophy,[16] or it could be called a multilevel philosophy. Kiblinger in 2009 offered an analogy that probably belongs in all health philosophies.[7] He stated, "In order to make the most of the present opportunity, it will be helpful if we can invoke what has been called the principle of charity as we approach new ways of looking at things."[7(p5)]

WRITING A HEALTH PHILOSOPHY

Many students do not know where to begin in entertaining a personal philosophy of health. The best advice is to look at other philosophies—and not just health philosophies. Find peer-reviewed articles concerning philosophy and take notes on those that strike a chord with your own personal views and correlate with your feelings about the health professional's role. What are you passionate about in the health profession? How could things change for the better? What efforts could significantly affect the health status in the population(s) you choose? What changes need instituting? Why hasn't this been tried before? How can this be solved efficiently and be cost-effectively. Is this the best solution to improve the quality of life of the people affected? These and many other salient questions should be roaming around inside your mind. Write down some ideas. Reflect on what you wrote. Revisit these ideas at a later time and expand your concept. Rethink the issue and pursue thoughtful decision making.

You could speak with a health professional to help you articulate and expand your views. This is the time for reflective thinking as promoted by Bandura in 1977.[27] Mull the idea over in your mind for several days. As you come up with new ideas, jot them down along with the first ideas. Speak with friends and acquaintances, and see if they can follow your line of thinking. Search the literature to see what other health professionals have done in the area you feel needs help. How did they try? What implications did they list at the end of the research? This research may provide evidence-based clues on how to go about formulating your philosophy of healthful change for a better world.

Everyone in a profession should leave a legacy that will be continued by future professionals. Perhaps you can find a health professional's philosophy that you can expand on. You may also want to construct a new philosophy based on past successes. It is not easy to reflect on the past and present and look to the future, but in doing so, you gain a sense of what it means to begin a legacy. What will you leave for other health educators to emulate and continue? Framing your objectives is the reason for this thoughtful process. It helps to solidify your health education values, to dictate the type of health professional you will become, and to indicate the path you will follow.

HEALTH PHILOSOPHY DEVELOPMENT

The first step in developing a health philosophy is to develop your statement of the philosophy. Reflect on the health profession and decide what has worked, what is needed, or what possible solution can be developed to a problem or concern that you are passionate about and would like to solve. What type of philosophy are you interested in formulating? Your focus could involve a change in policy, environment, professional practice, epidemiology, or other relevant health issues or problems. It may deal with specific health prevention, promotion, protection, maintenance, literacy, access to health services, maintenance, or enhancement. What is the focus of your philosophy? It could be related to child abuse, HIV/AIDS, childhood diabetes, or any other health problem that needs to be solved. Generating a personal philosophy works with concepts and principles but can be backed up by facts, which will aid understanding and reasoning. Develop a cause within the health profession for which you feel you could advocate with desire and passion. Try to devise a one sentence statement for your philosophy of health. Include what you believe and what is important to you about your profession. Then, describe your health philosophy in one sentence. Expand the meaning of the philosophy. Begin formulating an outline to help guide your philosophical paper. This helps you to change information as you find additions as well as categorize and organize your document in an efficient and logical manner as you proceed through the other steps and add professional references.

The second step involves developing the principles of the philosophy. This includes researching philosophic principles that seem congruent with your own from health professionals and different philosophers through the ages. Consider what is important to you about your philosophy. Because this is your own philosophy, you can combine established philosophies or use parts of philosophies to formulate your own. Reflect on the values, beliefs, attitudes, and habits that define the profession. Think critically and make connections within the profession and your understanding of a general or specific philosophy. You also need to consider how many principles or points belong with your philosophy while researching other philosophies. Explain each item in the philosophy, including the main principle or points in detail. You may need to add several points once your main philosophy is explained to further expand the meaning. Continue formulating an outline to help guide your philosophical paper. This helps you to change information as you find additions and categorize and organize your document in an efficient and logical manner.

A third step is to explain and justify the philosophy. Justify your philosophy and state the efforts need to help solve this health problem. Validate your opinion. You could interview or talk to health professionals about their personal views. See if their views seem similar to yours and let them guide you in the direction you have pursued. Become like a private investigator trying to solve a health problem or improve the nation's health. Give factual information and cite any statistics and reference articles available on the subject. Be sure to include the Code of Ethics (Appendix B) portions that are relevant to your philosophy. All issues must conform to and stand for principles in the professional Code of Ethics for the health profession. State the specific and relevant Responsibilities and Competencies for Health Educators and include the subcompetencies that are established for the profession that relate to your philosophy (see Appendix A). Give a plausible explanation of how the problem could be solved. These may help steer your efforts. Refrain from biased or prejudicial opinions that are not part of a true health philosophy. The fourth step is to explain how this philosophy could be applied to health and contribute to the health profession. State how this philosophy, if implemented, could improve health and create progress in heath educator practices. Justify and state specifically why this philosophy is necessary. Describe how this contributes to improving health for those involved and the health profession. Justify each principle and section of your philosophy thoroughly, and use internal documentation such as quotes and citations from professional journal articles and sources to back up the main points of your philosophy. Include as many main points as necessary under that philosophy that are relevant to the explanation. Use a thesaurus liberally to help you adjust your word choices and improve the flow of the philosophy. Be careful to avoid repetitive information.

Use documented professional health references to back up your philosophy. Describe why this philosophy is necessary and how it could help solve the health problem. Cite other relevant philosophers who may think similarly to you. Elaborate on the philosophy statement and cite other philosophies that are similar to your own beliefs and personal opinions about the profession. State how it would contribute to the health profession. Short quotes or citations from relevant health philosophies or other philosophers give credibility to your own philosophy.

Finish your philosophy with a conclusion—a paragraph that sums up or concludes what you have been discussing. Use relevant references that back up your philosophical statement. Read through it again, checking the flow, sequence, grammar, and spelling, and make sure you use complete sentences. Show it to another student or a health professional to critique. After another reading, polish any troublesome areas, and make sure that the title accurately reflects the philosophy discussed.

Develop a rough draft of your proposed philosophy. Read over the philosophy several times for proper flow and sequence. Also, you may need to reorder the information. Double-check your references. Health professionals uses two different types of reference formats for professional publications—American Psychological Association and the American Medical Association. Check the format prescribed for the philosophy paper. Format the references in the style requested by your instructor. Finally, print a hard copy. It should be double-spaced, with correct margins, numbered pages, headings correctly placed and formatted, and no more than 27 lines of text per page.

Your philosophy should be adequately researched and organized with a logical sequence. Accurate health principles should reflect your personal philosophy. Also, your personal philosophy should be ethical, responsible, moral, and culturally correct. Check your philosophy for correct grammar and spelling. Make sure you use accurate health principles. Check over it again and make sure you back up the statements, beliefs, and points with relevant references. Just remember that a philosophy is not a research effort to determine something; rather, it states your belief about how things could be better and suggests change for the future. Just because something has not been implemented does not mean you cannot offer a proposal. **Table 6–1** offers a sample outline to follow to formulate your philosophy. This is only a template to get you started, and the format is flexible. You can adjust the format to fit your particular philosophy. And remember, your philosophy can and will change as time progresses, the health profession and new practices evolve, and unfortunately, new problems emerge.

According to Kiblinger, a philosophy involves concepts and reasoning, and a person should engage in reasoned inquiry and self-reflection in contemplating the values, beliefs, attitudes, and habits that define the nature and quality of life.[7] This description applies to formulating a health philosophy. Keep your philosophy in a safe place, and revisit it from time to time. It is about interrelations between different philosophical viewpoints.

Your philosophy can change after you have written it. As your knowledge base increases and you become more aware of additional health issues in your health studies, you may want to modify or change

Table 6-1   TEMPLATE FOR FORMING A HEALTH PHILOSOPHY*

Title of Philosophy:

1. Statement
   a. My philosophy of health is: (list the basic problem and the premise of the philosophy and use citations)
   b. Type of health philosophy (prevention, promotion, protection, education, literacy, access to healthcare, enhancement, maintenance, or other)
   c. Focus of the philosophy (problem, disease, participants, etc.)

2. Principles
   a. List the principles or main points of the philosophy (list as many points as necessary for the philosophy). Explain in detail each point of the philosophy.
      1). The first point of the philosophy is: (use citation)
      2). The second point of the philosophy is: (use citation)
      3). The third point of the philosophy is: (use citation)
      4). The fourth point of the philosophy is: (use citation)

3. Explanation and justification
   a. Justify and state specifically why this philosophy is necessary for health
   b. State how this may contribute to solving the health problem
   c. Reinforce and validate this philosophy's principles with citations
      1). Give specific examples of factual information by using other philosophers' or health practitioners' citations from professional journals and references concerning this or a similar philosophy
      2). Include interviews from health professionals
   d. State how this philosophy relates to and is justified in the professional Responsibilities and Competencies for Health Education for Entry and/or Advanced Levels.
   e. State how this philosophy is justified and applied in the Code of Ethics for the profession

4. Application and contribution
   a. List the many different ways the philosophy has been applied in health and to the health profession
   b. State applications and situations where this philosophy or a similar philosophy has been applied specifically to health and/or to the health profession
      1). Give specific examples and an explanation of how it was applied and use internal citations
      2). Find research journal articles and references with similar principles for the contribution of the philosophy or similar philosophies and use internal citations

5. Conclusion
   a. Provide a summary statement of why this philosophy would promote health and the health profession now
   b. Give an explanation of its feasibility in the future

6. References (list in appropriate format)

*Note: Internal citations from professional journals or resources by other health professionals are necessary for each section to give credibility and justification to your philosophy, and they help back up the main points and principles of the philosophy. Investigating professional sources is necessary to help you to formulate your philosophy, to see philosophical reflections from other health professionals, and to extend your knowledge base.

your philosophy. New and emerging health issues may shift your philosophy. In addition, many health educators develop more specific philosophies during their internship and once employed in the health field. Experience helps solidify your philosophy. However, it should always be a work in progress, as professional health issues change and new issues surface. Most health educators will tell you that with proven empirical research, technological advances, and improved preventive techniques and treatment options, a personal health philosophy can and should change over time.

Think of your philosophy as malleable, to be massaged, rethought, and constantly contemplated. Reflect on it often, for this is how you feel about professional practice efforts and is an indication of your own personal beliefs and ideas about promoting healthier lives for people. This is your belief statement and involves ethics, aesthetics, and personal values. The philosophy may involve something that could be changed with revisions, or it may propose a new professional practice that, although not easily implemented, could be achieved with proper resources, access, trained professionals, and environmental and policy changes. Revisit your philosophy frequently and make changes or additions as necessary.

With vision and the ability to effect change, you may actually see that your health philosophy was solved or conditions changed suddenly in the health profession. A new cure, a new methodology, availability of adequate resources, and increased access may result from improved legislation or policy, or societal or environmental changes. Historic events, forming of coalitions, pooling of resources, and other scenarios can change the face of global health overnight. This is a good outcome and provides the foundation for future investigations of related problems or emerging issues. At that point, however, you will need to look to the future for new philosophical statements about health education and find a new position that you are passionate about.

Since a philosophy is a way of thinking, it is important to note that not all philosophies are ethical and fair. People sometimes distort their view to thrust their own biases and views at others framed as a philosophical viewpoint. You should be able to discern if a philosophy is sound, methodical thinking or a corrupted viewpoint. It is wise to know the difference. Having the ability to formulate your own philosophy will give you the ability to decipher and understand other philosophies. You can examine other health philosophies and determine their worth by critical thinking and reflection.

> **Thought Concept**
>
> *Give an example of how attitudes or values of others can influence people in health-related situations. Describe some positive examples and some negative examples.*

PHILOSOPHICAL VIEWS FROM HEALTH PROFESSIONALS AND ORGANIZATIONS

The American Association for Health Education's position statement on philosophy says that a "contemporary concept of health embraces the entire being."[24(p1)] Health education is unique. It influences and seeks improvement in individual, family, community, and societal development, knowledge, attitudes, and behavior. Individuals are multidimensional entities with many complex interrelationships. Good health requires active participation of individuals and society in the promotion of wellness. Health education literacy enables individuals to use knowledge that moves them to optimal stages of health. It enables individuals to gain skills for judging and using health-enhancing skills. The end is the achievement of societal well-being. Lifestyles should reflect the scope of health-enhancing lives.

It is important to equip individuals with an understanding of current realities so they can make healthy choices. Health education learning is of great value to individuals in the promotion of health-enhancing lifestyles. Knowing how to evaluate and access health knowledge and make wise choices concerning health can actually save a life or promote a higher-quality and longer life.[24]

The Ottawa Charter stated that there are fundamental conditions and resources for health that we must advocate, mediate, and enable for health. The necessary resources are: education, food, income, peace, shelter, a stable ecosystem, sustainable resources, social justice, and equity. These are reflected in the strategies and programs adapted to suit individual countries and regions including the social, economic, and cultural systems involved. Good health is a major resource, achieves equity, and the health sector alone cannot achieve this. Improvement in health requires a secure foundation of all entities in a country and a word wide commitment. This charter called for a global commitment to health and an international call to action.[13]

Dr. Lawrence Green

Dr. Green (see **Figure 6–5**) is best known for his many books and articles on the PRECEDE–PROCEED model (see Chapter 3). He is the author, along with Marshal Kreuter of the PRECEDE-PROCEED model that revolutionized program planning models in health. This definitive program model is responsible for more than 950 published applications in case studies, research, and books. Dr. Green is currently an adjunct professor in the Department of Epidemiology and Biostatistics and co-director of the Society, Diversity and Disparities Program, Comprehensive Cancer Center at the University of California at San Francisco. His previous university experiences were at the University of Maryland, College Park, University of California at Berkely, Rollins School of Public Health at Emory University, and the University of British Columbia, to name a few. He worked as the director of the Office of Science and Extramural Research at the CDC. He was a distinguished fellow/visiting scientist and director of the CDC World Health Orgnizaition Collaborating Center on Global Tobacco Control, in addition to many other prominent positions.

Besides authoring the PRECEDE-PROCEED model, his current research focuses on primary prevention of diabetes, randomized and other controlled trials on the PolyPill, and works on strengthening practices-based evidence to evidence-based practices. He has had a numerous research publications and is a world reknowned health researcher and investigator.[28]

If you follow the PRECEDE-PROCEED model, you will see all health issues addressed. It is based on the attitude that if health educators want more evidence based practice, then more practice based evidence is necessary. Dr. Green and the other authors' attempts to explain health related behaviors and environments, and to design and evaluate the interventions necessary, has caused a significant change in the way that health educators practice, address, and evaluate environmental issues. Every influential factor in the behaviors and living conditions of an individual must be examined when designing and evaluating programs, plans, and interventions. This approach is educational and ecological.[28]

In a conversation with Dr. Green, he stated, "There needs to be recognition of the broader upstream determinants of health. Community health should focus on additional determinants outside the person that influence individual behavior change and health." He further related that he felt that health deter-

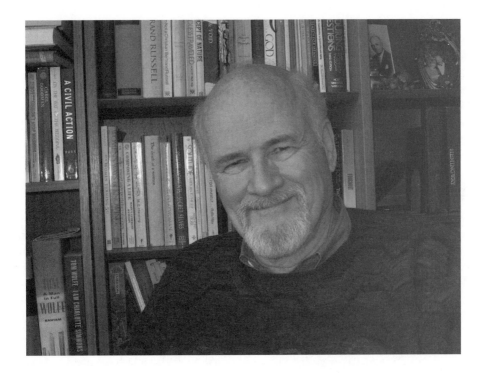

Figure 6–5   Dr. Lawrence Green

minants focused on behavior change should include the social, environmental, policy, and regulatory issues that impact health (L. Green, pers. comm., March 25, 2009).

Dr. Becky Smith

Dr. Smith is the former executive director of the American Association for Health Education (AAHE), vice president of the American Alliance for Health, Physical Education, Recreation, and Dance, and the executive editor of the *American Journal of Health Education* and the *International Electronic Journal of Health Education*. Dr. Smith completed her doctoral studies at the University of Illinois. She received the Professional Service Award and Presidential Citation from the American Association for Health Education. She is a certified association executive, certified health education specialist, and a certified K–12 educator in New York and Illinois.

Dr. Smith directed a diversity of projects in health education and health promotion funded by government, corporation, and foundation sources. She is the author of numerous publications and papers presented at national and international meetings.

Her leadership abilities at AAHE helped to establish it as a leading health authority and supporter in the health field. In an interview with Dr. Smith, she stated, "Health proposes to help people formulate healthy behaviors or change behaviors that aren't healthy." Behavior formulation is a key ingredient to this philosophy. If you decide how you want to be, whatever helps you toward that behavior is the "pusher." She also said that health behavior formulation is necessary at a much younger age. "There are points in the life span that young adults and adults need that formulation. Early childhood education, health education, and parenthood education should go hand in hand. We should do more high school electives in parenthood education" (B. Smith, pers. comm., April 3, 2009).

Dr. Collins Airhihenbuwa

Dr. Airhihenbuwa (see **Figure 6–6**) is currently professor of behavioral health in the Department of Biobehavioral Health, College of Health and Human Development, at The Pennsylvania State University. He was the former department chair of the College of Health Education, Department of Health and Human Development at the same university. His classic book, *Health and Culture: Beyond the Western Paradigm* (1995), secured his place in the health profession as a promoter of considering culture in approaching health promotion programs. His belief of health behavior as a cultural construct has spurred research on HIV/AIDS and work in underdeveloped countries. His publications have included American Indian populations, Nigerians, New Guineans, and Africans on such diverse subjects as first aid, global health, alcohol abuse, sexuality education, race and gender, and contraceptive use. His well known PEN-3 model is widely used as a cultural model for health programs and it has been recognized worldwide for its cultural entity and unique approach to cultural influences on health. He is a widely respected author and speaker and a prominent health professional. In an interview with Dr. Airhihenbuwa, he stated that a health science philosophy works in conjunction with evaluation. This approach includes fairness, social justice, and a slant toward utopia. Social and political philosophy deals with issues that affect society at a qualitative level. He said, "My approach to studying behavior is from a cultural standpoint and from broad areas of theory." He further stated that you have to strike a balance to find ways of applying principles of fairness and social justice that are grounded in experiences in society and qualitative contextual culture.

Dr. Airhihenbuwa said that you learn about experiences from the past by studying how people relate today. We need to prepare the current generation for working within relationships, the social context, and institutionalizing culture. This focus stems not from the individual, but from individual societies, promoting individual relationships, not individual differences. We need to institutionalize behavioral resources. For example, smoking bans saw remarkable results and we should see the same with obesity and diabetes. We need institutional and cultural changes. He said that two critical areas in food consumption are portion size and the content of the food. Portion size is the problem, as well as the size of the plates, dishes, and cups. Supersizing has started to influence what is normal.

He further stated that energy expenditures and exercise should be built into the environment. Dr. Airhihenbuwa is a strong advocate of restructuring the environment to encourage walking and include places where people can walk safely. This initiative requires walk-friendly sidewalks, proper lighting, park-like settings, and planned events that are family oriented. Food consumption and energy expenditure go together, so we must plan prudently. He concluded by saying that health professionals need

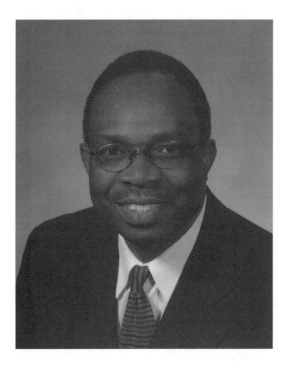

Figure 6–6   Dr. Collins Airhihenbuwa

to look at a philosophy in the social-cultural and environmental-structural context that shapes individuals' decisions (C. Airhihenbuwa, pers. comm., May 8, 2009).

Dr. Bob Blackburn

Dr. Blackburn (see **Figure** 6–7) is the Past President of the American Association for Health Education and former Executive Director of North Carolina AAHPERD.

He was a professor for 24 years and chair of the Department of Health Education and Physical Education at Gardner-Webb University. Bob received two Distinguished Service Awards and three Presidential Citations from the American Association of Health Education. He received the National Association of Local Boards of Health (NALBOH), Everett I. Hageman Award for public health leadership, commitment, and enthusiasm in 2009. Currently, he is vice-chair of the North Carolina Local Health Department Accreditation Board. Bob is the current president of the Foundation for the Advancement of Health Education. He was a member of the DHHS Secretary's Council on Health Promotion and Disease Prevention and he continues his advocacy work with the American Heart Association. Even after retiring, his service contributions to the health profession continued

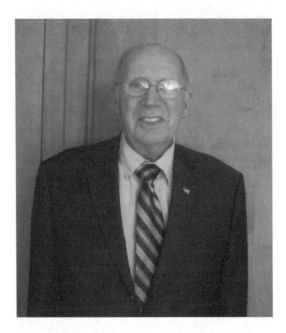

Figure 6–7   Dr. Robert Blackburn

through his interest in health societies and health advocacy. His quiet leadership abilities and charismatic personality have helped many doubters move to his philosophical viewpoint concerning health. He is not only a state leader, but a nationally admired, legendary professional, and a consummate health promoter.

He said in an interview, "Early training is imperative in health." He added that integrity is the key component of the profession and communication skills are paramount. Success also involves having the necessary human relations skills to work with people. In school, health and also in the public health realms, even more so, you are only as good as your work and behavior.[2]

He stated that as a grandfather, he believes in the "Bob the Builder" philosophy, adapted from the popular children's television show in the United States.[29] Dr. Blackburn said that this show's philosophy for children communicates the health philosophy that we should adopt. In the Bob the Builder philosophy, Bob and his Can-Do-Crew (tools) hammer out solutions and are ready to tackle any project. According to the show's Web site, the crew demonstrates the power of "...positive thinking, problem solving, teamwork and follow through" that lead to solutions for a job done well.[28] When Bob the Builder is asked by the "tools" in this cartoon whether they can accomplish a particular task, the answer is always "Yes, we can."And so, Dr. Blackburn summed up the idea of pursuing a health philosophy by saying, "As health educators, we must continue to pursue professional practice in a positive light, so we can continually move forward instead of resigning to defeat if all is not accomplished." As Bob the Builder says, "Yes, we can." In order to continue in Dr. Blackburn's footsteps, health professionals should always keep moving forward and not take defeat as a sign of never achieving the goal (R. Blackburn, pers. comm., April 4, 2009).

SUMMARY

- A philosophy is a foundation or basic set of beliefs and involves attitudes, values, behaviors, and true perceptions.
- The study of philosophy works with concepts rather than facts. Philosophy seeks understanding.
- John Dewey struggled with morality and ethical philosophies. Later philosophers contemplated goodness, knowledge, character, truth, and other moral issues.
- The four types of philosophies are logic (scientific methods), epistemology (study of knowledge), metaphysics (reality), and axiology (reality).
- Different authors espouse different philosophies.
- The philosophies examined for deriving a personal health philosophy include the holistic approach, empowerment, behavior change/modification, behavioral intention, cognitive-based healthy decision making, macro-perspective, and utilitarian, egalitarian, and universal philosophies.
- The Ottawa Charter supports a global environmental health promotion philosophy of cooperation and help among nations and people.
- Students of health and health educators need to determine a personal health philosophy based on their own ideas and opinions; backup with reputable sources gives credibility to a philosophy.
- A personal health philosophy is an investigation by a person to arrive at the true meaning of health practice as he or she sees it.
- Health philosophies can change through the years as emerging issues and health needs occur, as health advances solve problems, and as new challenges present themselves.

CONCEPTUAL TERMS

Philosophy

Constructivist

Utilitarianism

Pragmatism

Existentialism

Formalist

Logic

Epistemology

Metaphysics

Axiology

Holistic

Behavior change/modification

Functional/utilitarian philosophy

Egalitarian philosophy

Cognitive-based and healthy decision making

REFLECTIVE THINKING

Maria recently had her first professional job interview. She tried to prepare herself by reviewing the basic models and theories used in health programs. The agency with whom she interviewed had a Web site, and she visited it to find out as much about the organization as she could and to familiarize herself with the names of the people in the agency. She went to the bookstore and bought several books on how to interview for employment opportunities. She asked other health educators to provide her with some sample questions that she might be asked. She felt prepared and thoroughly reviewed everything before arriving at the interview. After a short conversation, the employer asked her several salient questions, and she felt she answered them successfully and showed her knowledge of the health profession. Then, the employer asked her for her philosophy of health. She hesitated, stammered a little, and spat out something she remembered one of her graduate instructors telling her about holistic health. When she left the interview, she realized she had neglected one of the major concepts of the profession.

What would your answer be for this prospective employer? Have you developed and formulated your own philosophy for the health profession that you believe in and can articulate to others? Can you back it up with reliable and research-based references? Not having a philosophy is like traveling without a compass. You need to solidify a health philosophy that is congruent with your career goals and beliefs. You need to formulate references that show you are not the only one who feels that this philosophy is worthy to the health profession. A solid, research-based health philosophy is as important as a degree in the health profession.

CONCEPTUAL LEARNING

1. Identify and describe the term *philosophy*.
2. Compare a constructivist and utilitarian approach to philosophy.
3. Summarize and explain the pragmatic philosophy.
4. Compose your own definition of existentialism.
5. Differentiate between the four basic types of philosophies: logic, epistemology, metaphysics, and axiology.
6. Examine and contrast between the different types of health education philosophies: the holistic approach, empowerment, behavior change/modification, cognitive-based and healthy decision making, changing attitudes, functional/utilitarian philosophy, and egalitarian philosophy.

REFERENCES

1. Parker, P. N. (2009). *Webster's online dictionary*. Philosophy. Retrieved March 7, 2010, from http://www.websters-online-dictionary.org/definition/philosophy
2. Longman Group Limited. (1993). *New concise Webster's dictionary: A comprehensive guide to the English language for home, office, and school*. New York: Modern Publishing.
3. MaGill, Frank N., & McGreal, I. P. (Eds.). (1961). *Masterpieces of world philosophy in summary form*. New York: Harpers and Brothers.
4. Archie, L., & Archie, J. G. (2004). *Reading for philosophical inquiry: A brief introduction to philosophical thinking*. Retrieved March 7, 2010, from philosophy.lander.edu Web site at http://philosophy.lander.edu/intro/intro-book-links.html
5. *Stanford encyclopedia of philosophy*. (2008, September 25). Concepts of disease and health. San Jose, CA: Stanford University.
6. Stotz, K. (2009). Philosophy in the trenches: From naturalized to experimental philosophy (of science). *Studies in history and philosophy of science*, Part A, 40(2), 225–226.
7. Kiblinger, W. P. (2009, Spring). *Philosophy 302: History of philosophy: Modern period*. Rock Hill, SC: Winthrop University.

8. Vardey, L. (1995). *Mother Teresa, a simple path.* New York: Ballantine Books.

9. Dewey, J. (1938). *Experience and education* (p. 51). New York: Macmillan.

10. Smith, B. J. (2006). Connecting a personal philosophy of health to the practice of health education. *The Health Education Monograph, 23*(1), 11–13.

11. von Glasersfeld, E. (1989). Constructivism in education. In T. Husen & N. Postlewaite (Eds.), *International encyclopedia of education* (Suppl., pp. 162–163). Oxford, England: Pergamon Press.

12. Haglund, B. J. A., & McDonald, G. (2000). A global Internet survey of health promotion training. *European Journal of Public Health, 10*(4), 304–306.

13. World Health Organization. (1986, November 21). *Ottawa charter for health promotion.* First International Conference on Health Promotion, Ottawa, Ontario, Canada.

14. Koop, C. E. (1982, October 20). *United States Public Health Service Luther Terry lecture.* Seventeenth Annual Meeting of the Commissioned officers of the United States Public Health Service. Orlando, Florida.

15. O'Rourke, T. (2006). Philosophical reflections on health education and health promotion: Shifting sands and ebbing tides. *The Health Education Monograph, 23*(1), 7–10.

16. Cottrell, R. R., Girvan, J. T. & McKenzie, J. F. (2008). *Principles and foundations of health promotion and education* (4th ed). San Francisco: Addison Wesley & Benjamin Cummings.

17. Greenberg, J. S. (1985). Health and wellness: A conceptual differentiation. *Journal of School Health, 55*(10), 403–406.

18. Wallerstein, N., & Bernstein, E. (1988). Empowerment education: Freire's ideas adapted to health education. *Health Education Quarterly, 15*, 379–394.

19. Minkler, M., Thompson, M., Bell, J., & Rose, K. (2002). Contributions of community involvement to organizational level empowerment: The Federal Health Start Experience. *Health Education & Behavior, 28*(6), 783–807.

20. Tai-Seale, T. (2001). Understanding health empowerment. *The Health Educator, 33*(1), 23–29.

21. McGuire, W. J. (1984). Public communication as a strategy for introducing health-promoting behavioral change. *Preventive Medicine, 13*(3), 299–313.

22. Prochaska, J. O., & Velicer, W. F. (1997). The transtheoretical model of health behavior change. *American Journal of Health Promotion, 12*, 38–48.

23. Ajzen, I., & Fishbein, M. (1980). *Understanding attitudes and predicting social behavior.* Englewood Cliffs, NJ: Prentice Hall.

24. American Association for Health Education. (2009). *Philosophy of health education: AAHE position statement.* Retrieved July 15, 2009, from http://aahperd.org/aahe/advocacy/positionStatement/upload/philosophy-2009.2pdf

25. Rothman, J., & Tropman, J. E. (1987). Models of community organization and macro practice perspectives: Their mixing and phasing. In F. M. Cox, J. L. Erlich, J. Rothman, & J. E. Tropman, (Eds.), *Strategies of community organization: Macro practice* (pp. 3–26). Itasca, IL: F. E. Peacock.

26. U. S. Department of Health and Human Services. Office of Disease Prevention and Health Promotion. (2000). *Healthy people 2010* (2nd ed.). Retrieved March 7, 2010, from http://www.healthypeople.gov/default.htm

27. Bandura, A. (1977). *Social learning theory.* Englewood Cliffs, NJ: Prentice Hall.

28. Green, L. W., & Kreuter, M. W. (2005). *Health program planning: An educational and ecological approach* (4th ed.). Boston: McGraw-Hill.

29. HIT Entertainment Limited and Keith Chapman. (2008). *Bob the builder.* Retrieved March 7, 2010, from http://www.bobthebuilder.com

ENHANCED READINGS

American Alliance for Health, Physical Education, Recreation and Dance. (2009). Available at: http://www.aahperd.org/aahe/aahe_main.html. Retrieved March 23, 2010, from http://aahperd.org/aahe/advocacy/positionStatement/upload/philosophy-2009.2pdf (Read the American Association for Health Education Philosophy.)

Welle, H. M., Russell, R. D., & Kittleson, M. J. (1995). Philosophical trends in health education: Implications for the 21st century. *Journal of Health Education*, 26(6), 326–333. (Read the 1995 article about philosophical trends in a research study.)

RELEVANT WEB SITES

UCSF Library. (2010). Tobacco control archives. Available at: http://www.library.ucsf.edu/tobacco/cigpapers/about .html. (Read the *Tobacco Papers* sponsored by the American Legacy Foundation. This is a collection of tobacco industry documents on scientific research, manufacturing, marketing, advertising, and sales. The philosophy promulgated by the tobacco industry is shown in the papers. As a result of these documents being published on the Internet, complaints were filed by the Attorney Generals of many states. The federal litigation and similar actions involving the tobacco industry are on this Web site.)

World Health Organization. (1986, November 21). *Ottawa charter for health promotion*. First International Conference on Health Promotion, Ottawa, Ontario, Canada. Available at: http://www.who.int/healthpromotion/ conferences/previous/ottawa/en/

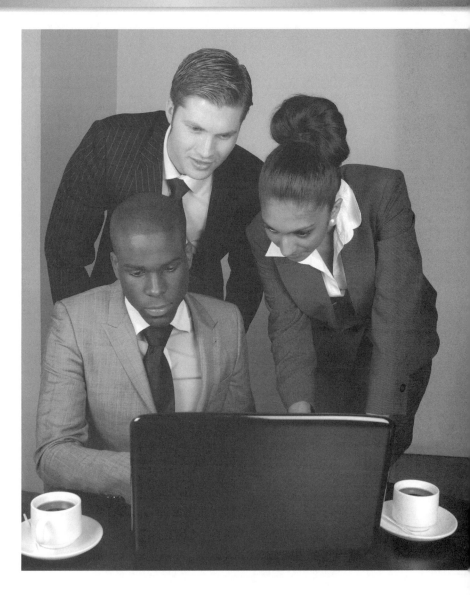

CHAPTER 7

Professional Tenets in Certifications, Standards, Ethics, and Competencies

OBJECTIVES AND ASSESSMENTS

This chapter meets the following National Commission for Health Education Credentialing, Inc., Society for Public Health Education, and American Association for Health Education Competency-Based Framework for Entry Level and Advanced Level Health Educator Competencies.* The learner will:

6. Serve as a health education resource person.

This chapter meets the following general learning objectives. The learner will:
   1. Identify and define the history of role delineation and certification.
   2. Compare the difference between model standards, objectives, and certifications.
   3. Examine and construct a rationale for the Code of Ethics and summarize professional conduct.
   4. Describe the 7 major undergraduate health educator responsibilities and competencies.
   5. Compare the 10 major graduate health educator responsibilities and competencies to the 7 major undergraduate health educator responsibilities and competencies.
   6. Develop a definition of a profession.
   7. Examine why the standard occupational classification in 2001 of a designated health educator by the United States Department of Labor was important to the profession.
   8. Compare the differences between accreditation, licensure, certification, registration, and credentialing.
   9. Review the history of the Certified Health Education Specialist (CHES) credentialing movement and the new designation, MCHES.

*Source: Reprinted with permission of NCHEC.

   National Commission for Health Education Credentialing, Inc. (NCHEC), Society for Public Health Education (SOPHE), & American Association for Health Education (AAHE). (2006). *A competency-based framework for health educators-2006.* Whitehall, PA: NCHEC.

10. Discuss the professional ethics principles of autonomy, nonmalfeasance, beneficence, justice, respect, utilitarianism, and paternalism.
11. Summarize professional conduct and the need for certain ethical principles that health educators should enforce in programs and research as defined by the Code of Ethics for health professionals.
12. List examples of a breach of ethics for each of the following: misconduct, questionable research practices, and unethical behavior.

INTRODUCTION

When we were in elementary school, the derogatory term used for someone informing the teacher about another student's inappropriate behavior was "tattletale." A more polite term is "social informer." An even more hideous one is "company spy." In industry and business, many people are also called "whistle-blowers" when reporting unethical practices, procedures, or manufacturing safety issues. Society denotes many names for people who tell it like it is. Some have lost their jobs reporting these inaccuracies or incompetent business and industrial practices. Being an ethical person requires tenacity, sacrifice, and even suffering.

Let's imagine that you are performing your health internship at a local community agency. You observe one of the project managers make an inappropriate racial remark to one of the subjects in the program. The subject speaks up in rebuttal but does not report it to anyone at the agency. What should you do? This is a question of ethics. Most people consider the repercussions if they become a whistle-blower and report unethical conduct. What you are bound and morally responsible to report should never be a consideration if you are a true professional person. As a health educator, there are codes of ethics you should obey. Moreover, human beings are responsible for all assumed honor and moral codes and should always respond swiftly and accurately when another professional or person exhibits unethical conduct.

The right to good health is a right of all human beings, regardless of gender, race, religion, socio-economic status, geographic location, or disease status. This chapter delineates the standards, certifications, codes of ethics and responsibilities, and competencies present in the health education profession. Each element represents a standard of excellence for health and health education practitioners for helping persons achieve a higher quality of life. Global examples are included concerning human subjects in health research and programs. All concepts covered here influence health education practice and are important for aspiring health educators to understand. Global documents are also included concerning human subjects in health research and programs. These documents affect health and human rights around the world.

PROFESSIONAL PREPARATION FOR THE PROFESSION

We all want to be "professional" in our career. Some professions are distinguished by certain signs, such as a barber pole, attorney's scales of justice, and the physician's staff symbol. There are certain requirements to being called a profession and certain designations for each. A *profession* is defined by the *New Concise Webster's Dictionary* as "an employment that needs special learning."[1(p225)] The role of a professional is to carry out the obligations of that profession. Patterson and Vitello state that professional preparation is an "educational opportunity for persons seeking specialized knowledge, skills, and/or training in a particular field of study or discipline."[2(p15)] The Coalition of National Health Education Organizations explain that the health education profession promotes, supports, and enables healthy lives and communities.[3]

Part of the evolution of health education was a process for establishing professional goals. A common framework for academic preparation of health educators was needed, as was a process for undergraduate credentialing and advanced levels to assure that all have a common set of skills.[4] Significant documents and certifications resulted from the work of many health professionals.[5] Included in these are the major four, including: (1) The National Commission for Health Education Certification that resulted in the credentialing esignation of the Certified Health Educational Specialist (CHES);[6] (2) *A Competency-Based Framework for Health Educators* (2006),[7] which was an update of *The Responsibilities and Competencies for Undergraduate Health Educators* (1996);[8] (3) *A Competency-Based Framework for Graduate-Level Health Educators* (1999),[9] which resulted in graduate-level competencies (the last two documents were standards of practice for academic preparation of health educators); and (4) *The National Health Education Standards*,[10] which provided a framework for standards for students in grades K–12.

ESSENTIAL CHARACTERISTICS OF A PROFESSION

Professions delineate themselves by setting minimum criteria and possibly testing requirements to assure competence. There are different ways to ensure professional competence in professions and education. Licensure, certification, credentialing, accreditation, standards, responsibilities, registries, and competencies are terms used.

According to Helen Cleary in 1995, "**Licensure** is concerned with protection of the public. It is a process by which an agency of government (usually a state) grants permission to become an active individual in a given profession by certifying that those licensed have attained specified standards of competence."[5(p42)] Patterson and Vitello explain that it is often a condition of employment or a mandatory process of submitting documents under government domain.[2]

Cleary states, "**Certification** is a process by which a professional organization grants recognition to an individual who, upon completion of a competency-based curriculum, can demonstrate a predetermined standard of performance."[5(p42)] The certification is a procedure by which an organization identifies and distinguishes an individual who has met certain predetermined qualifications.[11] Health educators teaching in the public schools are certified to teach by states, which vary greatly in their certification requirements. Certification for professions other than teaching could be administered by a professional organization. **Credentialing** can take the form of licensure, certification, or registration.[5] It includes

---

Licensure: Certified permission given by a governmental body to a person to practice a given profession after the person has produced documented evidence and achieved a specified competence level.
Certification: When a professional organization identifies a person who completes a competency-based curriculum and predetermined standard of performance and can practice the given profession.
Credentialing: A process by professional organizations that involves individual and/or programs and includes processes of licensure, certifications, and/or registration.

individual and.program credentialing. **Individual credentialing** involves regulation of persons.[4] It improves professional preparation and practice. In contrast, "**Program credentialing** is accreditation of a program in which certain standards are met."[4(p23)] An example is program credentialing of academic professional preparation programs at universities. Accreditation is "a process by which a professional body evaluates an entire program against predetermined criteria or standards."[5(p42)] It is a measure of quality assurance with adherence to a minimum set of stands.[2] **Registration**, however, has less formal requirements where standards are set for members. To register as a member of a profession, individuals must participate in certain practices.

Educational standards are the basic skills a person should possess after a period of education. **Professional standards** for individuals in a profession are defined by certification and licensure, while program standards are found in accreditation.[2]

There are many challenges for health professionals today. **Informatics** (information technology), genomics, communication, cultural competence, community-based participatory research, global health, policy and law, and public health ethics are critical educational components for the 21st-century health workforce. In addition, issues such as bioterrorism emergency preparedness, refugee health care, post-traumatic stress disorders as a result of wars, HIV/AIDS, and health disparities are prominent in the headlines.[2] School health issues involve working toward mandatory requirements of coordinated and comprehensive health education in the public schools, grades K–12, taught by certified health educators.

> **Career Concept**
>
> *Do you enjoy solving puzzles and following evidence to the original source? You may want to consider a career in epidemiology.*

NATIONAL HEALTH EDUCATION STANDARDS: ACHIEVING EXCELLENCE (K–12 EDUCATION)

In the early 1900s, there was a movement to improve the level of education. The National Education Goals[12] (1994) and the HR 1804 Goals 2000: Educate America Act[13] (1994) by the U.S. Office of Education and Research Information and the U.S. Department of Education created model standards in the core subjects. Recognizing a need for continuity, health education organizations formed the Joint Committee on National Health Education Standards and wrote the National Health Education

---

Individual credentialing: A process that involves the regulation of a professional by requiring predetermined, specific professional preparation and practice, academic standards, and achievement of standards of performance.

Program credentialing: A process that involves the regulation of professional programs by requiring that specific standards.

Registration: A process involving less formal requirements for a person to become registered and accepted within a profession.

Education standards: The basic skills a person should possess after a period of education.

Professional standards: The specific academic and other requirements that must be met for individuals in a profession in the form of certification and licensure.

Informatics: Information availability and accessibility via technology.

Standards (NHES) in July 1993, publishing them in 1995.[14] These were adopted or adapted by many states and school districts.

In 2004, the standards were revised due to research related to the health education field. The revised NHES aligned instructional, curriculum, and assessment practices for state and local education agencies and offered many state departments of education a basis for their state health standards for students.[10] Teachers, administrators, and policy makers use these standards as a template for their own programs and for evaluation of student achievement. The new standards focused on education and theory, inclusion, and assessment, emphasizing collaboration and partnerships.[10]

The NHES consist of three parts, including the standards, rationale statements, and performance indicators.[10] Standard 1 deals with health promotion and disease prevention. Standards 2–8 pertain to key processes and skills for healthy living. The rationale delineates clarity, importance, direction, and understanding. The performance indicators are provided by these grade ranges: pre-K through grade 2, grades 3–5, grades 6–8, and grades 9–12. The performance indicators relate to the cognitive domain including knowledge and skills, but the indicators are developmentally appropriate and include application, analysis, synthesis, and evaluations. While standards are minimum criteria indicators, they set a level for what most students should achieve and, hopefully, help education bodies embrace these standards as well as contribute additional indicators of students adopting and maintaining healthy behaviors. The basic health content areas identified in the NHES are community health, consumer health, environmental health, family life, mental/emotional health, injury prevention/safety, nutrition, personal health, prevention/control of disease, and substance use/abuse.[10] These standards are part of the Comprehensive School Health Program, which are the content areas taught in the classroom, ideally as part of the core curriculum. The eight basic NHES standards are:

Standard 1: Students will comprehend concepts related to health promotion and disease prevention to enhance health.
Standard 2: Students will analyze the influence of family, peers, culture, media, technology, and other factors on health behaviors.
Standard 3: Students will demonstrate the ability to access valid information, products, and services to enhance health.
Standard 4: Students will demonstrate the ability to use interpersonal communication skills to enhance health and avoid or reduce health risks.
Standard 5: Students will demonstrate the ability to use decision-making skills to enhance health.
Standard 6: Students will demonstrate the ability to use goal-setting skills to enhance health.
Standard 7: Students will demonstrate the ability to practice health-enhancing behaviors and avoid or reduce health risks.
Standard 8: Students will demonstrate the ability to advocate for personal, family, and community health.[10]

The Health Education Curriculum and Analysis Tool (HECAT) has identified basic topic modules for K–12 similar to those included in the list with the standards, but the differences are that physical activity is added, tobacco is separate from substance use/abuse, and safety sexual health is included. The HECAT was authored by the CDC's National Center for Chronic Disease Prevention and Health Promotion in 2007. The additional topic modules include alcohol and other drugs, healthy eating, mental and emotional health, personal health and wellness, physical activity, safety sexual health, tobacco, and violence prevention.[15]

There is now a push to include and align the risk behaviors identified by the Youth Risk and Behavior Surveillance Survey (YRBSS) data[16] from the National Center for Chronic Disease Prevention and Health Promotion Data and Statistics (2008) with the content standards. The risky behaviors identified by surveillance data include alcohol and other drug use, injury and violence, tobacco use, poor nutrition, inadequate physical activity, and risky sexual behaviors.

The goal of health education is to adopt and maintain healthy behaviors for life. It contributes to students' successful practice of health protection and promotive behaviors and helps them reduce and/ or avoid risks. We know from program research and theory that behavior change does not take place in a vacuum. Outside influences help shape changes to healthy behaviors. Other school-based services also support healthy outcomes for students. The Coordinated School Health Program (CSHP) is a planned, sequential, and integrated set of courses, services, policies, and interventions to meet the health and safety needs of students in kindergarten through grade 12 according to the CDC's National Center for Chronic Disease Prevention and Health in 2008.[17] This model consists of eight interrelated components, including: (1) health education, (2) physical education, (3) health services, (4) nutrition services, (5) counseling, psychological and social services, (6) healthy school environment, (7) health promotion for staff, and (8) family/community involvement.[10] There is a direct relationship between the NHES, the health content areas,[10] and the CSHP.[17] To see the interrelationships of the Coordinated School Health Program, see Figure 1–4.

THE CERTIFIED HEALTH EDUCATION SPECIALIST CREDENTIALING HISTORY AND FUTURE

The CHES designation, administered by the National Commission for Health Education Credentialing, Inc., is available to qualified health educators in the public schools and public and community health settings who meet the qualifications and testing requirements.[6] It emerged from the First Bethesda Conference in 1978, with impetus by the leadership efforts of Helen Cleary and the Coalition of National Health Education Organizations.[18] Efforts resulted to define health education standards of practice and to develop a credentialing system by the National Task Force on the Preparation and Practice of Health Educators in 1978.[5]

The work progressed, and a *Framework for the Development of Competency-Based Curricula for Entry-Level Health Educators* was born in 1985.[19] The National Task Force was replaced by the National Commission for Health Education Credentialing in 1988. The charter certification phase was initiated in 1989, and 1,558 individuals became the first CHES group through document examination. A division board of directors and at-large commissioners were elected in 1989, and their terms began in 1990. This proceeded to an examination construction workshop in 1989 where the first certification exam for CHES was produced. In 1990, 644 candidates in 16 U.S. cities became CHES certified. At the same time, job descriptions began to include "CHES preferred," and in 1991, an executive director was employed full time. By 1992, there were 3,713 professionals designated as CHES certified. Different health organizations became CHES single providers for professional development and additional designations were added for multiple providers. NCHEC now has a full board of directors that is elected and a full-time executive director. While this was a national movement to improve the profession, it ultimately led to the establishment of the undergraduate competencies and the CHES designation for health professionals.[18]

On May 19, 2009, the National Commission for Health Education Credentialing passed a policy statement by the Board of Commissioners regarding an advanced credential known as **Master Certified Health Education Specialist (MCHES)**.[20] Many health organizations applauded the implementation of an advanced credential as a result of the Competencies Update Project verifying health educator at the advanced practice level.[4] The exam will be based on a scientific approach verifying the advanced roles and responsibilities of health educators. Implementation of the MCHES examination is scheduled to occur in October 2011.[4] Eligibility requirements for taking the exam are CHES and non-CHES health educators with 5 current consecutive years of health education practice and active CHES status. The MCHES experience documentation opportunity will be offered for a limited time to active CHES with 5 years of active status. Other eligibility requirements are available for those without 5 years of active CHES experience with current and consecutive practice in health education.[20]

REVISIONS FOR A COMPETENCY-BASED FRAMEWORK FOR HEALTH EDUCATORS-2006

The Responsibilities and Competencies for Undergraduate Health Educators were born in 1985 as a result of the National Task Force on the Preparation and Practice of Health Education to identify health skills and practices.[19] The original undergraduate standards of the health profession were adopted by many universities and associations/organizations. This version outlined seven basic responsibilities and competencies for undergraduate health educators and additional ones for advanced level health educators.

Competencies are defined as broad skills and minimum standards that generic health educators should be able to accomplish. They involve the ability to apply specific skills in working with health subject matter. As a result of a nationwide survey, some competencies were revised and additions were made. The National Health Educator Competency Update Project (CUP) from 1998 to 2004 re-examined the competencies and defined the health practice settings in an updated edition.[8] The seven basic updated health education competencies according to the 2006 CUP model include:[8]

1. Assess individual and community needs for health education
2. Plan effective strategies, interventions, and programs
3. Implement effective strategies, interventions, and programs
4. Conduct evaluation and research related to health education
5. Administer effective strategies, interventions, and programs
6. Serve as a health education resource person
7. Communicate and advocate for health and health education

These entry level standards and the advanced level competencies described are currently being revised from the 2006 version.[7] New competencies are expected in the future, according to Linda Lysoby,

---

Master Certified Health Education Specialist (MCHES): An advanced credential and practice level available for CHES health professionals, passed by the National Commission for Health Education Credentialing in 2009 by the Board of Commissioners.

Executive Director for the NCHEC (pers. comm. Linda Lysoby, March 2010).The present *Competency-Based Framework for Health Educators* are included in Appendix A.

DEVELOPMENT OF GRADUATE-LEVEL HEALTH COMPETENCIES

The Joint Committee for Graduate Standards was created in 1992 by the Society of Public Health Education (SOPHE) and the American Association for Health Education (AAHE), which together formed the SOPHE/AAHE Baccalaureate Approval Committee, or SABPAC. The task was to determine advanced-level training and the possibility of additional entry-level competencies. The consensus was that if a health educator possessed the entry-level responsibilities for undergraduate preparation and competencies, there should be newly developed ones for graduate-level preparation. This marked the beginning of "A Competency-Based Framework for Graduate-Level Health Educators."[9] According to the AAHE, the standards should improve the consistency of graduate training programs in health education, which is beneficial for students and professional academicians. The standards would specify for employers the unique roles and services of graduate-prepared health educators.[21]

This document specifically outlined the responsibilities of a graduate-level health educator. Graduate programs and health education professionals can use these guidelines for training, certification, and accreditation. The first seven competencies from the undergraduate competencies were incorporated into the document. New competencies and subcompetencies for advanced-level practitioners were added and revised in 1999. In addition, three competencies were added.[9] The levels of practice for health educators in the field were addressed for each competency and were designated as community setting, medical care setting, school setting, workplace setting, and college/university setting.[9]

A COMPETENCY-BASED FRAMEWORK FOR ADVANCED-LEVEL HEALTH EDUCATORS

Advanced-level students must possess all competencies delineated by the National Commission for Health Education Credentialing, Inc. in the updated 2006 document along with the entry level competencies. The competencies and subcompetencies are included in Appendix A. The advanced competencies were developed along with the entry level competencies. The competencies for the advance 1 level includes persons with baccalaureate and master's degree and 5 years of experience or more, and the advanced 2 level includes persons possessing doctoral degrees and 5 years or more experience. These competencies are currently being updated for the MCHES designation and new revisions should be released with the revisions for the entry level health competencies.[7]

ACCREDITATION

The Council for Higher Education Accreditation defines accreditation at the higher education level as "a collegial process of self-review and peer review for improvement of academic quality and public accountability of institutions and programs."[22(p2)] Accreditations is the primary way by which higher education institutions ensure quality programs in the United States. Accreditation is a form of self-regulation with self-examination and judgment by peers. Colleges, universities, and programs work cooperatively to develop standards, policies, and procedures.[22] It is measure of quality assurance and adherence to a minimum set of standards.[2] Accreditation is normally voluntary; however, state departments of higher education or student financial aid assistance can mandate that only accredited institutions and students receive funding.

There are several accrediting bodies for institutions or programs. The Association of Schools of Public Health was established in 1974, and its accreditation entity, the Council on Education for Public Health (CEPH) accredits schools and graduate programs of public health, as they train physicians who may become leaders for public health departments. The six guiding principles of CEPH are external peer review, self-evaluation, centrality of mission, focus on outcome, objectivity, and fairness to enhance quality in education.[22] The National Council for Accreditation of Teacher Education (NCATE) accredits a higher education unit or school, college, or department that has a preparatory program for school health educators. NCATE works in coordination with Specialty Professional Associations, which are the AAHE groups for reviewing health education programs in institutions that prepare and certify school health educators.[2] Outside of school health education, a coalition of national organizations, called the National Public Health Performance Standards Program, is undertaking strategies for implementing a voluntary accreditation for public health departments in higher education.

Accreditation seems to give recognition to higher education institutions by including an external review process. It could provide an advantage in recruitment of students and faculty, as well as grants and state funding. Also, some states mandate accreditation for institutions. Accreditation is a form of accountability because it demonstrates that students have acquired certain skills and that programs are high quality, incorporating competency and evidence-based practices.[2]

Although there is not a single entity for programs seeking accreditation, ways of developing such an entity are being examined. The SOPHE and AAHE professional organizations established the National Task Force of Accreditation for developing a more unified accreditation system for health programs at the undergraduate and graduate level.[2] While they established many goals, a new initiative is to make only students of accredited programs eligible for CHES certification. These discussions continue as they plan to establish a unified health education accreditation system.[2]

There are other accreditation agencies for universities and schools of education. The Southern Association of Colleges and Schools baccalaureate approval program for health is coordinated by SOPHE and AAHE.[23] SABPAC approves baccalaureate programs for undergraduate community health education programs. It will eventually be phased out by the SOPHE and AAHE association boards. The original task force recommendations specify that the new system of health education accreditation should occur through the CEPH for both undergraduate and graduate community health education programs. There would not be a new SABPAC program approval.[24]

Currently, CEPH accredits programs with masters' degrees in public health and community health. The NCATE is the standard of excellence for accreditation of teacher preparation programs at universities.[25] Once the new system is in place, NCATE will become the preferred and recommended accrediting entity for school health education programs at the undergraduate and graduate levels.[25]

ETHICAL CONSIDERATIONS FOR PROFESSIONAL COMPETENCE _____

Ethics is "the philosophy of morality" and includes "that part of philosophy that deals with questions concerning the nature and source of value, rightness, duty and related matters."[26(pxxii)] Ethics refers to values or standards of professional conduct. It is also that branch of philosophy that helps to discover if a conduct is right or wrong. Professional ethics are the expected moral and righteous behavior of professionals for the betterment of the clients and/or persons directly affected by these decisions in practice. Priorities are influenced by decision makers abiding by a professional code that in essence deciphers right from wrong. This basic principle guides many professions. Whether there are formal codes of ethics or unwritten codes of ethics, practitioners should always consider what is best for the client, the profession, and the common good.

In ethical studies, moral responsibility is defined by a person's ability to make moral decisions and answer to a moral authority. There is also a view that moral theory helps individuals know their duties, reflect on their own moral conduct, and value the adequacy of accepted standards.[26] Ethics is important in specifying a code of conduct that defines the profession. It establishes boundaries between appropriate and inappropriate health education practices. Ethical codes establish continuity of ethics. To be morally responsible, an intelligent person, capable of making moral distinctions, must not be coerced; rather, this person must be actively involved in a situation whereby his or her behavior is predicted in advance. Self-realization or aiming at a high level of unity through social cooperation defines a moral person.[26] There seems to be a lack of ethical unity in the health profession. There are always unresolved and controversial issues inherent to health education, research, and practice, but we are all obligated as professionals to police unethical conduct.

PRINCIPLES OF ETHICS _____

Certain values are inherent in codes of ethics, including autonomy, nonmalfeasance, beneficence, justice, utilitarianism, respect, and paternalism. These **principles of ethics** are described as follows:

1. *Autonomy.* The principle of autonomy is equality and respect for others. It requires respecting the individual freedom, liberty, and privacy of others.[27]
2. *Nonmalfeasance.* This principle means, above all, do no harm.[28] Inflicting or causing more problems, especially adversarial health problems, does not necessitate extreme measures. It is a respect for and avoidance of others' pain and suffering.
3. *Beneficence.* This principle means doing what is best or benefits the clients/patients/participants the most in a research setting, medical setting, university setting, health program, or other health settings. This is respect for a person's welfare.
4. *Justice.* This word originally meant conforming to the law. But evolving, this principle means impartiality and giving all individuals their due. Distributive justice requires that each person

---

Ethics: The values or standards of professional conduct.
Principles of ethics: The eight values of ethics: autonomy, nonmalfeasance, beneficence, justice, utilitarianism, respect, and paternalism.

be treated according to merit. All are treated fairly and in the same manner with prudence and benevolence. Justice is described as "the appropriate name for certain social utilities by which the general good is realized."[26(p654)] It is closely associated with utilitarianism. The true idea of justice, according to John Mill,[26(p658)] is to examine objects in the concrete to discover their common features. Justice is respect for the legal and moral rights of others. It implies that taking another's moral rights by illegal or legal means is wrong. It involves equality and impartiality in the treatment of persons and claims.[26]

5. *Utilitarianism.* As stated by McLeroy, Bibeau, Steckler, and Glanz, "According to this principle, persons should perform the individual act or implement the social policy among the alternative policies which will result in the best balance of benefits over harms for all affected parties."[27(p314)] This definition recommends that we make judgments concerning the most reliable means available to promote the general welfare and respect for all participants. It requires weighing the bad over the good and choosing the best alternative for benefit versus harm.[27] An act is judged on its righteousness and or fairness from the utility principle, not from its basic form in a societal setting. John Mill, in 1863, said acts are right or good if they ensure and produce the greatest happiness for the largest number of persons.[26]

6. *Respect.* Respect relates to self-autonomy and deferring to patient and/or client choices and following their wishes for treatment options and care. It refers to humane consideration for personal decision making without being judgmental or condescending.

7. *Paternalism.* Paternalism means that clients have the right to be protected and treated with kindness and caring. This principle defines exactly how all participants should be treated and is a major responsibility for health practitioners.

ETHICAL PRINCIPLES IN HEALTH PROGRAMS AND RESEARCH

The provisions of a democratic society include the use of informed consent, decisions on how policy changes affect people, and the idea of personal decision making or free will. Morals are social, and social institutions have a responsibility to consider these provisions. They are part of the social environment— ever-changing, ever-present actualities. Ideal principles influence values, decision making, and obligations and provide humans with a foundation or moral code of conduct.[26] There are certain ethical principles that health educators should globally enforce in programs and research. Health educators discuss and espouse many principles that are vital to the profession, including but not limited to the following:

1. Voluntary and informed consent of all clients (participants) is required, and all participants are free to withdraw at any time.
2. All risks must be communicated and revealed ahead of time to the participants. The degree of risk cannot exceed the importance of the problems solved; the results must justify the methods— but not at the expense of the clients or participants.
3. Unnecessary suffering/injury must be avoided. Extensive prevention efforts are made to protect against injury, disability, or death. Investigators must terminate the program if any injury, disability, or death occurs.

4. The research must be conducted by qualified persons, and confidentiality and anonymity is preserved always. Confidential files are locked and secured. Files no longer relevant are destroyed after 5 years unless it is a longevity study.
5. The results must not help some participants at the expense of the other participants.
6. There must be meaningful results expected, and these must be a contribution to the health profession.
7. Using control groups is recommended for comparison of groups and providing proof that the program results were actual and not caused by an unmeasured variable.
8. Investigators must not compromise the participants' health status, religious practices, or cultural mores to perform the research.
9. Investigators must be moral and ethical at all times when approaching and working with clients or participants. Investigators must not be biased in assuming causes of behavior change. There must be no "victim blaming," or blaming the clients for their health problems or socio-economic levels even if the behavior or condition was self-inflicted, caused by an unhealthy lifestyle or behavior, and/or a result or an addiction. The investigator must realize that behavior change can be affected by other personal and/or societal factors, access to services, cultural and religious beliefs, poverty (SES), education, literacy, environment, and/or policy.
10. Investigators must not verbalize or be prejudicial in any way to the participants and must refrain at all times from any individual biases about participants, outcomes, or results.
11. Investigators may not use coercion or coerce compliance from any client or participant at any time.
12. Investigators must not be biased in assuming causes of behavior change bias and no assumptions that a change in behavior is the only factor involved. The investigator must realize that behavior change can be affected by other factors such as personal factors, society, access to services, environment, or policy
13. Investigators must always protect the confidentiality and anonymity of the participant and/or client at all times.

ETHICAL DOCUMENTS

The Nuremberg Code of 1947 outlined specific research and human rights principles in medical research.[29] It also paved the way for requiring **human subjects review boards** for governmental agencies, universities, research labs, and other research entities involving human subjects. It states, "The voluntary consent of the human subject is absolutely essential."[29(p1)] It was spurred by horrific war crimes and medical experiments against human subjects during World War II. However, quarantine laws for patients of certain diseases, such as Hansen's disease, in the United States and other countries still existed, and human rights violations occurred as a result of these medical quarantine laws.[30]

> **Human subjects review boards:** These are governments, agencies, universities, medical centers, and other institutional review boards that monitor all programs and research involving human subjects.

The abuses during wartime motivated a movement by the United Nations in 1948 to pass the Universal Declaration of Human Rights for the protection of human subjects in medical research. It states the following:

> Now, therefore the General Assembly proclaims this Universal Declaration of Human Rights as a common standard of achievement for all peoples and all nations, to the end that every individual and every organ of society, keeping this Declaration constantly in mind, shall strive by teaching and education to promote respect for these rights and freedoms and by progressive measures, national and international, to secure their universal and effective recognition and observance, both among the peoples of Member States themselves and among the peoples of territories under their jurisdiction.[31(p1)]

The Helsinki Declaration of 1964 by the World Medical Association was another document pertaining to governmental monitoring of all funded medical research. It is "a statement of ethical principles for medical research involving human subjects, including research on identifiable human material and data."[32(p1)]

In 1974 the U.S. government passed a law, PL 93-348, The National Research Act. It resulted in human subjects review boards for the U.S. government and formed the National Commission for the Protection of Human Subjects for Biomedical and Behavioral Research and the Office for Human Research Protections.[33] The Code of Federal Regulations, Title 45, Public Welfare, and Part 46, Protection of Human Subjects, were the U.S. legislative efforts supporting this office.

CODES OF ETHICS

For the health profession, there were two codes of ethics for several years in the United States. The Society for Public Health Education in 1983 and the AAHE in 1994 each established a separate code of ethics for health. The National Commission for Health Education and the Coalition of National Health Education Organizations (CNHEO) cosponsored a conference in 1995 entitled The Health Education Profession in the Twenty-First Century: Setting the Stage.[34] Participants were members of the CNHEO in 2001. The associations met at the conference and agreed to work on a unified code of ethics. A National Ethics Task Force was established with individuals from all representative health organizations to review the two existing codes of ethics and comprise a common code. A first draft of the Unified Code of Ethics was presented in 1997, and several more drafts occurred. **A Code of Ethics for the Health Education Profession** was approved by the coalition delegates in 1999.[35] This code is still in use today but is currently being revised according to CNHEO (see Appendix B) (C. Ledingham, pers. communication, Jan. 22, 2010).

Code of Ethics for the Health Education Profession: A document outlining the ethical standards of conduct and rights and protection of human subjects health research, teaching, and programs.

CONFLICTS OF INTEREST AND ETHICAL ISSUES IN RESEARCH, PROGRAMS, AND TEACHING

Ethical disagreements involve belief and attitude, but attitude is the distinctive element in the question of ethical behavior or conduct. Ethical judgment should be justified by the reason of the action. According to the National Academy of Sciences, three principles constitute ethical problems: misconduct, questionable research practices, and unethical behavior.[36] There are several areas of ethics breaches in university research relating to conflicts of interest, research, and teaching.

Conflicts of interest in unethical behavior involve cases in which the research serves the professor's ends and not the student goals, contracts with vendors or manufacturers that could lead to research bias, and the use of students as test subjects without informed consent or information. Questionable research practices involve plagiarism, date or data fabrication, inaccurate documentation, failure to report discrepancies and insignificant results, citations of fraud, publication bias, inaccurate data recording or changing statistical data for more favorable results, and submission of a manuscript to numerous journals at the same time.

Misconduct in teaching includes not involving students in the research process; setting one's own agenda; not returning students' work in timely fashion; not providing critique of students work; using different standards for students based on gender, race, religion, disability or other factors; allowing student plagiarism or cheating; not giving students appropriate authorship; biased and nonobjective presentation of information; and selection of readings that are dated, biased, or inaccurate. These are the main unethical practices that professionals in higher education need to be aware of and strictly avoid. A health professional must always act ethically; and ethical decision making is paramount for all health professionals.

HUMAN SUBJECTS REVIEW BOARDS

Health professional agencies and organizations, medical research centers, and higher education institutions need to monitor research efforts and report any unethical conduct or misconduct to the proper authorities. Every university or college is required to have an institutional human subjects review board, which should act as a deterrent to unethical behavior. Health agencies and organizations including those affiliated with governments, countries, states, or cities should also have human subjects review boards to monitor all health programs involving human subjects.

Medical research centers also have review boards. The boards review requests and grant approvals, require modifications of grants, or disapprove the research activities covered by this policy. The boards require faculty and students in universities or professionals in health agencies/organizations and medical research centers to submit a formal request to use human subjects in research before conducting any research and/or experiments. The request is reviewed by the board, and permission may be given or denied, or revisions may be requested before re-reviewing. This process requires information on human subjects and informed consent and protects the rights and welfare of subjects, analyzing if the degree of risk is appropriate. The request and the notification are in writing. Any questions or explanations for denial are addressed in writing. The investigator(s) is normally given an opportunity to respond. This process enables monitoring of the research, and reviews are usually required after 1 year if the research continues. A sample human subjects review board form is provided in **Table 7–1**.

Table 7–1   SAMPLE HUMAN SUBJECTS REVIEW FORM

Lamar University

Human Subjects Review Board

Cover Sheet for

Approval of Research Using Human Subjects

Date: _____

Title of research project: _____

Principal Investigator: _____

Department: _____   Email: _____

Campus Mailing Address: _____   Campus Phone: _____

If this is a student proposal, name of faculty advisor: _____

Requested Review: __ Exempt Review

                         __ Expedited Review

                         __ Full Board Review

Does this project involve minors, pregnant women, prisoners, or other special populations?

__ Yes __ No

Comments:

_____

_____

_____

_____

Research Office

Date Received: _____

To Be Reviewed by: _____

···

Lamar University

Request for Approval from Human Subjects Review Board

1. Description of Project (attach additional information as needed)

   a. Briefly describe the population of human subjects involved (e.g., university students, community members, school children, prisoners, pregnant women). Indicate if participation is voluntary or not.

TABLE 7–1   *(Continued)*

b. Briefly describe research procedures and data collection techniques (e.g., interview, questionnaire, observation).
c. Briefly present the objectives of the research (e.g., present in lay terms hypothesis to be tested).
2. Subject recruitment (in addition to the information requested below, submit verbatim copies of all letters, notices, advertisements, etc., with an outline of all oral presentations to be used):
   a. Direct person-to-person solicitation   _____
   b. Telephone solicitation   _____
   c. Newspaper solicitation   _____
   d. Letters of solicitation   _____
   e. Posted notices of solicitation   _____
   f. Other (explain)   _____
   g. List all criteria for including subjects.
   h. List all criteria for excluding subjects.

3. Benefits and costs to subjects:
   a. Indicate what, if any, benefits may accrue for each of the following (note: financial payment to subjects is considered a benefit).
      i. Benefits to human subjects involved
      ii. Benefits to individuals who are not subjects and generalized benefits to society
   b. If subjects are to be paid, present financial details (amount, method of disbursement, payment schedule, financial effect on subjects who withdraw from participation)
   c. Estimated participation costs to each subject
      i. Time (total time commitment for duration of project)
      ii. Money

4. Basis of claim for exemption or expedited review: To qualify for an exemption from a full evaluation by the Lamar University Human Subjects Review Board, at least one of the following must apply:
   ____ a. The research will be conducted only in established or commonly accepted educational settings (e.g., classrooms) and involves normal educational practices such as research on regular and special education instructional strategies, or research on the effectiveness of, or the comparison among instructional techniques, curricula, or classroom management methods.
   ____ b. The research will be conducted using only questionnaire or interview survey methods, and the subjects are elected or appointed by public officials or candidates for public office.
   ____ c. The research is limited to the collection and study of existing data, documents, records, or pathological or diagnostic specimens available to the public.
   ____ d. The research is limited to the collection and study of data obtained using only the following techniques, and the data or information obtained will be recorded in such a manner that subjects cannot be identified, directly or indirectly, through identifiers linked with the subjects. Check below the technique(s) that apply:
      ____ The data will be obtained through the use of educational tests (cognitive, diagnostic, aptitude, achievement, etc.).
      ____ Data will be obtained by observing the public behavior of subjects.
      ____ Data will be obtained through survey or interview procedures.
      ____ The data will be obtained from existing documents, records, or pathological or diagnostic specimens.

(Continues)

TABLE 7–1   *(Continued)*

___ e. The research is limited to the collection and study of data obtained by:
    ___ Observing the public behavior of the participants using survey or interview procedures and (both of the following must apply if this basis is to qualify for an exemption):
        ___ The information collected about the subjects' behavior does not involve sensitive subjects such as illegal or immoral conduct, drug or alcohol use, sexual behavior, mental illness, or other possibly embarrassing subjects.
        ___ The information collected, if it became known to outsiders, could not reasonably be expected to place the subjects at risk of civil or criminal liability, or be damaging to the subjects' social or financial standing or employability.

5. Statement of risk, request/recommendation for exemption:
The undersigned certify that they believe that the conduct of the above described research constitutes no more than minimal risk of physical or emotional harm, or social or legal embarrassment to participating human subjects and request that the above described research be considered exempt from full review by the Lamar University Human Subjects Review Board:

_____   _____
Principal Investigator(s)   Date

_____   _____
Principal Investigator(s)   Date

_____   _____
Principal Investigator(s)   Date

_____   _____
Faculty Sponsor (if the research is carried out by students)   Date

_____   _____
Department Chair   Date

Source: Courtesy of Lamar University, Research and Sponsored Programs Administration, Beaumont, TX.

Health programs involving human subjects should adhere to the same type of review boards as other professionals. The WHO monitors health and human rights, as well as treaty negotiations. The WHO includes in *Key Elements of Research Ethics and Guidelines* that all health and biomedical research must conform to the national and international scientific and ethical standards. A series entitled Health and Human Rights by WHO is published with updates and new information.[37] The "25 Questions in Health and Human Rights" document, series 1, discusses trends in globalization and concern with protection of the vulnerable members of society. The document calls for compatibility of programs and policies among government entities to protect the rights of humans. Free trade, international markets, deregulations, industrial developments, reduction of state involvement in economic affairs, and global markets for prescription medication mean governments cannot control all health-related factors and must pass laws and policies to protect their citizens from exploitation. As such, exploitations endangering health such as lack of access, conflicts of war, disease, emergencies, natural disasters, women's rights, economic rights, social rights, racial rights, children's rights, and other international problems must be addressed to protect global health and human rights.

Health practices for assessing, planning, implementing, and evaluating need to be grounded within the laws and regulations that frame health human rights and respect for human dignity without discrimination. The United Nations guidelines say that human rights violations must be promptly and confidentially transmitted to the Office of the United Nations High Commissioner for Human Rights.[37]

The U.S. Department of Health and Human Services also requires review boards for all research and/or experiments using humans. The National Institutes of Health has a review board guidebook for institutions, and there is a designated Office for Human Research Protections in the U.S. government.[33] All agencies and organizations where health educators practice should have a human subjects review board to protect the rights of the participants in health programs.

Each health professional should also abide by the Code of Ethics for the Health Education Profession[35] and hold other colleagues accountable to that code. The rights of human subjects should be protected no matter what happens in health research, teaching, and programs.

A classic 1989 article by Roland Lamartine, entitled "First, Do No Harm," provides a statement concerning human subjects research—one that every health educator should adopt.[28] Health educators also have a professional responsibility to abide by the Code of Ethics and human subjects review boards and to report any breach of ethics to the proper authorities. While there is no national professional body that reviews ethics for health educators, they are subject to the ethics professed in legal documents for all researchers. As a profession, perhaps a professional review board needs to be established worldwide to protect human participants in research, police unethical health conduct, and enforce authorized penalties.

HEALTH EDUCATION AS A STANDARD OCCUPATIONAL CLASSIFICATION

Health education meets the definition of a profession based on the criteria listed for a profession. According to the 2001 progress report of the Coalition of National Health Education Organizations, these criteria include "a common body of knowledge, a research base, a code of ethics, a common set of skills, quality assurance, and standards of practice."[3] The U.S. Department of Labor, Bureau of Labor Statistics, designated health educator as a **Standard Occupational Classification (SOC)**, identified as SOC 21-1091, in 2001 and revised it in 2009.[38] This means it can be listed as an IRS designation as an occupation. As a result, the federal government and states will be obliged to collect data on geographic locations, salaries, and data for the health profession. This designation will give credibility to the profession and allow for more detailed information on practicing health educators in the United States. The designation also includes a description of the skills a health educator must possess. The U.S. Department of Labor, Bureau of Labor Statistics (2010–2011), describes a health educator in the SOC 21-1091 document as follows: "Health educators work to encourage healthy lifestyles and wellness through educating individuals and communities about behaviors than can prevent disease, injury, and

---

Standard Occupational Classification (SOC) for health educators: A designation of health education as an occupation with a description of the skills necessary according to the U.S. Department of Labor, Bureau of Labor Statistics (2001); identified as SOC 21-1091.

Thought Concept

Why are certain standards of practice necessary in a profession? How does conformity to these practices involve ethics?

other health problems."[38(p1)] The document expands on the assessment, planning, implementing, and evaluation skills that are possessed by the profession. It includes training, employment, projections, and earnings. While there are many more responsibilities for health educators than are mentioned here, this designation gives credibility to the profession and puts a professional "face" on the designation of health educator.

PROGRESS IN HEALTH EDUCATION

While many strides have been taken toward stability, ethical practice, and standardization of practice and ethics, many more are anticipated in the future. The new CHES designation and continued movements by health educators and professional organizations must continue.[39] Ethics and health education research and practice need to continue to be monitored and evaluated. Research articles discuss ethics in the service of students;[40] changing risky behaviors in uncooperative participants;[41] research issues confronting professionals;[42] and biomedical, clinical, school, worksite,[43] and informed consent.[44] Article II of the Code of Ethics for Health Educators states that health educators are responsible for professional behavior and promoting ethical conduct.[35] The responsibilities and competencies for entry and advanced health educators raised the bar for professional preparations, and CHES improved and gave credibility to the profession and the MCHES designation is a milestone.[7,10] Approximately 15,000 professionals have earned the CHES credential since 1989 in almost 300 different institutions.[18] Some health accreditation agencies are in transition for the betterment of the profession as quality assurance methods are explored and put in place. The National Task Force on Accreditation in Health Education called for a profession-wide consensus for the implementation of a unified, coordinated accreditation process with key partners such as professional associations/organizations, governments, and interested philanthropic orgnizations.[45]

The WHO defines health education as facilitating "consciously constructed opportunities for learning involving some form of communication designed to improve health literacy, including improving knowledge, and developing life skills which are conducive to individual and community health."[46] To continue this quest requires professionals committed to quality standards of practice and evidence-based evaluations of the health professionals, the profession, the practice settings, and the institutions of higher education. Challenges and concerns to the profession will continue to surface, and health educators must continue the quest for improvement, quality research, revisions, constant monitoring, stringent ethical codes, increased quality assurance, and continued upgrades. Ensuring a standard of excellence for health professionals, preparatory institutions, and the practice is an ongoing process.

SUMMARY

- A profession is an employment that requires specific learning and training.
- The U.S. Department of Labor designated health educator as a standard occupational classification in 2001 and expanded this in 2009.
- There are many ways to certify professions, professionals, and organizations, including accreditation, licensure, certification, registration, and credentialing.

- Standards identify the expected characteristics of a profession.
- The CHES credentialing movement is solidified and is a preferred criterion for employment. A new designation, MCHES, is in progress.
- There are 7 basic responsibilities of entry-level health educators and advanced level health educators as identified by the National Commission for Health Education Credentialing, Inc. For each responsibility, competencies and subcompetencies are designated.
- Professional preparation for health educators at the undergraduate level and graduate level differs in degree programs and degree designations.
- Professional ethics include the principles of autonomy, nonmalfeasance, beneficence, justice, respect, utilitarianism, and paternalism. There are certain ethical principles that health educators should enforce in programs and research.
- The Code of Ethics for the Health Education Profession was approved by the coalition delegates in 1999 and is the designated code of ethics for the profession.
- Ethical issues in research and teaching should be of concern to professional health educators.
- A breach of ethics such as misconduct, questionable research practices, and unethical behavior should be reported.
- The health profession needs an agency to police unethical practices.

CONCEPTUAL TERMS

Licensure
Certification
Credentialing
Individual credentialing
Program credentialing
Registration
Education standards
Professional standards
Informatics

Master Certified Health Education Specialist
   (MCHES)
Ethics
Principles of ethics
Human subjects review boards
Code of Ethics for the Health Education
   Profession
Standard Occupational Classification (SOC) for
   health educators

REFLECTIVE THINKING

Ethical dilemmas are always the most difficult to solve. They not only involve facts, but human emotions and differences in beliefs for some. As a health educator, you will face many ethical and moral dilemmas. An administrator once told me that was why she decided to return to full-time teaching. She said the ethical dilemmas were becoming more and more complex, and she was tired of using all her efforts on a situation that someone could have resolved or not even started if they were ethical.

Consider the following scenario. You are a program manager in a new community health program that started in your hometown. It is an exercise and dietary program with pain management techniques for persons diagnosed with rheumatoid arthritis. Your friend's mother has been diagnosed with the disease. The participants are randomly selected from people 65–75 years of age and identified by their physicians as patients who could benefit and possibly manage their pain better with this program. Even though you know this person's mother applied for the program, the identities of the actual participants in the program have not yet been released. Your friend calls you and says she really wants her mother in the program. You explain how the participants are chosen, but she contends that you could "pull some strings" to get her mother enrolled in the program. What do you say to someone who is trying to coerce you to go against your ethical principles? Even if you knew her mother was or was not chosen for the program, can you tell her? Are you obligated to stand by the ethical code even if it risks losing a friendship? Do you try to get her mother into the program if she is not accepted? Do you notify your supervisor of the conversation with your friend?

Consider another scenario. You are a health teacher in the public schools. A child comes to school with a black eye and gives you two different versions of how the injury occurred. You go to the principal's office to file a formal report and notify authorities. The principal says that this child's father is a physician and he knows the family well. The principal reminds you that the parents are outstanding citizens of this community and regular churchgoers. The principal asks that you forego the usual procedure of filling out a formal report, and he says he will discuss it with the parents and that you have no further responsibility in this matter. Your principal also says that you would not want to embarrass yourself if you were wrong. Besides, the principal states, "I may retire in the near future, and I don't want any major problems at this point." You know that teachers are legally bound to report suspected child abuse of any kind in a formal written school district report and report it to the proper authorities (i.e., the Department of Child and Family Services). If you risk going against your principal, it could mean a transfer to another school the next year, a bad review, or you could be fired. Because this principal is also a good friend of the school board president, it could mean there will be future problems for you if you seek other employment in another district. What would you do in this case? Are you ethically and legally bound to report this? Can we judge persons suspected of child abuse differently if they are from a "good and religious family"? How do you counter the statement about being "embarrassed" if you are wrong? Why is being wrong about child abuse a bad thing? Don't you want to be wrong? Can you handle the pressure if you are wrong? Would the alternative be better (this means a child is being abused and no adult is intervening for the minor child)?

CONCEPTUAL LEARNING

1. Identify the characteristics of a profession.
2. Discuss the CHES credentialing movement. Defend the need for an advanced credential, the MCHES.
3. Compare the professional preparation for health educators at the undergraduate level and graduate level for two different universities.
4. Assemble a list of professional preparation skills needed for all health educators.
5. Explain the basic principles defined in the code of ethics for the profession.
6. Evaluate two different ethical issues in health education. Why should they be of concern to professional health educators?
7. Perform an Internet search for national laws that were passed to protect human subjects. Devise any modifications you feel may be needed. Demonstrate the reason(s) these national laws were necessary.

REFERENCES

1. Longman Group Limited. (1993). *New concise Webster's dictionary: A comprehensive guide to the English language for home, office, and school.* New York: Modern Publishing.

2. Patterson, S. M., & Vitello, E. M. (2006). Key influences shaping health education: Progress toward accreditation. *The Health Education Monograph, 23*(1), 14–19.

3. Coalition of National Health Education Organizations. (2001). *The health education profession in the 21st century progress report 1995–2001.* Retrieved March 8, 2010, from www.cnheo.org/PDF%20files/21stCentury.pdf

4. Dennis, D. (2009). Health educators comment about the upcoming MCHES credential. *The CHES Bulletin, 20,* 2–3.

5. Cleary, H. P. (1995). *The credentialing of health educators: An historical account 1970–1990.* Whitehall, PA: The National Commission for Health Education Credentialing, Inc.

6. National Commission for Health Education Credentialing, Inc. (2002). *Main menu.* Retrieved March 8, 2010, from http://www.nchec.org/

7. National Commission for Health Education Credentialing, Inc., Society for Public Health Education, & American Association for Health Education. (2006). *A competency-based framework for health educators–2006.* Whitehall, PA: NCHEC.

8. National Commission for Health Education Credentialing, Inc. (1996). *A competency-based framework for professional development of certified health education.* New York: Author.

9. American Association for Health Education, National Commission for Health Education Credentialing, Inc., & Society for Public Health Education. (1999). *A competency-based framework for graduate level health educators.* Reston, VA: Author.

10. Joint Committee on National Health Education Standards. (2007). *National health education standards: Achieving excellence* (2nd ed). Athens, GA: American Cancer Society.

11. Taub, A. (1993). Credentialing: The basics. *Journal of Health Education, 24*(5), 261–262.

12. United States Office of Education and Research Information. (1994). *National Education Goals archived information.* Retrieved March 8, 2010, from http://www.ed.gov/bulletin/summer1994/goals.html

13. United States Office of Education and Research Information. (1994). *H.R. 1804 Goals 2000: Educate America Act archived information.* Retrieved March 8, 2010, from http://www.ed.gov/legislation/GOALS2000/TheAct/intro.html

14. Joint Committee on National Health Education Standards. (1995). *National health education standards: Achieving health literacy.* Athens, GA: American Cancer Society.

15. National Center for Chronic Disease Prevention and Health Promotion, Centers for Disease Control and Prevention. (2007). *Health education curriculum analysis tool (HECAT).* Retrieved March 8, 2010, from http://www.cdc.gov/nccdphp/dash/rtc/index.htm

16. National Center for Chronic Disease Prevention and Health Promotion Data and Statistics. (2008). *YRBSS: Youth Risk Behavior Surveillance System.* Retrieved March 8, 2010, from http://www.cdc.gov/HealthyYouth/yrbs/index.htm

17. National Center for Chronic Disease Prevention and Health, Centers for Disease Control and Prevention. (2008). *Healthy youth! Coordinated School Health Program.* Retrieved March 8, 2010, from http://www.cdc.gov/HealthyYouth/CSHP/

18. McKenzie, J. F., & Seabert, D. M. A retrospective review of those who hold the certified health education specialist (CHES) credential. *American Journal of Health Studies, 24*(2), 2009.

19. National Task Force on the Preparation and Practice of Health Education. (1985). *A framework for the development of competency based curricula for entry-level health educators.* New York: National Commission for Health Education Credentialing, Inc.

20. National Commission for Health Education Credentialing, Inc. (2009). *Press release: NCHEC board of commissioners pass policy statement regarding the advanced level credential.* Retrieved May 15, 2009, from http://www.nchec.org/

21. American Association for Health Education. *Graduate health education. Standards.* Reston, VA: Author.

22. Council for Higher Education Accreditation. (2006). *About CHEA: CHEA at a glance.* Retrieved March 8, 2010, from http://www.chea.org/default.asp?link=7

23. Southern Association of Colleges and Schools. (2006). *SOPHE, AAHE Baccalaureate Program Approval Program.* Retrieved August 27, 2009, from http://www.sacs.org/

24. Society of Public Health Educators. (2005). *Update on SABPAC and accreditation progress in health education.* Retrieved August 20, 2009, from http://www.sophe.org/Acrobat/sabpac statement_mar25_2.doc

25. National Council for Accreditation of Teacher Education. (1997–2009). *NCATE: The standard of excellence in teacher preparation* (In *About NCATE*). Retrieved March 8, 2010, from http://www.ncate.org/public/aboutN-CATE.asp

26. MaGill, F. N., & McGreal, I. P. (Eds.) (1961). *Masterpieces of world philosophy in summary form.* New York: Harpers and Brothers.

27. McLeroy, M. W., Bibeau, D., Steckler, A., & Glanz, K. (1988). An ecological perspective on health promotion programs. *Health Education Quarterly, 15,* 351–377.

28. Lamarine, R. (1989). First, do no harm. *Health Education,* August/September, 22–25.

29. United States Department of Health and Human Services. (1949). *Trials of war criminals before the Nuremberg Military Tribunals under Control Council Law* (10[2]). Washington, DC: U.S. Government Printing Office.

30. Hernandez, B. L. M., Vengurlekar, R., Kelkar, A., & Thomas, G. (2009). The legacy of Carville: A history of the last leprosarium in the U.S. *American Journal of Health Studies, 24*(2).

31. United Nations. (1948). *The Universal Declaration of Human Rights.* Retrieved March 8, 2010, from http://www.un.org/en/documents/udhr/

32. The World Medical Association. (1964). *The Helsinki Declaration of 1964.* Retrieved May 13, 2009, from http://wma.net/en/20activities/10ethics/10helsinki/index.html

33. United States Department of Health and Human Services, Office for Human Research Protections. (2009). *IRB registration and assurance filing procedures general information.* Retrieved July 25, 2009, from http://www.hhs.gov/ohrp/

34. Coalition of National Health Education Organizations. (2001). The health education profession in the twenty-first century: Setting the stage. *Journal of Health Education, 27*(6), 3, 357–364.

35. Coalition of National Health Education Organizations. (1999). *Code of ethics for the health education profession.* Retrieved March 8, 2010, from http://www.cnheo.org/

36. Swazey, J., Anderson, M., & Louis, K. (1993). A survey of doctoral candidates and faculty raises important questions about the ethical environment of graduate education and research. *American Scientist,* November/December.

37. World Health Organization. (2009). 25 questions in health and human rights. *Health and Human Rights,* series 1. Retrieved July 26, 2009, from http://www.who.int/hhr/information

38. Bureau of Labor Statistics, United States Department of Labor. (2009). Standard Occupational Classification, 21-1091.00 health educators. In *Occupational outlook handbook 2010–2011.* Retrieved March 8, 2010, from http://www.bls.gov/oco/ocos063.htm#nature

39. Dennis, D. L., & Lysoby, L. (2006). Credentialing and professional preparation in health education: From yesterday into tomorrow. *The Health Education Monograph, 23*(1), 22–27.

40. Price, J. H., Dake, J. A., & Teljohann, S. K. (2001). Ethical issues regarding service: Perceptions of health education faculty. *American Journal of Health Education, 32*(4), 208–215.

41. Sciaccca, J., Dennis, D. L., & Black, D. R. (204). Are interventions for informed, efficacious, precontemplators unethical? *American Journal of Health Education, 35*(6), 322–327.

42. Elliott, D., & Stern, J. E. (1997). *Research ethics: A reader.* Hanover, NH: University Press of New England.

43. Pigg, M. R. (1994). Ethical issues of scientific inquiry in health science education. *Eta Sigma Gamma Monograph, 12*(2), 1–162.

44. Price, J. H., Drake, J. A., & Islam, R. (2001). Selected ethical issues in research and publication: Perceptions of health education faculty. *Health Education and Behavior, 28*(1), 51–64.

45. Allegrante, J. P., Airhihenbuwa, C. O., Auld, M. E., et al. (2004). Toward a unified system of accreditation for professional preparation in health education: Final report of the National Task Force on Accreditation in Health Education. *Health Education and Behavior, 31,* 668–683.

46. World Health Organization. (1998). List of basic terms. *Health promotion glossary*. (p.4) Retrieved March 8, 2010, from http://www.who.int/hpr/NPH/docs/hp_glossary_en.pdf

ENHANCED READINGS

American Association for Health Education, National Commission for Health Education Credentialing, Inc., & Society for Public Health Education. (1999). *A competency-based framework for graduate-level health educators*. Reston, VA: Author.

Joint Committee on National Health Education Standards. (2007). *National health education standards: Achieving excellence* (2nd. ed). Athens, GA: American Cancer Society.

National Commission for Health Education Credentialing, Inc. (1996). *A competency-based framework for professional development of certified health education specialist*. New York: Author.

National Center for Chronic Disease Prevention and Health Promotion, Centers for Disease Control and Prevention. (2007). *Health education curriculum analysis tool (HECAT)*. Retrieved April 27, 2009, from http://www.cdc .gov/nccdphp/dash/rtc/index.htm

National Center for Chronic Disease Prevention and Health, Centers for Disease Control and Prevention. (2008). *Healthy youth! Coordinated School Health Program*. Retrieved March 8, 2010, from http://www.cdc.gov/ HealthyYouth/CSHP/

National Center for Chronic Disease Prevention and Health Promotion Data and Statistics. (2008). *YRBSS: Youth Risk Behavior Surveillance System*. Retrieved March 8, 2010, from http://www.cdc.gov/HealthyYouth/yrbs/ index.htm

RELEVANT WEB SITES

Bureau of Labor Statistics, United States Department of Labor. (2009). Standard Occupational Classification, 21-1091.00 health educators. In *Occupational outlook handbook 2010–2011*. Retrieved March 8, 2010, from http://www.bls.gov/oco/ocos063.htm#nature

National Center for Chronic Disease Prevention and Health Promotion, Centers for Disease Control and Prevention. (2007). *Health education curriculum analysis tool (HECAT)*. Retrieved April 27, 2009, from http://www.cdc .gov/nccdphp/dash/rtc/index.htm

National Center for Chronic Disease Prevention and Health, Centers for Disease Control and Prevention. (2008). *Healthy youth! Coordinated school health program*. Retrieved March 8, 2010, from http://www.cdc.gov/ HealthyYouth/CSHP/

National Center for Chronic Disease Prevention and Health Promotion Data and Statistics. (2008). *YRBSS: Youth Risk Behavior Surveillance System*. Retrieved March 8, 2010, from http://www.cdc.gov/HealthyYouth/yrbs/ index.htm

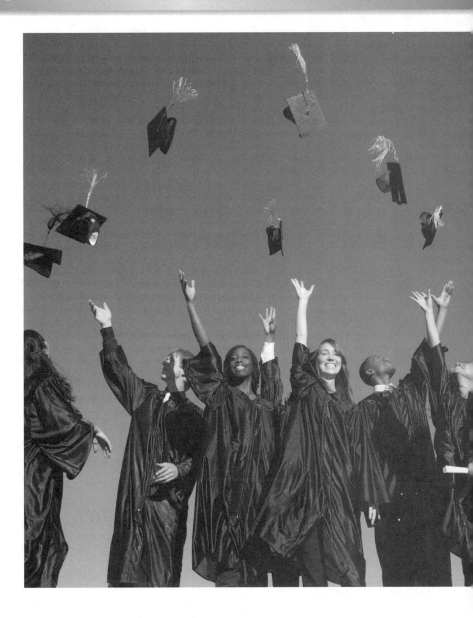

CHAPTER 8

Predictions, Technology, and Future Health Professional Career Objectives

OBJECTIVES AND ASSESSMENTS

This chapter meets the following National Commission for Health Education Credentialing, Inc., Society for Public Health Education, and American Association for Health Education Competency-Based Framework for Entry Level and Advanced Level Health Educator Competencies.* The learner will:

6. Serve as a health education resource person
7. Communicate and advocate for health and health education.

This chapter meets the following learning objectives:
1. Define health education career practice settings.
2. Describe the current and future status of health education as an up-and-coming profession.
3. Write a resume, and design and construct an e-portfolio.

INTRODUCTION

Deciding on a degree in community or public health takes time and may involve considering the career options you wish to pursue. There are different bachelor-, master-, and doctoral-level degrees available. It may seem confusing. However, an informed decision ensures that your career goals are reached with

---

*Source: Reprinted with permission of NCHEC.

National Commission for Health Education Credentialing, Inc. (NCHEC), Society for Public Health Education (SOPHE), & American Association for Health Education (AAHE). (2006). *A competency-based framework for health educators-2006*. Whitehall, PA: NCHEC.

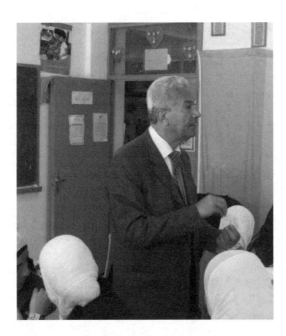

FIGURE 8–1   Dr. Muhammad Antaki at a Community-Based Initiative at Suf Camp (Palestinian Refugee Camp at Jordan)

the proper professional preparation, training, and **education**. An e-resume and e-portfolio are necessary in today's technological world to present your skills and expertise to a future employer.

The health education profession is in constant transition, with new opportunities and improvements; unfortunately, new threats may cause a paradigm change at any given time. The ability to adjust and reach salient resources to understand new changes or build new research-based programs for effective practice is necessary. Researching online requires a methodical and analytical approach to determine the best information on health programs.

What is the job of health practitioners? According to the AAHE:

> Health educators plan, implement and evaluate the effects of educational programs and strategies designed to improve the health of individuals, families and communities. Health educators work in schools and universities; federal, state and local public health departments; hospitals and managed care settings; voluntary groups; businesses; international organizations; and other settings.[1(p1)]

See Dr. Mohammad Antaki, of the United Nations Relief and Works Agency (UNWRA) in Amman, Jordan for a sample health program led by a health practitioner (**Figure 8–1**). He is shown

---

Education: Formal knowledge training and skills provided in grades K–12 and higher education settings.

speaking at a community-based refugee camp. This program is an example of a health practitioner and administrator making a difference. Dr. Antaki is president of the Jordanian Gaucher Association and chairman of the CBRC Marka and was instrumental in formulating the "Disabled Persons Camp Campaign" at the Suf Camp in Jordan on January 6, 2010. This program was successful in facilitating an educational campaign and an environmental modification for children with disabilities. The "Integrated Community Based Initiative Awareness Plan" (ICBIA) at the Suf Camp was a community based initiative supported by the Social and Relief, Education Departments and Headquarters of the UNRWA, Jordan, and by the WHO/EMRO, and the Jordanian Department of Palestinian Affairs Jerash Governate, Municipality and Private Sector. This awareness plan focused on the cause and prevention of disability, with an emphasis on children. The main goal of the ICBIA is to improve personal quality of life by community empowerment. The opening ceremony began a month-long series of activities organized by the advisory committee. The march was organized to raise community awareness to the issue. Under the Integrated Community Based Actions (ICBA), a series of 15 awareness workshops related to disability, treatment, care and rehabilitation were offered by specialists for the community. Along with the month long campaign, environmental modifications for children with disabilities were installed in the homes to facilitate access. The campaign also focused on disabled human rights, preconception care, antenatal care, postnatal care, PKU tests, healthy and safe schools, and awareness workshops conducted by specialists for the community on different subjects. This successful campaign not only empowered the community but gave medical workers training and assisted physical modifications in the homes of disabled children. This is community health action at work (pers. comm. Dr. Antaki, March 25, 2010).

UNDERGRADUATE HEALTH DEGREES

Bachelor degrees available in health include **Bachelor of Arts (BA)** or **Bachelor of Science (BS)**. The BA degree is often granted in the humanities, requires general education courses[2] along with a foreign language, and is sometimes considered more traditional education. The BS health degree normally requires more major courses, fewer electives, and a formal minor or research paper.[3]

GRADUATE HEALTH DEGREES

Master of Health Degrees

Graduate degrees awarded in health are **Master of Arts (MA)**, **Master of Science (MS)**, **Master of Science in Public Health (MSPH)**, and **Master of Public Health (MPH)**. There are two types of

---

Bachelor of Arts (BA): A degree granted in the humanities, requiring general education courses, along with a foreign language; it is sometimes considered a more traditional education.

Bachelor of Science (BS): A degree requiring more major courses, fewer electives, and often a formal minor and/or a research paper.

Master of Arts (MA): A degree focused on one area and awarded in the liberal arts to prepare students for the application of theory to health issues.

master's degrees in health: academic master's degrees and science master's degrees. The MA and the MS degree are awarded in the liberal arts and sciences, respectively. They prepare students for application of theory to health issues and focus on one area. The master's degrees with a public health designation (MPH and MSPH) are considered professional degrees. These two are for professionals with required practical work experience and other graduate requirements. The MPH provides a generalized preparation for public health work. The MSPH tends to focus on one particular public health topic.[3]

Doctorate of Health Degrees

Typically there are three terminal degrees in health education and public health, including the **Doctorate of Education (EdD)**, **Doctor of Public Health (DrPH)**, or the **Doctor of Philosophy (PhD)**. The EdD is normally practice-focused and includes specific education requirements. The DrPH is a professional degree that encompasses a broad spectrum in public health and can focus on one specific aspect of public health. Applied or action research and administrative skills are emphasized. The PhD degree is the highest academic degree and is normally the terminal degree in health. It requires mastering health knowledge and conducting research. It normally requires original research and a dissertation.[3]

You career goals and choices determine your degree designation. Your background and preparation are important because they give you the appropriate skills and educational knowledge to pursue a particular professional health career. Research and knowledge is important in choosing the correct degree and the correct program emphasis to meet your career goals. Individual program reputation and professional affiliations are important considerations when pursuing a professional health degree. Visit several universities you are interested in attending, and talk with a departmental representative about your career goals and the type of health career you wish to pursue. Academic counselors can advise you on proper choices and will honestly tell you what programs seem a good fit for your career goals.

Also, you need to consider the prerequisites for each institution. Many have stringent grade point average (GPA) requirements as well as graduate record exam (GRE) requirements. Some entrance requirements use formulas combining the GPA and GRE. You may also be asked to submit a paper, attend an interview with faculty, submit letters of recommendation, or perform other specific requirements to gain admission. It is always best to apply for admission to more than one university to increase

---

Master of Science (MS): A degree focused on one area and awarded in sciences to prepare students for the application of theory to health issues.
Master of Science in Public Health (MSPH): A degree that tends to focus on one particular public health topic.
Master of Public Health (MPH): A degree that provides a generalized preparation for public health work.
Doctor of Education (EdD): A terminal degree that is normally practice-focused and includes specific education requirements.
Doctor of Public Health (DrPH): A terminal degree that focuses on one specific aspect of public health and emphasizes research and administration.
Doctor of Philosophy (PhD): A terminal degree encompassing a broad spectrum in public health emphasis.

your options. It is also a good idea to meet with a financial aid counselor to determine if there are any income sources to assist you in your education, such as grants, graduate or research assistantships, scholarships, stipends, or incentives. You need to take into account out-of-state fees, tuition fees, textbook costs, and lab fees for certain courses. Deciding what degree to pursue involves meeting your career goals and economic feasibility, a task that requires good common sense and good decision making. A proper education, degree, and training are valuable commodities in the health profession to pursue a meaningful, fulfilling career in your area of health emphasis.

CAREER OPTIONS IN HEALTH

Once you receive your degree in health, you need to concentrate on the particular career options that suit your degree and training. Your career preparation should assist you in mastering the research and development skills for planning, implementing, administering, and evaluating health programs. You should possess the skills necessary for undergraduate and/or graduates as designated by the professional competencies as well as the ethical codes of the profession. There are many career opportunities for health educators and more opportunities are opening every day because of the diverse training and skills that health educators possess.

Some sample career titles for health educators include health educator, manager, supervisor, director, researcher, consultant, administrator, grant and fund developer, specialist, sales person, patient educator, evaluator, journalist, coordinator, advisor, editor, health officer, and chief executive officer. This list is not exhaustive; the different job titles and career options available are too numerous to list.

Many diverse settings offer career options for health educators. While the list is only a sampling of settings and types of jobs and titles, there are many more types available. Many authors list different job titles, but those discussed here are in an effort to define more clearly the varied and different job opportunities available today. Listings of worldwide agencies and organizations that employ health educators appear in Appendix C. Global opportunities for health educators are emerging and offer possibilities of working in different areas of the world with diverse populations. The different career **settings for health educator** include, but are not limited to:[3–6]

1. Education settings (K–12 and higher education)
2. Research organizations
3. Medical care settings
4. Worksite healthcare settings
5. Nontraditional health settings
6. Private voluntary or nonprofit organizations
7. Philanthropic foundations

Settings for health education: The 11 diverse settings for career options for health educators: education settings (K–12 and higher education), research organizations, medical care settings, worksite healthcare settings, nontraditional health settings, private voluntary or nonprofit organizations, philanthropic foundations, professional or technical associations/organizations/societies, private industrial companies, governmental/public health agencies, and intergovernmental organizations.

---

8. Professional or technical associations/organizations/societies
9. Private industrial companies
10. Governmental/public health agencies
11. Intergovernmental organizations

MAJOR TYPES OF CAREER SETTINGS AND JOB TITLES

1. Education Settings

Teaching and faculty positions and administrative positions are available in all educational settings.[5] These include working in a K–12 public, private, or religious school setting or in higher education settings such as universities and colleges.[7] Some sample jobs include K–12 health teacher in the public, private, religious, or charter schools; faculty member; professor; instructor; school administrator; principal or supervisor; school superintendent; health librarian; health media specialist; and state director for school health.

2. Research Organizations

These jobs involve health research conducted at medical centers, universities,[5] hospitals, private companies, and medical-based companies.[6] A wide range of research in behavioral science takes place from low-level to very high-level and sensitive activities. Some sample jobs include health researcher, laboratory director, laboratory assistant, research assistant, research coordinator, primary investigator, evaluator; epidemiologist, behavioral investigator, and researcher. See the example of a health practitioner working in a research/medical setting in **Figure 8–2** and **Table 8–1**.

3. Medical Care Settings

These types of jobs involve working along with medical professionals in assisting the organization and the patients in education, information, advocacy, and health communications.[5,6] Some health professionals are patient educators and communicate with patients on progress and report to a physician. Settings include practitioner's offices, clinics, hospitals, outpatient and ambulatory care facilities, rehabilitation centers, and long-term care facilities. Some sample jobs include consultant, patient advocate, patient educator, public relations representative, and trainer.

Education setting (K–12 and higher education): A setting for health education that includes teaching and faculty positions and administrative positions in educational settings.
Research organization: A setting for health education that includes health research conducted at medical centers, universities, hospitals, private companies, and medical-based companies.
Medical care setting: A setting for health education that includes working along with the medical professionals in assisting the organization and the patients in education, information, advocacy, and health communications.

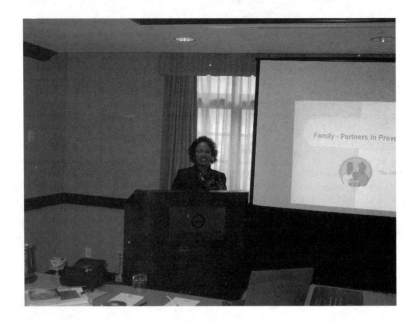

FIGURE 8–2   Cassandra Harris, MS, CHES, MD   Cassandra Harris, MS, CHES, MD is facilitating a trainer session at the regional conference of the 100 Black Men, Inc., for partners in a family health education program at the University of Texas M.D. Anderson Cancer Center, Houston, Texas.

4. Worksite Healthcare Settings

Working in many different settings, this field mainly involves creating and managing a wellness center and health promotion and prevention program for employees in a company.[5] Corporate fitness centers not only include fitness and workout facilities; they coordinate programs for weight reduction, nutrition, and prevention; take vital signs; record measurements; offer personal training and prescriptive exercise programs; and manage the facility and employees. Many services include health risk assessments, screening tests, access to health services, and other employee programs. Some sample jobs include fitness instructor, manager, program coordinator, personal trainer, and director.

> **Worksite healthcare setting:** A setting for health education that includes corporate fitness centers in many different settings and involves creating and managing wellness centers and programs for employees in a company.

TABLE 8–1   JOB DESCRIPTION FOR HEALTH PRACTITIONER CASSANDRA HARRIS, MS, CHES, MD

Name and Degrees: Cassandra Harris, MS, CHES, MD

Title: Manager, Health Education

Employer: The University of Texas M. D. Anderson Cancer Center

Job Description: Manages the Minority and Women Clinical Trial Recruitment Program's collaborations that address barriers to increase participation and retention of minorities and women in clinical trials at M. D. Anderson Cancer Center.

Qualifications: Required: Master's degree in public health, social science, health education, or health-related field

Licensure/Certification: Preferred: Certification as a Certified Health Education Specialist (CHES)

Skills Needed:

1. Seven years community health education, outreach, and collaboration experience, with a minimum of 2 years of supervisory/management experience

2. Course work in planning, marketing, and health education program evaluation

3. Program management

4. Community education, planning, and implementation

5. Communications and outreach

Technology Skills Needed:

• The ability to use information technology for personal productivity

• The ability to operate standard office equipment such as computer, laser printer, calculator, fax machine, photocopier, etc.

• Functional proficiency and literacy in the use of standard word-processing software (i.e., Word and other off-the-shelf or customized software packages specific to job functions such as Excel, PowerPoint, Access, SPSS)

• A strong understanding of Internet technology

Professional Memberships:

Society for Public Health Education

Texas Society for Public Health Education—National Delegate

The Most Rewarding Part of the Job: Helping community organizations implement, evaluate, and replicate their efforts to improve the health of the communities in which they serve.

Health Philosophy: Awareness leads to action, and action leads to change.

Quote: "Join a professional organization and get involved. The information, contacts, and professional development will help guide your career."

Source: Courtesy of Cassandra Harris, MS, CHES, MD. Anderson Cancer Center. Used by permission.

5. Nontraditional Health Settings

These jobs involve working in sales or other sales-related jobs marketing health and health products. Duties include sales and marketing for all types of medical and pharmaceutical companies, fitness equipment and sportswear companies, health food and vitamin stores, and booksellers; writing health/fitness articles; and editing health publications. Some sample jobs include pharmaceutical, medical, fitness equipment, and textbook sales person; editor; journalist;[7] and communication specialist.

6. Private Voluntary or Nonprofit Organizations

These jobs involve working with voluntary health organizations formed by citizens and/or groups to fulfill a need. Their goal may be educating and/or distributing information to the public advocating for preventing and understanding a particular health condition.[5] Diverse institutions and supported missions, including those of religious and secular groups, are for "international relief, cooperation and understanding."[4(pp326–327)] This includes religious, nonreligious, and nonprofit organizations. The nonprofit organizations are not affiliated with a professional association or organization but may partner with them. Day-to-day operations include designated programs, a specific focus, and outsourced efforts. Some sample jobs include program manager, executive director, chief executive officer, grant consultant, and evaluation consultant. A list of agencies is available from the Global Health Council (formerly the National Center for International Health) and the International Council of Voluntary Agencies.

7. Philanthropic Foundations

These organizations are privately funded and have a specific health interest in making meaningful contributions to solving particular health-related problems in international health work and other causes.[4] These organizations have a specific disease or problem focus dictated by the foundation. They are organized and function similarly to nonprofit organizations, but they are privately funded. A designated program focus is delivered. Some sample jobs include program manager, program coordinator, fund developer, executive director, chief executive officer, and grant consultant.

Nontraditional health setting: A setting for health education that includes sales, marketing, or other sales-related jobs marketing health and health products.

Private voluntary or nonprofit organization: A setting for health education that includes working in organizations founded by citizens and/or groups to fulfill a need, education, and/or public information and involves advocating for a particular health condition.

Philanthropic foundation: A setting for health education that includes privately funded foundations with a specific health interest contributing to solving health-related problems in international health work and other causes.

8. Professional or Technical Associations/Organizations/Societies

These jobs involve working with privately owned and formed and/or public-professional and technical associations serving in the "dissemination of information; in the provision of expert consultation, training, and fellowships; [and] in the maintenance of professional standards and conditions of employment."[4(p330)] These organizations consist of professionals who organize and meet for professional development, advocacy, and promotion of the profession, certification, licensure, and other reasons. They can also function as a nonprofit organization. Some sample jobs include program manager, executive director, chief executive officer, and fund developer.

9. Private Industrial Companies

Commercial industries provide investments, employment, and market access in international health enterprises for altruistic enterprises. It is in the form of multinational or transnational approaches.[4] While these companies operate similarly to nonprofits, they do not necessarily have this designation because they are run by companies. Some sample jobs include company liaison, intermediary, director, assistant director, program manager, program consultant, and health specialist.

10. Governmental/Public Health Agencies

While most operate in the country of origin or unilaterally, these agencies can include bilateral and multilateral agreements among governments to form organizations to influence the well-being and health of populations.[4,7] The specific areas governmental and public health agencies serve can be defined by country, city, and region. These agencies are usually multipurpose, not focused on one particular disease or area but instead serving many purposes. With environmental health threats and preparedness for intentional health threats emerging, these jobs are becoming more prevalent.[6] Some sample jobs include epidemiologist, health director, health officer, academic policy advisor, legislative policy advisor, management policy advisor, environmental advisor, homeland security advisor, and health specialist. There is an example of a health practitioners working in a governmental agency in **Figure 8–3** and **Table 8–2**.

Professional or technical association/organization/society: A setting for health education that includes organizations and nonprofits that consist of professionals who meet for professional development, advocacy, and promotion of the profession, certification, licensure, and other reasons.
Private industrial company: A setting for health education that includes commercial industries providing investments, employment, and market access in international health enterprises for altruistic enterprises with multinational and/or transnational approaches.
Governmental/public health agency: A setting for health education that includes the country of origin or unilateral, bilateral, and/or multilateral agreements among governments to form organizations that influence the well-being and health of a population.

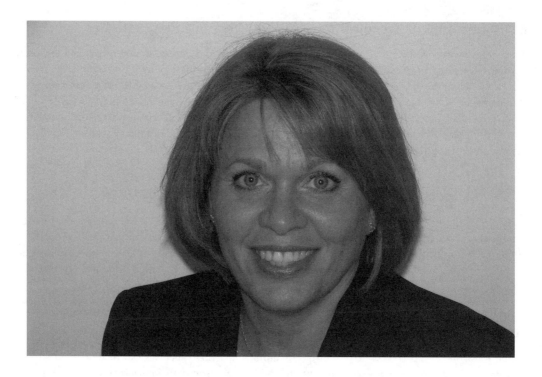

FIGURE 8–3   Kelly Bishop Alley, MA, CHES, FASHA   Health Practitioner Kelly Bishop Alley, MA, CHES, FASHA, Centers for Disease Control and Prevention, Team Leader in the Division of Adolescent and School Health (DASH), Program Development and Services Branch, Atlanta, Georgia.

11. Intergovernmental Organizations

Career Concept

Do you love politics and the law? You may enjoy a career in government/public agencies or intergovernmental agencies, advocating for health-related laws and policies.

These organizations are regional and global and have an interest in international health working along with a government agency. These can be established because of geographic locations, political implications, economic reasons and disease problems, and other reasons.[4] These are sometimes partnership efforts with large organizations and governments working together for a common cause. They also function somewhat as nonprofits, but may or may not have this designation. Some sample jobs include program manager, program coordinator,

> **Intergovernmental organization:** A setting for health education that includes regional and global organizations with an interest in international health and working in conjunction with a government agency.

TABLE 8–2   JOB DESCRIPTION FOR HEALTH PRACTITIONER KELLY BISHOP ALLEY, MA, CHES, FASHA

Name and Degrees: Kelly Bishop Alley, MA, CHES, FASHA

Title: National Nongovernmental Organization Partners Team Lead

Employer: Division of Adolescent and School Health, Centers for Disease Control and Prevention

Job Description: Serves as a team leader in the Division of Adolescent and School Health (DASH), Program Development and Services Branch (PDSB). Ensures that the organization's strategic plan, mission, vision, and values are communicated to the team and integrated into the team's strategies, goals, objectives, work plans, work products, and services. Articulates and communicates assignments, projects, problems to be solved, actionable events, milestones, and/or program issues under review, and deadlines and time frames for completion. Coaches the team in the selection and application of appropriate problem-solving methods, practices, and procedures, and assists the team and/or individual members in indentifying the parameters of a viable solution. Leads the team in identifying, distributing, and balancing workload in accordance with established priorities to ensure timely accomplishment of individual and team tasks, and ensuring that each employee has an integral role in developing the final team product. Trains or arranges for the training necessary for accomplishment of individual and team tasks. Maintains program and administrative reference material. Serves as coach, facilitator, and/or negotiator in coordinating team initiatives and consensus-building activities. Provides technical assistance to assigned national, state, and local organizations in assessing and documenting the implementation of coordinated school health education, including targeted chronic disease education, HIV prevention education, physical activity and healthy eating, prevention of tobacco use, and management of asthma for school-aged youth. Aggregates and analyzes data from multiple sources to define school health education needs and achievements. Performs other duties as assigned.

Qualifications: BS Health and Safety Education, MA Counseling Psychology, and Certified Health Education Specialist (CHES)

Skills Needed:

1. Program administration
2. Supervision/management
3. Coaching, mentoring
4. Strategic problem solving
5. Project management

Technology Skills Needed: Experience with Microsoft Office products, live meeting, CDC-specific budgeting and program monitoring applications

Professional Memberships:

Society for Public Health Education (SOPHE)

American School Health Association (ASHA)

American Association for Health Education (AAHE)

Eta Sigma Gamma (ESG; National Health Education Honorary)

Indiana Society for Public Health Education (InSOPHE)

The Most Rewarding Part of the Job: Empowering others. I absolutely love it when staff or partners realize they have the capacity to achieve something they didn't think was possible.

Health Philosophy: I believe that as health educators we all have the responsibility to help grow and nurture our profession by being CHES certified, mentoring others, and actively promoting our profession.

Quote: "In all facets of life, set your goals, make your plans, and make it happen!"

Source: Courtesy of Kelly Bishop Alley, CHES, FASHA, of CDC. Used by permission.

fund developer, executive director, chief executive officer, and grant consultant. See the job description of a sample health practitioner in Israel working in a governmental organization along with a health services agency for intersection cooperation (see **Table 8–3**).

HEALTH EDUCATOR JOB ANALYSIS

The National Health Educator Job Analysis Project was conducted to meet the National Organization for Competency Assurance recommendations. A periodic analysis validates the practice of health educators. Procedures based on credentialing, standards, and best practices that were established by the American Psychological Association, National Council on Measurement in Education, and the American Educational Research Association. Beginning in August of 2008, Professional Examination Services (PES) representatives and a steering committee worked with volunteer health educators to develop a job analysis survey instrument. The PES is working with a steering committee of representatives from the American Association for Health Education, the National Commission for Health Education Credentialing, and the Society for Public Health Education. The survey will produce valuable information about the practices of work settings. A stratified random sample of health educators selected from members of health organizations belonging to the Coalition of National Health Education Organizations were surveyed in March through April of 2009. The results are being tabulated, and valuable information about health education practice in work settings will provide a detailed job analysis and pertinent information relevant to the profession.[8]

RESUMES AND COVER LETTERS

Resumes are essential documentation of what you have achieved in your career. They are written documents that display your credentials to potential employers or could be used for professional development requirements. They should be printed on 100% cotton paper and printed on off-white or light-grey paper. No staples are used, which helps keep them environmentally friendly. Do not mail resumes in a regular legal envelope. Resume folders are recommended or white envelopes of 8½ × 11 inches. Do not include a photo image or personal information in the resume. It should be a summary of your education and experience and how you achieved the responsibilities and competencies.

A cover letter should accompany the **resume or vita**. The cover letter expresses how you meet the skills needed for the job based on the job description listed. It can give a short history of additional skills and experiences not related in the job description that may be useful. For instance, the CHES designation is important to list if you have acquired it. A cover letter should never exceed more than two pages, but one page is preferred. Do not forget to add your signature to the cover letter, and check spelling and grammar before you mail it.

There are basic elements to include in a resume/vita/portfolio. However, for new graduates or students without significant publications or professional service, you should not list these or any other

---

Resume or vita: A written document of what you achieved in your career; it displays your credentials when searching for employment or for professional development.

TABLE 8–3 JOB DESCRIPTION FOR HEALTH PRACTITIONER DIANE LEVIN-ZAMIR, PhD, MPH

Name and Degrees: Diane Levin-Zamir, PhD, MPH

Title: Director, National Department of Health Education and Promotion

Employer: Clalit Health Services, Israel

Job Description: Provides professional management of a department whose function is to develop and implement methodology in health promotion, promote intersectoral cooperation, and promote integration of health promotion in the functioning of primary care and hospital health services.

Qualifications: Academic background in health promotion and public health, personal skills for promoting teamwork in an interdisciplinary approach

Skills Needed:

1. Program planning, implementation, and evaluation

2. Department management

3. Intersectoral collaboration

4. Resource development and management

Technology Skills Needed: Experience with Microsoft Office programs

Professional Memberships:

International Union of Health Education and Promotion

Israel Association of Health Education and Promotion

Israel Association of Public Health

Israel Association for Family Planning

Israel Association for Quality in Medicine

The Most Rewarding Part of the Job: Watching successful initiatives become sustainable through healthy public policy.

Health Philosophy: Health promotion should be included in all policies.

Quote: "If you want to go fast, go alone. If you want to go far, go together." —Margaret Chan, WHO

Source: Courtesy of Diane Levin-Zamir, PhD, MPH, Director, National Department of Health Education and Promotion, Clalit Health Services, Israel. Used by permission.

items that you do not possess. List only the items that you can document. Use a basic font such as Times New Roman in 12-point size, and print with black ink only. You can apply boldface type to the following divisions shown herein. Do not italicize information in the cover letter or resume unless it is a publication.

1. **Contact Information.** Your name should go at the top, centered and boldfaced. The second line contains your e-mail address, flush to the left margin, and your cell phone number and fax number flush to the right margin. Do not include your address or home phone number on a resume posted online, even if you pay to have it password protected. You can be contacted via your cell phone, e-mail, or fax, and this information cannot be traced to your personal home address and phone.

2. **Occupational Objective Statement.** Provide a statement of your career goals and the type of environment in which you are most successful. Construct it carefully and succinctly without using a long compound sentence. It should be precise and express clearly what you want to achieve.

3. **Computer Literacy Skills.** Include a statement about computer skills, or simply a statement that you are computer literate. If your work involves specific computer skills, such as competency with computer research software or health software (e.g., CDCynergy or EMPOWER), these should be listed.

4. **Professional Profile.** List the undergraduate or graduate responsibilities and competencies achieved using a superscript number, and key each to the work experience, education, publications, professional memberships, professional service, honors, and awards with the same superscript number.

5. **Work Experience.** List your work experience with your job title and a brief description of duties and dates employed, if desired. Start with the most recent work experience and work backward. Internships (especially paid internships) can be listed. While full-time positions are always listed, part-time positions may also be listed, especially if they are significant to health education. For teaching experience, list the course title, semesters, and years you taught each course.

6. **Education and Certifications.** Start with your most advanced degree, listing the exact wordage of the degree, the school where the degree was acquired, and the date received. List any other degrees acquired. List all certifications received, especially CHES.

7. **Scholarship and Research.** Scholarship and research includes publications and presentations. If you do have publications, you should list them in a standardized format such as American Psychological Association (APA) format or American Medical Association (AMA) format, as these are the ones used by health research journals.[9,10] List peer-reviewed journal articles first, books, online courses taught, and any other significant publications. List any professional presentations given in the same format.

8. **Professional Memberships.** List any professional memberships, with each on a separate line, and include the dates you were a member. Any honor societies, even if not health related, should be mentioned here.

9. **Professional Service.** If you served as an officer for a university health club or Eta Sigma Gamma Professional Honor Society, you should list them here along with the dates. You should also list any offices held, committees you served on, or any other volunteer work for any professional associations or organizations. Write out the full name of the organizations and the dates you were an officer or performed other services.

10. **Grants, Honors, Awards, Fellowships, and Scholarships.** Any significant grants, honors, awards, fellowships, and scholarships should be listed here. Grant applications should list the title, funding source, amount requested, and duration of the grant funding. All grants should

be listed in a consistent format. While grants acquired are listed here, any research as a result of the grant that was published should go in the publications section.

11. **Community Service and Volunteer Work.** Many employers want to see that they are hiring a well-rounded and altruistic individual. Volunteer and community service work, especially if health related, can sometimes make the difference in whether you are hired over someone with similar qualifications. List all community service work or other volunteer work.

12. **Statement of Health Philosophy.** Include only your personal health philosophy statement (see Chapter 6). The complete philosophy paper will be used in the e-portfolio as a link.

13. **Professional References.** List people who can attest to your work experience (e.g., former employers), your personal character (e.g., a clergy or religious leader or a mentor), and, if you have graduated within the last 5 years, your professors, instructors, or advisors. List the person's name, title, phone number, e-mail address, and fax number. Three to five references is normal. Receive permission from the references to print their contact information on your resume. Better yet, ask them what you can list. There are some who feel that personal references should not be listed on a resume. However, if you have notified your references and they are aware that you are applying for the job, it may save time for the employer to have the contact information for your references readily available. The references should be listed on a separate sheet of paper following the resume. However, if you do not want to include these with the resume, it is appropriate to simply state at the end of the resume that references are available upon request.

PORTFOLIOS: HARD COPY AND ELECTRONIC

Hard copy **portfolios** are those containing not only the resume but documentation showing a diversity of experiences and study.[11] While these are required in some professions for job interviews and continually charting progress such as for tenure and promotion reviews, the new trend is electronic portfolios (or e-portfolios).[12] While hard copy portfolios and e-portfolios contain the same elements, the same criteria should be included in each but be displayed in a different format.

Portfolios are a selective and specific collection of work made available in hard copy format or in electronic format as a Web site or saved on a CD. Portfolios document abilities and records and provide evidence of achievements. The Internet, with its multimedia capabilities, has opened a new medium for e-portfolios. Many teacher education programs are requiring e-portfolios for students.[13,14]

E-portfolios contain many of the same elements as hard copy portfolios but are available online for prospective employers and companies to view via a Web site, html document, CD-ROM, or e-mail attachment. While the basic content is similar to a resume, this electronic medium allows the user an experience of sight and sound through streaming videos, dictated PowerPoint slides, animated sessions, and other technological advances. The e-portfolio also demonstrates the individual's technological skills.

Electronic portfolio or hard copy portfolio: A selective and specific collection of work made available in hard copy format or on a Web site. It documents abilities and records and provides evidence of achievements.

Imagine the difference in reading a PowerPoint slide from a piece of paper and viewing it online with voice-over, sound, or visual effects. A video showing a health promotion program that the prospective employee carried out or was involved in, with the prospective employee applying a philosophy or engaging with individuals in a practice setting, working with a focus group, or presenting to a community forum, is a more definitive measure of skills than a hard copy portfolio.

Provide a description of a health standard and a hyperlink to a Web site that demonstrated a project, a diary entry, or work in a multicultural and/or diverse setting. An e-portfolio is a powerful tool that shows reflection, knowledge, evolution of thought, and professional development. It demonstrates how a person applies practice in the field or the real world and can demonstrate professional health standards in action. It is an interactive presentation that engages the viewer in a multimedia showcase of the person's talents, knowledge, skills, and abilities.

An e-portfolio provides links to the most relevant materials using documents that are supported and made real by artifacts. Do not use too many images or gimmicks. It should provide an indexed list to the most relevant materials. E-portfolios can include an Excel spreadsheet that demonstrates how these electronic documents meet the professional health standards.

In the professional world, there are different types of portfolios, whether hard copy or electronic. *Showcase portfolios* allow artists, architects, engineers, and other career individuals to showcase their produced works. *Formative portfolios* are ongoing and help health professionals showcase professional development when applying for tenure or promotion. *Summative portfolios* occur within the context of a formal evaluation process and are used by professionals practicing in the health field. *Marketing portfolios* are useful for persons seeking employment or by companies to showcase products and services. The marketing portfolio is the type explained here.

The e-portfolio should contain some common elements and sections found in any professional portfolio, including examples of work completed and documentation of what is cited in the resume. If you do not have experience in one of the elements listed below, then do not list it on the document. Assessing the elements you cannot list may help you gauge what skills you need to acquire to show you are a well-rounded candidate. You can use bold typeface for each heading below, but use regular typeface for the elements listed for each. If it is a linked element, you will also want to include a hyperlink to that document. The elements of an e-portfolio include:

- Home page (contact information, occupational objective statement, and table of contents link)
- Current vita or resume (as explained previously)
- Computer literacy skills
- Professional profile
- Work experience
- Education and certifications
- Publications and presentations
- Professional memberships
- Professional service
- Grants, honors, awards, and scholarships
- Community service and volunteer work
- Health philosophy
- Professional references

CRITERIA FOR AN ELECTRONIC RESUME AND PORTFOLIO

Home Page

The **home page** is the first page of the Web site. It provides your contact information, including your name, your degree, and your occupational objective statement. You can link to a table of contents or list the table of contents with hyperlinks to the items provided (see the other criteria listed next for recommendations). You may include several links. The table of contents may link to scholarship and research. There may be a listing of relevant documents under that category link with additional links to the documents attached. Thus, a future employer can view the documents relevant to the job you are pursuing. The criteria listed may not all apply to you. Do not include any of the elements recommended as links if you do not have anything in that area. However, this may provide a clue to what you are lacking so you can try to increase your experiences for the future. Contact information includes name, cell phone number, e-mail address, and fax number. Do not post an image of yourself and do not list your home address and home phone if your e-portfolio is posted on a Web site. A secure Web site is also recommended as a protection of your information. You can give future employers only the username and/or password to access the Web site when requested.

Current Vita or Resume

Use the professional resume you developed in the previous section for the links that will be discussed next. Each section you developed is displayed as a resume document or linked to the items from your resume and to the documentation showing expertise. Thus, future employers can see items as they read the resume. You could also list a table of contents instead of the printed resume so viewers can scroll through the table of contents for certain items if they do not wish to view the entire resume. From each listing, the documentation listed next is linked for viewing.

Computer Literacy Skills

Include examples of your best technology skills. If your work involves specific computer skills, such as competency with research software or health software (e.g., CDCynergy or EMPOWER), that should be listed. Any PowerPoint presentations, Web sites developed, brochures, newsletters, or other computer-generated items should be included. Other examples to include are audiovisual materials, brochures, instructional videotape or slide shows, computer program software programs, and Web sites created. Include only documentation of the items you performed. This list is an example only and is not exhaustive. There may be other significant items that you feel are important enough to be included.

Home page of a Web site: The first page of the Web site with basic contact information and a menu bar or table of contents that links to other elements.

Professional Profile

Using the responsibilities and competencies listed in the resume, cite each competency in order after each of the following listed items to show that you are meeting them. For example, under work experience, you may list competencies after each experience.

Work Experience

List evidence of practice and how the health responsibilities and competencies were met. List the competencies and provide links to the documents that meet these competencies. Provide documents from programs, a well-constructed program plan or proposal, evidence of research and evaluation activities, internship or employer evaluations of field experiences or student teaching, and reflections on internships, field experiences, employment, or student teaching or teaching experiences. For teaching, list the courses taught and submit evidence of teaching excellence. Provide community workshops facilitated and list the program's title, place, audience, and date you facilitated. Suggestions are objective student or participant evaluations, course outlines or syllabi, agenda, and lesson plans. Include materials indicating course development or revision and innovative teaching strategies.

Education and Certifications

Provide copies of grade transcripts, test scores, evaluations, and certifications.

Scholarship and Research

This section provides a list and a link to publications and professional presentations given. It is a bibliography of your written work and creative projects. It is a description of scholarship/research projects completed and in progress. Provide full citations in a standardized format. Link and attach copies of published and in-press articles in refereed scholarly journals, book chapters, translations, manuscripts submitted for publication, published and press articles in nonrefereed publications, newspaper and/or magazine articles, and exemplary class term papers or projects.

Include documentation of presentations of scholarship/research findings at conferences or professional meetings. Indicate if the presentation was juried or invited. Service evidence could also include an editor or reviewer for a scholarly publication (list name of publisher). Descriptions of creative activities related to professional responsibilities such as exhibitions, performances, and critical review of books are included. A description of your participation in planning, developing, or implementing professional conferences or workshops is included. Continuing education, as documented by continuing education units, verifiable self-instruction, or other objective measure, should be included. Consider offering a brief description of committee reports or documents of substantial scope and depth for which you had the primary writing responsibility.

Professional Memberships

Membership cards, registrations for conferences, evidence of workshops attended, certificates received, a copy of the front page of the conference manual, or other evidence that you pursue professional memberships should be included.

Professional Service

This section involves documentable service related to your professional role. It includes offices in professional organizations and lists your major contributions. It may include a description of committee and administrative service, including your role (e.g., chair or member), dates of service, and major contributions. Provide documentation of service for any university committees, local and/or regional community committees, task forces, or commissions. Include any national, state, or regional committees, task forces, commissions. Document any internships or apprenticeships with professional organizations.

Grants, Honors, Awards, and Scholarships

Place supporting documentation of any grants received. Copies of honors, awards, and scholarships received as well as special recognition(s) are inserted. Undergraduate traditional students can include high school and college honors, awards, and scholarships.

Community Service and Volunteer Work

Provide a description of community service related to your professional role. This might include membership on an organization's advisory board, public education presentations, leadership in the area of expertise in community projects as a consultant, community service hours, and community volunteer activities. Another option is a summary narrative, which highlights major accomplishments related to your professional role with samples of completed projects and original work or letters of appreciation for volunteer work.

Statement of Health Philosophy

Provide a copy of your health philosophy, as discussed in Chapter 6. Include the complete document backed up by professional references.

Professional References

Provide at least one reference from an administrator or professor (if you are a student) in your area of expertise. Provide one reference from a community or religious leader who can attest to your character. Provide another from a colleague who has worked with you in the area of expertise. If you are a student without relevant job experience in an area, provide another reference from an administrator or professor in your areas of expertise.

Once you post your e-portfolio, you need to start searching Web sites to determine your career choices and the positions available. There are also some print resources that give salient information about job searching. It is a skill to search for employment in a professional field. Bardwell offers advice on how to evaluate job offers that may prove useful to you.[15] The National Association of Colleges and Employers has a guide for job searching that gives excellent advice for first-time job seekers.[16] Follow-up is also relevant. A phone call to make sure a possible employer received the materials you sent, whether by mail, fax, or e-mail, is recommended. A follow-up note after an interview is highly recommended. Thank the person for his or her time, and go over salient points identified or discussed in the interview. Highlight your main strengths that fit the particular job description.

TECHNOLOGY AND THE HEALTH PROFESSION

Technology and health education have a great marriage. Technology has impacted the way we plan, implement, and evaluate programs and deliver information. It has impacted health literacy, health education, distance education, response systems, emergency and basic education, service learning, information exchange, delivery of strategies, and extended communication of health information. Examples of how technology has affected health education include the following:

- Needs assessments and risk analysis software programs are easier to conduct and score.
- Epidemiological surveillance data is available instantaneously on a worldwide basis through health organizations and government Web sites.
- Surveys are conducted online and contact people not ordinarily within reach.
- E-mail provides instant communications between health educators and program participants and this medium assists professors in advising and mentoring for health students, including distance education courses.
- Various software program applications for planning and evaluating programs are available on CD-ROMs that are user friendly.
- Tool kits are available online for program information and analysis.
- Research journals published online via the World Wide Web and library online retrieval systems allow easy access and retrieval of published health articles.
- Surveillance information and other data and statistics are posted online from around the world are easily accessible and available for research and comparisons.
- Statistical programs are run through Excel and other statistical software making computations instantaneous and assists analysis, evaluation, and extrapolation in many different forms.[17]
- Programs and successful strategies are shared online for replication, research, and evaluation.
- Smart Boards, PowerPoint technology, DVD's and other technologies are used in classrooms to enhance visual learning and online courses.
- Conferencing is accessible online and aids communication between health educators.
- Technological strategies are conducted online for easier maintenance.
- Administrators use managerial software that makes record keeping for budgets, grants, and payroll smarter and efficient.
- Participant response systems are available and provide easy accessibility.
- Health public service announcements are proliferating the Internet and validated online Web sites are communicating health messages in many different mediums to meet a multitude of audiences.
- Analysis software and statistical programs are available for research and evaluation; these save time and analysis is conducted quicker and more efficiently.
- Health determinants and fitness scoring analysis software records self-reported data, gives results, and determines risk for participants with recommendations for improving health.

- Web-based tutorials and program strategies for health participants are available in packaged programs and on the Internet for easy access and education.
- Web-based courses have changed the way that training for undergraduate and graduate health degrees are delivered and have enhanced strategies for Web-based learning.
- Professional development opportunities are available through distance education and online webinars for training and information proliferation online.
- Blogs, list servs, and e-mail communications give access, communications, and discussion mediums between health professionals across the globe.

All these possibilities have greatly improved and widened the information received and have essentially changed and enhanced the way we train, plan, practice, deliver, research, and evaluate in health education. Many strategies are delivered through technology, and there are interactive tools, health risk assessments and research tools, physical activity software programs, Web-based tutorials, health software program authoring, PowerPoint presentations, and government and health department programs downloadable online for health education and a wealth of surveillance data available online.

Distance education is another new development in health education training and professional development. Many courses are delivered online and offer health career opportunities to students who may otherwise not have the ability to travel or live on campus. Many face-to-face courses are Web enhanced using technology for resources. Technology in the classroom for the K–12 school systems and higher education has improved the delivery of health education and health education training. Classroom technology has improved communications skills and made innumerable health resources available to teachers through the Internet or DVDs and CD-ROMS and lesson plans online. E-portfolios are posted online by both young and seasoned health professionals alike. Extensive computer literacy skills and information retrieval skills are a necessity for graduating health students. Professional development opportunities such as evaluating research articles online, attending online webinars and workshops online, using educational CD-ROM or DVD tools, and conferencing online are invaluable communication and access tools. Information sharing at conferences now includes technology such as PowerPoint presentations, Web sites, and authored technology materials (e.g., DVDs CD-ROMs, streaming videos, videotaped interviews, etc.). Many distance education instructors are advising and mentoring via e-mail and other technology resources.

There is valuable information on the Web and from other traditional resources, and many wonderful resource applications are available. As health professionals, we must be able to evaluate articles, especially research articles published online and through other resources. Students and professionals need to determine accurate, evidence-based, and pure research and detect misinformation or biased information. Technology has improved the profession, but we must not accept everything that is published on health as fact.

QUICK TIPS FOR EVALUATING CREDIBLE ARTICLES AND RESEARCH ON THE INTERNET AND BEYOND

As mentioned at the beginning of this chapter, the health education profession is constantly in transition, with new opportunities and improvement; unfortunately, new threats may cause a paradigm change at different times. The ability to adjust and reach salient resources to understand new changes or build new research-based programs for effective practice is necessary. Researching online for information requires a methodical and analytical approach to determine the best information health programs. Researching through university or local library information retrieval systems or obtaining hard copy information still means that all articles must be thoroughly analyzed.

When evaluating articles on the Internet and beyond, remember that there is an incredible amount of information out there with no regulation. Determining if something is accurate or inaccurate can be confusing. Obtaining articles by other means also takes skills to determine correct information and true research. There are many available retrieval resources online and through university and public library information retrieval systems. These include bibliographies, abstracts, indexes, research reviews, journals, conference publications, and computerized information retrieval.[18] Whether these sources were obtained online, through a search index at your university or local library, or as hard copy, there are specific items to examine.

There are six basic tips for evaluating articles individually via the Internet or other means. These tips offer a generalized look at the articles so you can eliminate the ones that are not as credible as you need. They include (1) consider the source, (2) identify the reason it was posted, (3) consider how current it is (date posted), (4) compare the information to other sources, (5) consider if there is propaganda or bias, and (6) use good common sense when evaluating the materials. A breakdown of the six tips follows to help you determine if information is genuine or fraudulent.

1. *Consider the source.* Check out the source or authority of the information. Government agencies, reputable universities, and major organizations like the American Cancer Society are clues to accuracy. If necessary, verify the source.
2. *Identify why it was posted.* Check out the reason for the Web posting or the publication. If it is advertising something, chances are it is slanted. Even some nonprofit organizations may not be credible. Scan the material first to get a good idea of what is in it before you take the time to read it. It may or may not be a waste of your time. There are many online international health journals that are excellent resources and wish to make the information readily available.
3. *Consider when it was posted.* Check out the date it was posted or published for determining whether or not the information is current. A good rule of thumb for determining currency for hard copy articles is if it was published within the past five years; for Internet or Web site articles the basic time is 1–2 years or less. Remember that medical and other health information can change daily. Historical information may not change and older sources could be reliable. There are also classic articles that may be timeless, and the information is sound and a worthwhile reference and information source.
4. *Compare the information to other sources.* If information is found at a Web site, compare it to other similar sites to see if there is consistency among the sources. Pay attention to content and details for coverage. Credible references and other links are a clue as to the accuracy of the information.
5. *Consider if there is propaganda or bias.* Beware of propaganda materials and those with only one viewpoint. Information without the support of reputable sources is a good indication that it is only an opinion. It is both good and bad that anyone can publish on the Internet, and some magazines allow anyone to publish an article on health. Sorting out the difference between real and opinionated information requires skill.

6. *Use good common sense.* Use your own good common sense. If information seems off-base, it probably is inaccurate. Remember, if you do not feel that a site or the information is authentic, then look for another source. There are many worthwhile sites to view. Once you determine these authentic and accurate sites, you will have access to a wealth of health information.

When evaluating articles online for participants or client usage, you must consider the literacy level(s) of the group. Some software computer programs for documents include readability-testing functions. There are several professional programs for evaluating literacy levels of reading materials as Fry, Flesch, FOG, SMOG, CLOZE, & WRAT Readability Formulas. You can view some of these sample programs on the National Cancer Institute Web site listed under Enhanced Readings.

ANALYZING RESEARCH PRACTICES IN JOURNAL ARTICLES AND PUBLICATIONS

If you have evaluated the information available using the above criteria, there are other criteria to use for analyzing research in journals or other professional publications. Peer-reviewed journals are excellent sources because a panel of professionals examined the accuracy and professionalism of the research before it was published, and proper research protocol was used. Many articles, not necessarily peer reviewed, are published as research. Many reputable government and other health agencies have credible online publications. The five-year rule of thumb for currency generally applies here unless it is a classic article or you are doing historical research.

Organizing and evaluating material takes time initially, but it saves time in the long run. Reading the abstract is a good way to determine relevance for the information you are retrieving and is a way to begin finding articles of interest and determine a credible source. Once you have applied the six basic tips for evaluating all articles retrieved and narrowed down the relevant research articles or program research, you will want to analyze each full-text article.

Berg recommends reading the current reviews of the literature, constructing a summary table of the studies, tallying the studies, showing the results (significant or insignificant), and using a meta-analysis to determine the studies to use.[18] While hard copy journals are still being published, many journals are published via the Internet. Some have membership log-ins, while others publish the journal online or make certain articles available without membership. University libraries purchase online databases to retrieve resources, and some health journals are available through online libraries and other databases.

Specific items for students to identify, examine, and interpret in peer-reviewed research journal articles are:

1. Rationale
2. Purpose
3. Participants (sample)
4. Research question
5. Methods, data collection techniques, variables, and theory
6. Measures (instruments)
7. Statistical analyses

8. Results
9. Discussion/Conclusions

Rationale qualifies a reason for the research or shows a need. The purpose tells you why the research was done. The participants are important for generalizability and randomness. The research question tells you what the researcher is asking. The methods are the procedures used in the research including all objectives, strategies, data collection techniques, and independent and dependent variables. The significance level is determined in the procedures and methods. The theory is the change agent employed in the research. The measures taken refer to the instruments used and how the data are collected and recorded, and in what form(s). The statistical analysis or analyses tell you what statistical principles were used to analyze the data. The results state exactly what was found in the research. The discussion and conclusions make summary statements of the meaning of the results to the research study, health research and the profession. The conclusions should be based on the facts presented in the results.

To interpret the research of the articles, remember that statistics and results can exaggerate the findings in the way they are presented, statistical significance is influenced by the sample size and may not be generalizable. You should consider the sampling procedure used to determine bias (e.g., convenience samples or grab samples cannot be generalized), figures can be deceptive in the interpretation, and correlation does not automatically mean there is a cause and effect relationship. You should examine these additional research indicators: internal and external validity (limitations and delimitations), accuracy of the measurements, variance, significance level, treatment effect, and post hoc errors.[18] Once you make these basic research determinations, you can decide on the quality articles that are useful for your purposes.

General health databases, search engines, and resources are listed at the end of this chapter and in Appendix C. If looking for a research project, read the implications at the end of the research journal article where the author has listed information that may precipitate more studies in this area.

HEALTH EDUCATION PRACTICE AND REFORM

We are the helping profession with an ideal of a higher quality of life and health for all individuals. Health education is a behavioral and social science that comes from many other disciplines including psychology, physical education, biology, environmentalism, sociology, anthropology, and the medical sciences. The profession's main goal is to support health and avoid disease, disability, and death through health prevention, promotion, literacy, protection, access to health services, maintenance, and enhancement of health for all peoples globally. Health education is the development of individual, institutional, community, group, and universal strategies for improving individual health and health conditions. Strategies include educational and theoretical behavior, policy, and environmental change using specific research-based strategies. Research has provided a strong theoretical base for health education interventions. The purpose of health education is to support the health of individuals, communities, and the environment and other conditions that influence health.

The National Commission for Health Education Credentialing (NCHEC) Web site states that a health educator works "to encourage healthy lifestyles and wellness through educating individuals and communities about behaviors that promote healthy living and prevent diseases and other health problems."[19] Health educators are professionals who develop, implement, conduct, and evaluate programs to improve the health of all people. These activities can take place in a variety of settings, from school settings to community agencies and many others. These professionals implement evidence-based practice to address needs, investigate social determinants of health, reduce risk, manage diseases, promote cultural competence, protect human rights, form partnerships, and promote health strategies with respect for all healthy lives within the globe.

As we move to the future for the profession, there are still major issues and work to be done. WHO's Web site states, "In the 21st century, health is a shared responsibility, involving equitable access to essential care and collective defense against transnational threats."[20] This can be done with six strategies: promoting development; fostering health security; strengthening health systems; harnessing research, information, and evidence; enhancing partnerships; and improving performance. Health reform legislation is needed globally to improve wellness, eliminate health disparities, and improve access to health care, especially for children and women. The World Health Report from WHO states that primary health care is needed now more than ever.[21] The Galway Conference of Ireland 2009 focused on closing the gap for child and adolescent health.[22] Child health promotion, research, best practices, networking, communication, and supporting international links were the aims of this conference. Many programs and entities are leading the efforts to promote a healthier world as well as human rights and the right to health.[23] But much work remains for health educators as we face new challenges, new disease threats, and unforeseen disasters and events that threaten society's health.

The right to the highest attainable standard of health was stated in the WHO constitution of 1947.[20] Governments and public officials need action policies and plans to improve health access and care within enabling environments. The latest promotion effort by the United Nations Committee was the International Covenant on Economic, Social and Cultural Rights of 2009 that advocated for protection of human rights, of which health is a basic right. Many other entities endorsed these efforts to improve global health, economic, social, cultural, and human rights.[24,25] The best answer to protect human rights and basic health needs is a global mechanism to ensure, enforce, and protect these rights. With this in mind, there needs to be a realization that environments, politics, infrastructures, and social/cultural patterns vary in many different countries and parts of the world. Recognizing these differences and working toward global health promotion is not without problems and barriers. The bar must be set high with continued evidence-based practice along with supportive laws, policies, regulations, and norms. It is not enough to change individual behaviors; environmental changes and supportive communities along with formal laws and policies are needed. Respecting differences that do not adversely affect health and embracing likenesses are strategies necessary to achieve this goal. Governmental health agencies, regional organizations, nongovernmental agencies, and other public and private partnerships, agencies, associations, and coalitions must work together in prevention, funding, and intervention efforts. Health educators are a part of this goal; we are the facilitators; we are the program developers; we are the program implementers; we are the program evaluators; we are the researchers; we are health and human rights advocates; and we are change agents for a healthier, improved, and enhanced global society (see **Table 8–4**).

LEADERS FOR TOMORROW

Leadership skills are a necessity as a health educator and especially as a health administrator. The successful characteristics you exhibit as a leader can help you become more effective in your practice. It

TABLE 8–4   GLOBALIZATION

What is it?

This refers to the way in which the operation of businesses, production, and markets are integrated across national boundaries.

Broader implications: In a broader sense, globalization refers not just to the integration of economic production and markets, but to the social and political consequences of this trend. There are many views about whether these consequences are positive or negative.

For public health, globalization has several implications, including the following:

• Increasing complexity in terms of ensuring work-place health and safety across globalized operations

• Increasing complexity in terms of ensuring environmental responsibility where facilities and production are segmented and located in different countries, under different regulations and conditions

• Much more rapid routes of transmission for infection disease around the globe

• Much more rapid avenues for communication and dissemination.

• Health problems occur due to variations in these ecological factors as:

  ○ environmental risks

  ○ inadequate system capacity and infrastructure

  ○ non-supportive socioeconomic conditions

  ○ political instability

  ○ issues in social patterns and cultural traditions

gives the profession credibility and helps build partnerships and liaisons with other groups. Effective leaders produce effective employees and effective practice. Janet Lapp's book *Dancing with Tigers* is about creating and managing change and overcoming resistance to change.[26] Effective leaders understand when change is needed and prioritize changes necessary for sustaining change in practice. This is especially true in a profession where change is the constant, as new discoveries, practices, and strategies are constantly researched and improved upon.

Sheila Bethel cites eight characteristics of leaders in her book *A New Breed of Leader: 8 Leadership Qualities That Matter Most in the Real World*.[27] These qualities are competence, accountability, openness, humility, language, values, perspective, and power. Competence is building a purpose. Accountability is building trust. Openness is formulating integrity. Humility is inspiring authenticity. Language is connecting relationships. Value is forging a sense of community. Perspective is establishing balance. Power, the last element, is mastering influence. Competence is the quality that seems to be in the forefront from most leadership literature. This is a characteristic that involves not only skills and being responsible, but the ability to demonstrate as a role model and delegate an appropriate workloads with integrity, clarity, and building on the strengths of the employees.

Thought Concept

Are you a born leader or do you think you can become a leader? Can all health leaders improve or increase their leadership skills?

FINAL REFLECTIONS

Building a healthier tomorrow means health educators, as leaders, must stay constantly alert, thwarting dangers to society by being proactive, consummate advocates and working as professional health practitioners and forward thinking leaders to improve the health status of as many persons as possible in the future. The expectations are high, the opportunities are there, and the possibilities are endless. Training, perseverance, dedication, continuing education, and honoring professional ethics and standards of practice are what it takes to be called a practicing health educator. Global cooperation, coalitions, intergovernmental cooperative efforts, linkages, and sharing are paramount for a global quality of life and improvement.

Continuance is important. We can preserve and work toward health literacy, prevention, promotion, protection, access, maintenance, and enhancement of the health status of all people and places and propose solutions on a global level. The right to attain the highest standard of health possible involves participatory decision making in health decisions at the community, national, and international levels. Working together in unison to solve the same goal through global strategic planning is a promising plan for improving global health for all health educators. This is the health educator's professional role, and a welcome to all future health educators is extended. Your chosen profession makes a difference in this quest for progressive, enhanced global health, and we need you—the future generations—to continue this stalwart effort as well as continuously improve the practice, the profession, and research-based evidence of success. Think outside of the box, design new paradigm changes that work, and share evidence-based results and knowledge gained with others. Together we can provide a healthier future for all persons on our globe. It will be an impressive and extraordinary legacy to leave for all future generations. Are you ready for the challenge?

SELECTED GENERAL HEALTH DATABASES AND INFORMATION RESOURCES

Achoo Health Directory: http://www.healthedia.com/sectors/directory/achoo-the-blog
American Cancer Society: http://www.cancer.org/
American Heart Association: http://www.americanheart.org/
American Medical Association: http://www.ama-assn.org/
BIOETHICSLINE: http://libweb.lib.buffalo.edu/pdp/index.asp?ID=258
Bio Research (International): http://www.intute.ac.uk/biologicalsciences/
CDC's Health A to Z: http://www.cdc.gov/az/a.html
CDC's WONDER: http://wonder.cdc.gov/
Centers for Disease Control and Prevention: http://www.cdc.gov/
Clinical Trials (U.S.): http://clinicaltrials.gov/
Combined Health Information Database (CHID): http://www.cehn.org/cehn/resourceguide/chid.html

Cumulative Index for Nursing and Allied Health Literature (CINAHL): http://www.cinahl.com/library/library.htm

Combined Health Information Database: http://www.nidcd.nih.gov/health/inside/spr05/pg3.asp

Consumer Gateway: http://www.consumer.gov/

Cumulative Index to Nursing and Allied Health Literature: http://www.library.pitt.edu/articles/database_info/cinahl.html

Current Index to Journals in Education: http://www.saintjoe.edu/library/Printindexes/CIJE.htm

Department of Health and Human Services: http://www.hhs.gov/

Education Index: http://www.educationindex.com/

Educational Resources Information (ERIC): http://www.acceseric.org

ERIC: http://www.ericfacility.net/extra/index.html

EU Health: http://www.euhealth.net/

Index Medicus: http://www.nlm.nih.gov/tsd/serials/lji.html

Institute of Medicine: http://www2.nas.edu/iom/

International health resources: http://www.pitt.edu/HOME/GHNet/GHKR.html

Global Health Council: http://www.globalhealth.org/

Go Ask Alice: http://www.goaskalice.columbia.edu/

Health A to Z: http://www.healthatoz.com/

Health Canada http://www.hc-sc.gc.ca/

Health database: http://chid.nih.gov/

Health education resources: http://www.nyu.edu/education/hepr/

Healthfinder: http://www.healthfinder.gov/

Health Information Resources (UK): http://www.library.nhs.uk/Default.aspx

Health journals: http://www.ki.se/phs/hprin/hprin_journals.html

Health science journals: http://www.mco.edu/lib/instr/libinsta.html

Index Medicus/MEDLINE: http://www.nlm.nih.gov/pubs/factsheets/jsel.html

Intellihealth: http://www.intelihealth.com

Internet Sleuth (Health): http://www.isleuth.com/heal/html

London School of Economics Health and Social Care (LSEHSC): http://www2.lse.ac.uk/LSEHealthAndSocialCare/Home.aspx

MedWeb: http://www.gen.emory.edu/MEDWEB/keyword.html

Melvyl: http://www.melvyl.ucop.edu/

Minority health resources: http://www.minority.unc.edu/

National Cancer Institute: http://www.nci.nih.gov/

National Institute for Allergy and Infectious Diseases: http://www.niaid.nih.gov/

National Institutes of Health: http://www.nih.gov/

National Library of Medicine: http://www.nlm.nih.gov/

Oxford University Press: http://oup-usa.org/

Population Index on the Web: http://popindex.princeton.edu/index.html

Ovid Healthstar: http://www.ovid.com/site/products/ovidguide/hstrdb.htm

Psychological Abstracts (PsycInfo): http://www.apa.org/psycinfo/

PubMed: http://www.ncbi.nlm.nih.gov/PubMed

Sociological Abstracts: http://www.csa.com/factsheets/socioabs-set-c.php

U.S. Food and Drug Administration: http://www.fda.gov/
UT Southwestern Medical Center at Dallas Library: http://www4.utsouthwestern.edu/library/
Yahoo! Health: http://www.yahoo.com//health
WebMD: http://www.webmd.com/

SEARCH PROGRAMS

Alta Vista: http://www.altavista.com/
Excite: http://www.excite.com/
Google: http://www.google.com/
Lycos: http://www.lycos.com/
WebCrawler: http://www.webcrawler.com/
Yahoo: http://www.yahoo.com/Health/Medicine/

LISTSERV

Health Education E-mail Directory (HEDIR) sponsored by AAHE at: http://www.hedir.org/

SUMMARY

- There are different bachelor-, master-, and doctoral-level degrees available in health. An informed decision is necessary so that career goals are reached with the proper professional preparation and training background available in the various degree programs.
- Bachelor's degrees available in health include the Bachelor of Arts (BA) or Bachelor of Science (BS).
- Master's degrees in health include Master of Arts (MA), Master of Science (MS), Master of Science in Public Health (MSPH), and Master of Public Health (MPH).
- The terminal or advanced degrees beyond the master's level include Doctor of Education (EdD), Doctor of Public Health (DrPH), or the Doctor of Philosophy degree (PhD).
- Some sample career titles for health educators include health educator, manager, supervisor, director, researcher, consultant, administrator, grant and fund developer, specialist, sales person, patient educator, evaluator, journalist, coordinator, advisor, editor, health officer, and chief executive officer.
- Health education career settings include, but are not limited to, education settings (grades K–12 and higher education), research organizations, medical care settings, worksite healthcare settings, nontraditional health settings, private voluntary or nonprofit organizations, philanthropic foundations, professional or technical associations/organizations/societies, private industrial companies, governmental/public health agencies, and intergovernmental organizations.
- Career goals should determine the degrees obtained along with the required training to pursue specific health careers.
- Evaluating research and other articles takes skill, and analyzing each source for competence and credibility is important.
- Health educators are change agents for an improving global health status.

CONCEPTUAL TERMS

Education
Bachelor of Arts (BA)
Bachelor of Science (BS)
Master of Arts (MA)
Master of Science (MS)
Master of Science in Public Health (MSPH)
Master of Public Health (MPH)
Doctor of Education (EdD)
Doctor of Public Health (DrPH)
Doctor of Philosophy (PhD)
Settings for health education
Education setting (grades K–12 and higher education)
Research organization

Medical care setting
Worksite healthcare setting
Nontraditional health setting
Private voluntary or nonprofit organization
Philanthropic foundation
Professional or technical association/organization/ society
Private industrial company
Governmental/public health agency
Intergovernmental organization
Resume or vita
Electronic portfolio or hard copy portfolio
Home page of a Web site

REFLECTIVE THINKING

Career goals are as important as your philosophy of health. Determining your goals for the future is an important step in planning a fulfilling and rewarding career. It also helps you to investigate job progress and advancement. You grow as you gain more experience in the field, and these experiences are valuable assets for gaining new administrative positions. You need a progression for yourself and your career "ladder" goals as you move up. When you are an administrator, you are responsible for solving personal and work problems for employees and participants.

You are a new administrator in a health agency. You are considering hiring a new young professional. The person meets the qualifications and is enthusiastic and bright. Her references are stellar. She is late for her first interview with you. While this is duly noted, she says she is not familiar with the neighborhood or parking and was inadvertently detained. You set up a second interview and she is on time. She is subsequently hired. For the first couple weeks, things go very well. The third week, however, she is 30 minutes late to work one morning with no explanation. The fourth week, she is 30 minutes late on Monday and calls in on Friday with "car trouble," showing up at noon.

What are your responsibilities as an administrator when someone is consistently late? What is your responsibility as an administrator after the first time the employee is late, or should you ignore the first time she is late? How long should you carry someone who is repeatedly tardy for work? What legal procedures do administrators use for documenting performance? What strategies could you use to encourage an employee who is faltering, or should you use strategies? What do you need to do legally if you need to terminate an employee? Is there a probationary period for employees in which you can terminate them for no reason? Is an employee manual and contract legally binding? What are employees' rights regarding termination? Do they get a warning or note? These and more questions need to be answered. From experience, firing someone is never easy and requires a great deal of paperwork. It must be done legally or you put your agency/organization in jeopardy of a lawsuit. Firing someone who you know is the family breadwinner is equally difficult. As an administrator, you may face these and other ethical dilemmas. What are some strategies to deter this employee's behavior and/or handle this dilemma? Would you have the guts to fire an incompetent employee?

CONCEPTUAL LEARNING

1. Describe and distinguish between the bachelor's degrees available in health, including the Bachelor of Arts (BA) and Bachelor of Science (BS).
2. Compare the different master's degrees in health, including Master of Arts (MA), Master of Science (MS), Master of Science in Public Health (MSPH), and Master of Public Health (MPH).
5. Defend why a terminal or advanced degree beyond the master's level is appropriate for a health educator.
6. Discuss the different terminal degrees and contrast their differences, including Doctor of Education (EdD), Doctor of Public Health (DrPH), or Doctor of Philosophy (PhD).
7. List some sample career titles for health educators, and include one of the career resources listed where they may be employed.
8. Analyze the different health education career settings, and describe the skills needed and the duties of one of the careers.
9. Examine the different health education career settings, and choose one that you would be interested in pursuing. Describe the degree(s) needed to pursue this specific health career.

REFERENCES

1. American Association for Health Education. *Health education careers*. Reston, VA: Author. Retrieved August 29, 2009, from http://www.aahperd.org/aahe/
2. Levine, A. (1978). *Handbook on undergraduate curriculum*. San Francisco: Jossey-Bass.
3. Hayden, J. (2002). The ABC's of health education degrees. *Health Promotion Practice, 3*, 352–354.
4. Basch, P. F. (1990). *Textbook of international health*. New York: Oxford University Press.
5. Eta Sigma Gamma. (2007). *The Health Education Monograph Series, 24*(1), 1–36.
6. DeBuono, B. A., & Tilson, H. (2003). *Advancing healthy populations: The Pfizer guide to careers in public health*. New York: Pfizer Pharmaceutical Groups.
7. Cottrell, R. R., Girvan, J. T., & McKenzie, J. F. (2008). *Principles and foundations of health promotion and education* (4th ed). San Francisco: Addison Wesley & Benjamin Cummings.
8. Health educator job analysis. (Spring, 2009). *The CHES Bulletin, 20*, 2, 1.
9. American Psychological Association. (2001). *Publication manual of the American Psychological Association* (5th ed). Washington, DC: Author.
10. Iverson, C., Christiansen, S., Flanagin, A., Fontanarosa, P. B., Glass, R. G., Gregoline, B., et al. (2007). *AMA manual of style: A guide for authors and editors* (10th ed). New York: Oxford University Press.
11. Cleary, M. J., & Birch, D. A. (1997). How prospective school health educators can build a portfolio to communicate professional expertise. *Journal of School Health, 67*, 228–231.
12. Young, J. R. (2002, March 8). "E-Portfolios" could give students a new sense of their accomplishments. *The Chronicle of Higher Education*, pp. A31–32.
13. Mullen, L., Bauer, W. I., & Newbold, W. (2001, Fall). Developing a university-wide electronic portfolio system for teacher education. Retrieved March 10, 2010, from http://english.ttu.edu/kairos/6.2/coverweb/assessment/mullenbauernewbold/main.htm

14. Wolf, K., Whinery, B., & Hagerty, P. (1995). Teaching portfolios and portfolio conversations for teacher educators and teachers. *Action in Teacher Education, 17*(1), 30–39.
15. Bardwell, C. B. (1998). How to evaluate a job offer. *The Black Collegian, 28*(2), 64–68.
16. The National Association of Colleges and Employers. (2003). *Job choices: A guide to the job search for new college graduates* (46th ed.). Bethlehem, PA: Author.
17. Kittleson, M. J. (2005). *Using excel to run statistics.* Carbondale, IL: HEDIR Publishing.
18. Berg, K., & Latin, R. (2008). *Essentials of research methods in health, physical education, exercise science and recreation* (3rd ed.). Baltimore, MD: Lippincott Williams & Williams.
19. National Commission for Health Education Credentialing, Inc. (2009). *Health/Education Profession.* Retrieved May 15, 2009, from http://www.nchec.org/
20. World Health Organization. (1947). *Constitution of the World Health Organization.* Chronicle of the World Health Organization, Geneva, Switzerland: Author.
21. World Health Organization. (2008). *The World Health Report 2008 primary health care, now more than ever.* Geneva, Switzerland: Author.
22. NUI Galway, OÉ Gaillimh. *Health promotion conference 2010.* Retrieved March 25, 2010, from http://www.hprcconference.ie/index.html
23. United Nations. (1948). *The universal declaration of human rights.* Retrieved March 10, 2010, from http://www.un.org/en/documents/udhr/
24. Office of the United Nations, High Commissioner for Human Rights. (2009). Committee on Economic, Social and Cultural Rights. In *International Covenant on Economic, Social and Cultural Rights (ICESCR).* Geneva, Switzerland: Author. Retrieved March 10, 2010, from http://www2.ohchr.org/english/bodies/cescr/index.htm
25. Krug, H. N. (2002, July). *25 questions and answers on health and human rights.* Geneva, Switzerland: World Health Organization.
26. Lapp, J. E. (2003). *Dancing with tigers.* Toronto: Demeter Press.
27. Bethel, S. M. (2009). *A new breed of leader: 8 leadership qualities that matter most in the real world.* New York: Penguin Group Incorporated.

ENHANCED READINGS

National Cancer Institute. (2008). *Making Health Communications Program Work.* Available at: http://cancer.gov/pinkbook
See:

Communication Research Methods
Look at examples of SMOG, CLOZE, & WRAT Readability Formulas
Appendix C: Information Sources

RELEVANT WEB SITES

Access and review the career resource Web sites in Appendix C. Choose three sources and find three job descriptions that interest you and fit your career goals. Examine the job description, credentials, work experience, and skills. See if you possess the right characteristics for the position. Are you missing some pertinent skills? If so, you may need to acquire these to be competitive in the search for employment in the health field.

A Competency-Based Framework for Health Educators

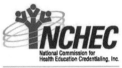

National Commission for Health Education Credentialing, Inc.

The Seven Areas of Responsibility are a comprehensive set of Competencies and Sub-competencies defining the role of a health educator. These Responsibilities were verified through the Competencies Update Project (CUP), conducted from 1998 to 2004. The entry level serves as the basis of the Certified Health Education Specialist (CHES) exam. The entry and advanced levels will be the basis of the Master Certified Health Education Specialist (MCHES) exam.

AREA I: ASSESS INDIVIDUAL AND COMMUNITY NEEDS FOR HEALTH EDUCATION

Competency A: Access existing health-related data

  Sub-competencies:

    Entry

      1. Identify diverse health-related databases

      2. Use computerized sources of health-related information

      3. Determine the compatibility of data from different data sources

      4. Select valid sources of information about health needs and interests

    Advanced 2

      1. Critique sources of health information.

Competency B: Collect health-related data

  Sub-competencies:

    Entry

      1. Use appropriate data-gathering instruments

      2. Apply survey techniques to acquire health data

      3. Conduct health-related needs assessments

      4. Implement appropriate measures to assess capacity for improving health status

Competency C: Distinguish between behaviors that foster and hinder well-being

  Sub-competencies:

Entry
1. Identify diverse factors that influence health behaviors
2. Identify behaviors that tend to promote or comprise health

Advanced 1
1. Explain the role of experiences in shaping patterns of health behavior

Competency D: Determine factors that influence learning
Sub-competencies
Advanced 1
1. Assess learning literacy
2. Assess learning styles
Advanced 2
1. Assess the learning environment

Competency E: Identify factors that foster or hinder the process of health education
Sub-competencies:
Entry
1. Determine the extent of available health education services
2. Identify gaps and overlaps in the provision of collaborative health services

Advanced 1
1. Assess the environmental and political climate regarding conditions that advance or inhibit program goals

Advanced 2
1. Investigate social forces causing opposing viewpoints regarding health education needs and concerns

Competency F: Infer needs for health education from obtained data
Sub-competencies:
Entry
1. Analyze needs assessment data

Advanced 1
1. Determine priorities for health education

Advanced 2
1. Predict future health education needs based upon societal changes

AREA II: PLAN HEALTH EDUCATION STRATEGIES, INTERVENTIONS, AND PROGRAMS

Competency A: Involve people and organizations in program planning
Sub-competencies:
Entry
1. Identify populations for health education programs
2. Elicit input from those who will affect or be affected by the program
3. Obtain commitments from individuals who will be involved
4. Develop plans for promoting collaborative efforts among health agencies and organizations with mutual interests

Reprinted by permission of the National Commission for Health Education Credentialing, Inc. (NCHEC), Society of Public Health Education (SOPHE), and American Association for Health Education (AAHE).

Advanced 1

1. Involve participants in planning health education programs

Competency B: Incorporate data analysis and principles of community organization

Sub-competencies:

Entry

1. Use research results when planning programs
2. Apply principles of community organization when planning programs
3. Suggest approaches for integrating health education within existing health programs
4. Communicate need for the program to those who will be involved

Advanced 1

1. Incorporate results of needs assessment into the planning process

Competency C: Formulate appropriate and measurable program objectives

Sub-competencies:

Entry

1. Design developmentally appropriate interventions

Advanced 1

1. Establish criteria for health education program objectives
2. Develop program objectives based upon identified needs
3. Appraise appropriateness of resources and materials relative to given objectives
4. Revise program objectives as necessitated by changing needs

Advanced 2

1. Develop subordinate measurable objectives as needed for instruction
2. Evaluate the efficacy of various methods to achieve objectives

Competency D: Develop a logical scope and sequence plan for health education practice

Sub-competencies:

Entry

1. Determine the range of health information necessary for a given program of instruction
2. Select references relevant to health education issues or programs

Advanced 1

1. Organize the subject areas compromising the scope of a program in logical sequence
2. Analyze the process for integrating health education into other programs

Advanced 2

1. Incorporate theory-based foundations in planning health education programs

Competency E: Design strategies, interventions, and programs consistent with specified objectives

Sub-competencies:

Advanced 1

1. Plan a sequence of learning opportunities that reinforce mastery of preceding objectives
2. Select strategies best suited to achieve objectives in a given setting

Advanced 2

1. Formulate a variety of educational methods
2. Match proposed learning activities with stated program objectives
3. Select appropriate theory-based strategies in health program planning

Reprinted by permission of the National Commission for Health Education Credentialing, Inc. (NCHEC), Society of Public Health Education (SOPHE), and American Association for Health Education (AAHE).

Competency F: Select appropriate strategies to meet objectives
  Sub-competencies:
    Entry
      1. Analyze technologies, methods and media for their acceptability to diverse groups
      2. Match health education services to proposed program activities
    Advanced 1
      1. Plan training and instructional programs for diverse populations
      2. Incorporate communication strategies into program planning
    Advanced 2
      1. Select educational materials consistent with accepted theory
Competency G: Assess factors that affect implementation
  Sub-competencies:
    Entry
      1. Determine the availability of information and resources needed to implement health education programs for a given audience
      2. Identify barriers to the implementation of health education programs
    Advanced 1
      1. Analyze factors (e.g., learner characteristics, legal aspects, feasibility) that influence choices among implementation methods
      2. Select implementation strategies based upon research results

AREA III: IMPLEMENT HEALTH EDUCATION STRATEGIES, INTERVENTIONS, AND PROGRAMS

Competency A: Initiate a plan of action
  Sub-competencies:
    Entry
      1. Use community organization principles to facilitate change conducive to health
      2. Pretest learners to determine baseline data relative to proposed program objectives
      3. Deliver educational technology effectively
      4. Facilitate groups
    Advanced 1
      1. Apply individual or group process methods as appropriate to given learning situations
Competency B: Demonstrate a variety of skills in delivering strategies, interventions, and programs
  Sub-competencies:
    Entry
      1. Use instructional technology effectively
      2. Apply implementation strategies
    Advanced 1
      1. Select methods that best facilitate achievement of program objectives
      2. Apply technologies that will contribute to program objectives

Reprinted by permission of the National Commission for Health Education Credentialing, Inc. (NCHEC), Society of Public Health Education (SOPHE), and American Association for Health Education (AAHE).

Advanced 2

    1. Use a variety of educational methods

Competency C: Use a variety of methods to implement strategies, interventions, and programs

    Sub-competencies:

    Entry

        1. Use the Code of Ethics in professional practice

        2. Apply theoretical and conceptual models from health education and related disciplines to improve program delivery

        3. Demonstrate skills needed to develop capacity for improving health status

        4. Incorporate demographically and culturally sensitive techniques when promoting programs

        5. Implement intervention strategies to facilitate health-related change

    Advanced 1

        1. Employ appropriate strategies when dealing with controversial health issues

Competency D: Conduct training programs

    Sub-competencies

    Advanced 1

        1. Demonstrate a wide range of strategies for conducting training programs

    Advanced 2

        1. Use instructional resources that meet a variety of training needs

AREA IV: CONDUCT EVALUATION AND RESEARCH RELATED TO HEALTH EDUCATION

Competency A: Develop plans for evaluation and research

    Sub-competencies:

    Entry

        1. Synthesize information presented in the literature

        2. Evaluate research designs, methods and findings presented in the literature

    Advanced 1

        1. Develop an inventory of existing valid and reliable tests and survey instruments

    Advanced 2

        1. Assess the merits and limitations of qualitative and quantitative methods

Competency B: Review research and evaluation procedures

    Sub-competencies:

    Entry

        1. Evaluate data-gathering instruments and processes

        2. Develop methods to evaluate factors that influence shifts in health status

    Advanced 1

        1. Identify standards of performance to be applied as criteria of effectiveness

        2. Identify methods to evaluate factors that influence shifts in health status

        3. Select appropriate methods for evaluating program effectiveness

Reprinted by permission of the National Commission for Health Education Credentialing, Inc. (NCHEC), Society of Public Health Education (SOPHE), and American Association for Health Education (AAHE).

Advanced 2

1. Establish a realistic scope of evaluation efforts
2. Select appropriate qualitative and/or quantitative evaluation design

Competency C: Design data collection instruments

Sub-competencies:

Entry

1. Develop valid and reliable evaluation instruments
2. Develop appropriate data-gathering instruments

Competency D: Carry out evaluation and research plans

Sub-competencies:

Entry

1. Use appropriate research methods and designs in health education practice
2. Use data collection methods appropriate for measuring stated objectives
3. Implement appropriate qualitative and quantitative evaluation techniques
4. Implement methods to evaluate factors that influence shifts in health status

Advanced 1

1. Assess the relevance of existing program objectives to current needs

Advanced 2

1. Apply appropriate evaluation technology
2. Analyze evaluation data

Competency E: Interpret results from evaluation and research

Sub-competencies:

Entry

1. Analyze evaluation data
2. Analyze research data
3. Compare evaluation results to other findings
4. Report effectiveness of programs in achieving proposed objectives

Advanced 1

1. Compare program activities with the stated program objectives
2. Develop recommendations based upon evaluation results

Advanced 2

1. Determine the achievement of objectives by applying criteria to evaluation results
2. Communicate evaluation results using easily understood terms

Competency F: Infer implications from findings for future health-related activities

Sub-competencies

Advanced 1

1. Suggest strategies for implementing recommendations that result from evaluation
2. Apply evaluation findings to refine and maintain programs

Advanced 2

1. Propose possible explanations for evaluation findings

Reprinted by permission of the National Commission for Health Education Credentialing, Inc. (NCHEC), Society of Public Health Education (SOPHE), and American Association for Health Education (AAHE).

AREA V: ADMINISTER HEALTH EDUCATION STRATEGIES, INTERVENTIONS, AND PROGRAMS _____

Competency A: Exercise organizational leadership

Sub-competencies:

Entry

1. Conduct strategic planning
2. Analyze the organization's culture in relationship to program goals
3. Promote cooperation and feedback among personnel related to the program

Advanced 1

1. Develop strategies to reinforce or change organizational culture to achieve program goals
2. Ensure that program activities comply with existing laws and regulations
3. Develop budgets to support program requirements

Advanced 2

1. Facilitate administration of the evaluation plan

Competency B: Secure fiscal resources

Sub-competencies

Advanced 1

1. Manage program budgets

Advanced 2

1. Prepare proposals to obtain fiscal resources

Competency C: Manage human resources

Sub-competencies:

Entry

1. Develop volunteer opportunities

Advanced 1

1. Demonstrate leadership in managing human resources
2. Apply human resource policies consistent with relevant laws and regulation
3. Identify qualifications of personnel needed for programs
4. Facilitate staff development
5. Apply appropriate methods of conflict reduction

Competency D: Obtain acceptance and support for programs

Sub-competencies

Advanced 1

1. Use concepts and theories of public relations and communications to obtain program support
2. Facilitate cooperation among personnel responsible for health education programs

Advanced 2

1. Provide support for individuals who deliver professional development courses

Reprinted by permission of the National Commission for Health Education Credentialing, Inc. (NCHEC), Society of Public Health Education (SOPHE), and American Association for Health Education (AAHE).

AREA VI: SERVE AS A HEALTH EDUCATION RESOURCE PERSON _____

Competency A: Use health-related information resources
  Sub-competencies:
    Entry
      1. Match information needs with the appropriate retrieval systems
      2. Select a data system commensurate with program needs
      3. Determine the relevance of various computerized health information resources
      4. Access health information resources
      5. Employ electronic technology for retrieving references
Competency B: Respond to requests for health information
  Sub-competencies:
    Entry
      1. Identify information sources needed to satisfy a request
      2. Refer requesters to valid sources of health information
Competency C: Select resource materials for dissemination
  Sub-competencies:
    Entry
      1. Evaluate applicability of resource materials for given audience
      2. Apply various processes to acquire resource materials
      3. Assemble educational material of value to the health of individuals and community groups
Competency D: Establish consultative relationships
  Sub-Competencies:
    Entry
      1. Analyze parameters of effective consultative relationships
      2. Analyze the role of the health educator as a liaison between program staff and outside groups
         and organizations
      3. Act as a liaison among consumer groups, individuals and health care providers
      4. Apply networking skills to develop and maintain consultative relationships
      5. Facilitate collaborative training efforts among health agencies and organizations
    Advanced 1
      1. Describe consulting skills needed by health educators

AREA VII: COMMUNICATE AND ADVOCATE
FOR HEALTH AND HEALTH EDUCATION _____

Competency A: Analyze and respond to current and future needs in health education
  Sub-competencies:
    Entry
      1. Analyze factors (e.g., social, cultural, demographic, political) that influence decision-makers
    Advanced 1
      1. Respond to challenges facing health education programs

2. Implement strategies for advocacy initiatives

3. Use evaluation data to advocate for health education programs

Advanced 2

1. Analyze the interrelationships among ethics, values, and behavior

2. Relate health education issues to larger social issues

Competency B: Apply a variety of communication methods and techniques

Sub-competencies:

Entry

1. Assess the appropriateness of language in health education messages

2. Compare different methods of distributing educational materials

3. Respond to public input regarding health education information

4. Use culturally sensitive communication methods and techniques

5. Use appropriate techniques for communicating health education information

6. Use oral, electronic and written techniques for communicating health education information

7. Demonstrate proficiency in communicating health information and health education needs

Competency C: Promote the health education profession individually and collectively

Sub-competencies:

Entry

1. Develop a personal plan for professional development

Advanced 2

1. Describe the state of the art of health education practice

2. Explain the major responsibilities of the health educator in the practice of health education

3. Explain the role of health education associations in advancing the profession

4. Explain the benefits of participating in professional organizations

Competency D: Influence health policy to promote health

Sub-competencies:

Entry

1. Identify the significance and implications of health are providers' messages to consumers

Advanced 1

1. Use research results to develop health policy

Advanced 2

1. Describe how research results influence health policy

2. Use evaluation findings in policy analysis and development

Reprinted by permission of the National Commission for Health Education Credentialing, Inc. (NCHEC), Society of Public Health Education (SOPHE), and American Association for Health Education (AAHE).

Code of Ethics for the Health Education Profession

PREAMBLE

The health education profession is dedicated to excellence in the practice of promoting individual, family, organizational, and community health. Guided by common ideals, Health Educators are responsible for upholding the integrity and ethics of the profession as they face the daily challenges of making decisions. By acknowledging the value of diversity in society and embracing a cross-cultural approach, Health Educators support the worth, dignity, potential, and uniqueness of all people.

The Code of Ethics provides a framework of shared values within which health education is practiced. The Code of Ethics is grounded in fundamental ethical principles that underlie all healthcare services: respect for autonomy, promotion of social justice, active promotion of good, and avoidance of harm. The responsibility of each Health Educator is to aspire to the highest possible standards of conduct and to encourage the ethical behavior of all those with whom they work.

Regardless of job title, professional affiliation, work setting, or population served, Health Educators abide by these guidelines when making professional decisions.

ARTICLE I: RESPONSIBILITY TO THE PUBLIC

A Health Educator's ultimate responsibility is to educate people for the purpose of promoting, maintaining, and improving individual, family, and community health. When a conflict of issues arises among individuals, groups, organizations, agencies, or institutions, Health Educators must consider all issues and give priority to those that promote wellness and quality of living through principles of self-determination and freedom of choice for the individual.

Section 1: Health Educators support the right of individuals to make informed decisions regarding health, as long as such decisions pose no threat to the health of others.

Section 2: Health Educators encourage actions and social policies that support and facilitate the best balance of benefits over harm for all affected parties.

Section 3: Health Educators accurately communicate the potential benefits and consequences of the services and programs with which they are associated.

Section 4: Health Educators accept the responsibility to act on issues that can adversely affect the health of individuals, families, and communities.

Section 5: Health Educators are truthful about their qualifications and the limitations of their expertise and provide services consistent with their competencies.

Section 6: Health Educators protect the privacy and dignity of individuals.

Section 7: Health Educators actively involve individuals, groups, and communities in the entire educational process so that all aspects of the process are clearly understood by those who may be affected.

Section 8: Health Educators respect and acknowledge the rights of others to hold diverse values, attitudes, and opinions.

Section 9: Health Educators provide services equitably to all people.

ARTICLE II: RESPONSIBILITY TO THE PROFESSION

Health Educators are responsible for their professional behavior, for the reputation of their profession, and for promoting ethical conduct among their colleagues.

Section 1: Health Educators maintain, improve, and expand their professional competence through continued study and education; membership, participation, and leadership in professional organizations; and involvement in issues related to the health of the public.

Section 2: Health Educators model and encourage nondiscriminatory standards of behavior in their interactions with others.

Section 3: Health Educators encourage and accept responsible critical discourse to protect and enhance the profession.

Section 4: Health Educators contribute to the development of the profession by sharing the processes and outcomes of their work.

Section 5: Health Educators are aware of possible professional conflicts of interest, exercise integrity in conflict situations, and do not manipulate or violate the rights of others.

Section 6: Health Educators give appropriate recognition to others for their professional contributions and achievements.

ARTICLE III: RESPONSIBILITY TO EMPLOYERS

Health Educators recognize the boundaries of their professional competence and are accountable for their professional activities and actions.

Section 1: Health Educators accurately represent their qualifications and the qualifications of others whom they recommend.

Section 2: Health Educators use appropriate standards, theories, and guidelines as criteria when carrying out their professional responsibilities.

Section 3: Health Educators accurately represent potential service and program outcomes to employers.

Section 4: Health Educators anticipate and disclose competing commitments, conflicts of interest, and endorsement of products.

Section 5: Health Educators openly communicate to employers expectations of job-related assignments that conflict with their professional ethics.

Section 6: Health Educators maintain competence in their areas of professional practice.

ARTICLE IV: RESPONSIBILITY IN THE DELIVERY OF HEALTH EDUCATION

Health Educators promote integrity in the delivery of health education. They respect the rights, dignity, confidentiality, and worth of all people by adapting strategies and methods to the needs of diverse populations and communities.

Section 1: Health Educators are sensitive to social and cultural diversity and are in accord with the law when planning and implementing programs.

Section 2: Health Educators are informed of the latest advances in theory, research, and practice, and use strategies and methods that are grounded in and contribute to development of professional standards, theories, guidelines, statistics, and experience.

Section 3: Health Educators are committed to rigorous evaluation of both program effectiveness and the methods used to achieve results.

Section 4: Health Educators empower individuals to adopt healthy lifestyles through informed choice rather than by coercion or intimidation.

Section 5: Health Educators communicate the potential outcomes of proposed services, strategies, and pending decisions to all individuals who will be affected.

ARTICLE V: RESPONSIBILITY IN RESEARCH AND EVALUATION

Health Educators contribute to the health of the population and to the profession through research and evaluation activities. When planning and conducting research or evaluation, health educators do so in accordance with federal and state laws and regulations, organizational and institutional policies, and professional standards.

Section 1: Health Educators support principles and practices of research and evaluation that do no harm to individuals, groups, society, or the environment.

Section 2: Health Educators ensure that participation in research is voluntary and is based upon the informed consent of the participants.

Section 3: Health Educators respect the privacy, rights, and dignity of research participants, and honor commitments made to those participants.

Section 4: Health Educators treat all information obtained from participants as confidential unless otherwise required by law.

Section 5: Health Educators take credit, including authorship, only for work they have actually performed and give credit to the contributions of others.

Section 6: Health Educators who serve as research or evaluation consultants discuss their results only with those to whom they are providing service, unless maintaining such confidentiality would jeopardize the health or safety of others.

Section 7: Health Educators report the results of their research and evaluation objectively, accurately, and in a timely fashion.

ARTICLE VI: RESPONSIBILITY IN PROFESSIONAL PREPARATION

Those involved in the preparation and training of Health Educators have an obligation to accord learners the same respect and treatment given other groups by providing quality education that benefits the profession and the public.

Section 1: Health Educators select students for professional preparation programs based upon equal opportunity for all and the individual's academic performance, abilities, and potential contribution to the profession and the public's health.

Section 2: Health Educators strive to make the educational environment and culture conducive to the health of all involved, and free from sexual harassment and all forms of discrimination.

Section 3: Health Educators involved in professional preparation and professional development engage in careful preparation; present material that is accurate, up-to-date, and timely; provide reasonable and timely feedback; state clear and reasonable expectations; and conduct fair assessments and evaluations of learners.

Section 4: Health Educators provide objective and accurate counseling to learners about career opportunities, development, and advancement, and they help learners secure professional employment.

Section 5: Health Educators provide adequate supervision and meaningful opportunities for the professional development of learners.

Source: Coalition of National Health Education Organizations. (1999). Available at: http://www.cnheo.org/. Used with permission.

Career and Health Resources

U.S. ASSOCIATIONS/ORGANIZATIONS/NONPROFITS

American Academy of Health Behavior (AAHB): http://www.aahb-temp.net/index.php

American Association for Health Education (AAHE): http://www.aahperd.org/

American Cancer Society: http://www.cancer.org/docroot/home/index.asp

American College Health Association (ACHA): http://www.acha.org

American College of Epidemiology: http://acepidemiology.org/

American College of Sports Medicine (ACSM): http://www.acsm.org/AM/Template.cfm?Section=About_ACSM

American Diabetes Association: http://www.diabetes.org/

American Evaluation Association: http://www.eval.org/

American Heart Association: http://www.americanheart.org/

American Psychological Association: http://www.apa.org/

American Public Health Association (APHA): http://www.apha.org/

American Red Cross: http://www.redcross.org/

American School Health Association: http://www.ashaweb.org

Association of Schools of Public Health: http://www.asph.org/

Association of State and Territorial Directors of Health Promotion and Public Health Education (AST-DHPPHE): http://www.astho.org/

Association of State and Territorial Health Officials: http://www.astho.org

Center for Advancing Health: http://www.cfah.org/

Center for the Advancement of Public Health: http://www.caph.gmu.edu/

Coalition of National Health Education Organizations (CNHEO): http://www.cnheo.org/

Directors of Health Promotion and Public Health Education: http://www.dhpe.org/about.asp

Eta Sigma Gamma (ESG) Health Education Honorary: http://www.etasigmagamma.org/

National Association of County and City Health Officials (NACCHO): http://www.naccho.org

National Association of Health Education Centers (NAHEC): http://www.nahec.org/

National Association of School-Based Health: http://www.nasbhc.org/

National Commission for Health Education Credentialing: http://www.nchec.org

National Coalition for Promoting Physical Activity: http://www.ncppa.org

National Coalition for Skin Cancer Prevention in Health, Physical Education, Recreation And Youth
Sports: http://www.cdc.gov/HealthyYouth/skincancer/facts.htm

National Wellness Institute: http://www.nationalwellness.org/

Partners in Information Access for the Public Health Workforce: http://www.phpartners.org

Society of State Directors of Health and Physical Education and Recreation: http://www.thesociety.org

Society for Public Health Education (SOPHE): http://www.sophe.org/

Society of State Departments of Health, Physical Education, and Recreation (SSDHPER): http://wg
.thesociety.org/default.asp

INTERNATIONAL ASSOCIATIONS/ORGANIZATIONS/NONPROFITS

Action for Global Health: http://www.actionforglobalhealth.org/

American International Health Alliance (AIHA): http://www.aiha.com/en/

Asociacion de Educacion para la Salud (Spain): http://www.adeps.org/

Center for Health and Gender Equity (CHANGE): http://www.genderhealth.org

Child Health and Nutrition Research Initiative: http://www.chnri.org/

Cooperative for Assistance and Relief Everywhere (CARE): http://www.care.org/

Equal Access: http://www.equalaccess.org/

European Clinical Research Infrastructures Network: http://www.ecrin.org/

European Public Health Association: http://www.eupha.org/

Family Health International: http://www.fhi.org

The George Institute for International Health: http://www.thegeorgeinstitute.org/

Global Health Action (GHA): http://www.globalhealthaction.org/

Global Health Council (GHC): http://www.globalhealth.org/

Grand Challenges in Global Health: http://www.grandchallenges.org/Pages/default.aspx

Health Metrics Network: http://www.who.int/healthmetrics/en/

International Committee of the Red Cross (ICRC): http://www.icrc.org/

International Council for Health, Physical Education, Recreation, Sport and Dance (ICHPER-SD):
http://www.ichpersd.org/

International Union for Health Promotion and Education (IUHPE): http://www.iuhpe.org

Archives of the Office International d'Hygiène Publique: https://www.who.int/archives/fonds_collec-
tions/bytitle/fonds_1/en/index.html

Pan American Health Organization (PAHO): http://new.paho.org/

Peace Corps: http://www.peacecorps.gov/

People's Health Movement: http://www.phmovement.org/

Population Index, Office of Population Research: http://www.popindex.princeton.edu

Population Reference Bureau (PRB): http://www.Prb.net

Project Concern International: http://www.projectconcern.org/site/PageServer

United National Education, Scientific and Cultural Organizations (UNESCO): http://www.unesco.org/
new/en/unesco/

United Nations Children Fund (UNICEF) and The NGO Working Groups on Girls: http://www
.girlsrights.org
United States Agency for International Development (USAID): http://www.usaid.gov/
The World Bank: http://www.worldbank.org
World Health Assembly (WHA): http://www.who.int/mediacentre/events/2005/wha58/en/
World Health Organization (WHO): http://www.who.int/en/
World Heart Federation (WHF): http://www.worldheart.org/
World Population Council (WPC): http://www.PopCouncil.org

INTERNATIONAL PRIVATE VOLUNTARY ORGANIZATIONS

ActionAid International (ACTIONAID INTERNATIONAL): http://www.actionaid.org/
Action by Churches Together International (ACT-INTL): http://www.act-intl.org/
Afghan NGOs Coordination Bureau (ANCB): http://www.ancb.org/
Africa and Middle East Refugee Assistance (AMERA): http://www.amera-uk.org/egypt/index_eg.html
Africa Humanitarian Action (AHA): http://www.africahumanitarian.org/home.aspx
All Africa Conference of Churches (AACC): http://www.aacc-ceta.org/en/
All India Disaster Mitigation Institute (AIDMI): http://www.aidmi.org/
Lebanese Association for Popular Action (AMEL): http://www.amel.org.lb/aasite/page.asp?pid=17&
lang=0
Anatolian Development Foundation (ADF): http://www.roldirectory.org/details.asp?Orgname=Anatoli
an+Development+Foundation
Austcare (AUSTCARE): http://www.austcare.org.au/
Australian Council for International Development (ACFID): http://www.acfid.asn.au/
BADIL Resource Center for Palestinian Residency and Refugee Rights (BADIL): http://www.badil.org/
Canadian Council for Refugees (CCR): http://www.ccrweb.ca/eng/engfront/frontpage.htm
Cooperative for Assistance and Relief Everywhere-CARE International Secretariat Geneva (CARE
INTL): http://www.care.org.eg/International/careintl.htm
Catholic Agency for Overseas Development (CAFOD): http://www.cafod.org.uk/
Christian Relief and Development Association (CRDA): http://www.crdaethiopia.org/aboutCRDA.php
Church World Service (CWS): http://www.churchworldservice.org/site/PageServer
Coastal Association for Social Transformation Trust (COAST): http://www.coastbd.org/Press_coco4_
021209/actitivity_photos.htm
Concern Worldwide (CONCERN): http://www.concern-worldwide.org/
Danish Refugee Council (DRC): http://www.drc.dk/
European Council for Refugees and Exiles: http://www.ecre.org/members/wrd_2009/dutch_council
Evangelical Foreign Missions Associations: http://www.emisdirect.com/
Frontiers—Ruwad Association (FRONTIERS): http://frontiersruwad.org/index.htm
Handicap International (HI): http://www.handicap-international.us/
HealthNet TPO: http://www.tpopom.org/HealthnetTPO(EN)
HelpAge International (HELPAGE): http://www.helpage.org/Home

Human Appeal International (HAI): http://humanappeal.org.uk/index.html

Human Rights First (HRF): http://www.humanrightsfirst.org/index.aspx

Human Rights Watch (HRW): http://www.hrw.org/

Individuell Människohjälp (IM) (Swedish Organisation for Individual Relief): http://www.manniskohjalp.se/sv/

InterAction (American Council for Voluntary International Action): http://www.interaction.org/

Interchurch Organisation for Development Co-operation (ICCO): http://www.icco.nl/delivery/main/en/

International Blue Crescent Relief and Development Foundation (IBC): http://www.ibc.org.tr/projekimlik/suriyeyardimeng.html

International Catholic Migration Commission (ICMC): http://www.icmc.net/docs/en

International Committee of the Red Cross (ICRC): http://www.icrc.org/

International Federation of Red Cross and Red Crescent Societies (IFRC): http://www.ifrc.org/

International Islamic Relief Organisation (IIRO): http://www.iirosa.org/

International Medical Corps (IMC): http://www.imcworldwide.org/

International Rehabilitation Council for Torture Victims (IRCT): http://www.irct.org/age.aspx?pid=183

International Rescue Committee (IRC): http://www.theirc.org/

Jesuit Refugee Service (JRS): http://www.jrs.net/home.php

Lutheran Immigration and Refugee Service (LIRS): http://www.lirs.org/site/c.nhLPJ0PMKuG/b.5537769/k.BFCA/Home.htm

Lutheran World Federation (LWF): http://www.lutheranworld.org/

Malaysian Medical Relief Society (MERCY Malaysia): http://www.mercy.org.my/

Marie Stopes International (MSI): http://www.mariestopes.org/

Mercy Corps (MERCY CORPS): http://www.mercycorps.org/

Norwegian Refugee Council (NRC): http://www.nrc.no/?aid=9160624

OXFAM Great Britain (OXFAM GB): http://www.oxfam.org.uk/

Plan International (PLAN): http://plan-international.org/

Refugee Consortium of Kenya (RCK): http://www.rckkenya.org/

Refugee Council of Australia (RCOA): http://www.refugeecouncil.org.au/

Refugee Council USA (RCUSA): http://www.rcusa.org

Refugees International (RI): http://www.refintl.org/

Refugee Studies Centre (RSC): http://www.rsc.ox.ac.uk/

Salvation Army International Headquarters (SALVATION ARMY): http://www.salvationarmy.org/ihq/www_sa.nsf

Save the Children Alliance (SAVE ALLIANCE): http://www.savethechildren.org/

Stichting Vluchteling (SV): http://www.vluchteling.org/pagina/6B7DF36C-39A2-4FFC-B229-D22518061417

Sustainable Environment and Ecological Development Society (SEEDS India): http://www.gdrc.org/uem/seeds.html

Thailand Burma Border Consortium (TBBC): http://www.tbbc.org/

Women's Refugee Commission: http://www.womensrefugeecommission.org/

World Council of Churches (WCC): http://www.oikoumene.org/

World Vision International (WVI): http://www.wvi.org/wvi/wviweb.nsf

INTERNATIONAL PHILANTHROPIC FOUNDATIONS

Carnegie Corporation: http://carnegie.org/
Hewlett Foundation: http://www.hewlett.org/
Milbank Memorial Fund of New York: http://www.milbank.org/
Nuffield Foundation: http://www.nuffieldfoundation.org/
Rockefeller Foundation: http://www.rockefellerfoundation.org/
Sasakawa Memorial Health Foundation: http://www.smhf.or.jp/e/index.html
Welcome Trust: http://www.wellcome.ac.uk/
W. K. Kellogg Foundation: http://www.wkkf.org/

International Private Industry

Essential Drugs Program: http://www.who.int/countries/eth/areas/medicines/en/
International Federation of Pharmaceutical Manufacturers and Associations (IFPMA): http://www
.ifpma.org/

GOVERNMENTAL AGENCIES

United States Governmental Agencies and Nonprofit Organizations

Advocates for Youth: http://www.advocatesforyouth.org
Agency for Healthcare Research and Quality (AHRQ): http://www.ahrq.gov
Agency for Toxic Substances and Disease Registry (STSDR): http://www.atsdr.cdc.gov/
Alliance for Curriculum Reform: http://www.acr.uc.edu
American Cancer Society (ACS): http://www.cancer.org
American Red Cross (ARC): http://www.redcross.org/
Center for the Advancement of Health: http://www.cfah.org/
Center for the Advancement of Public Health: http://www.caph.gmu.edu/
Center for Medicare and Medicaid Services: http://www.cms.gov/
Centers for Disease Control and Prevention (CDC): http://www.cdc.gov/
Child Health Coalition: http://www.cancer.org
Children's Defense Fund: http://www.childrensdefense.org
Department of Energy's Environment, Safety, and Health: http://www.energy.gov/safetyhealth/index
.htm
Environmental Protection Agency (EPA): http://www.epa.gov/
Families and Children (FACT): http://www.familiesandchildren.org/
Food and Drug Administration (FDA) 4Girls Health: http://www.girlshealth.gov/
Healthfinder (Consumer Health): http://www.healthfinder.gov/
National Alliance for Hispanic Health: http://www.Hispanichealth.org
National Alliance for Nutrition and Activity: http://www.cspinet.org/nutritionpolicy/nana.html

National Cancer Institute: http://www.cancer.gov/
National Center for Chronic Disease Prevention and Health Promotion: http://www.cdc.gov/nccdphp
National Center for Health Statistics (NCHS): http://www.cdc.gov/nchs/
National Coalition to Support Sexuality Education: http://www.siecus.org
National Health Information Center (NHIC): http://www.health.gov/nhic/
National Heart, Lung, and Blood Institute (NHLBI): http://www.nhlbi.nih.gov
National Institutes of Health (NIH): http://www.nih.gov/
National Institutes of Health Office of Women's Health Research: http://orwh.od.nih.gov/
National Resource Center on Aging and Injury (NRCAI): http://www.nrcai.org
Occupational Safety and Health Administration (OSHA): http://www.osha.gov/
Partners in Information Access for the Public Health Workforce: http://www.phpartners.org
President's Council on Physical Fitness and Sports: http://www.hoptechno.com/book11.htm
Roper Center for Public Opinion Research: http://www.roercenter.uconn.edu
Substance Abuse and Mental Health Services Administration—Center for Substance Abuse Prevention/
    National Clearinghouse for Alcohol and Drug Information (SAMHSA): http://www.samhsa.gov/
Social Statistics Briefing Room at the White House: http://nces.ed.gov/ssbr/pages/index.asp
Substance Abuse and Mental Health Services (SAMHSA): http://www.samhsa.gov/
The Surgeon General's Prescription for Health: http://www.surgeongeneral.gov/SGScripts/prescription
    .cfm
Trust for America's Health: http://www.tfah.org
U.S. Census Bureau: http://www.Census.gov
U.S. Department of Health and Human Services (USDHHS): http://www.os.dhhs.gov
U.S. Department of Labor: http://www.dol.gov/
U.S. National Library of Medicine (NLB): http://www.nlm.nih.gov/

International Governmental and Intergovernmental Agencies

American Red Cross: http://www.redcross.org/
Australia Department of Health: http://www.health.gov.au/
Public Health Agency of Canada: http://www.phac-aspc.gc.ca/hp-ps/index-eng.php
United Nations Children Fund (UNICEF): http://www.unicef.org/
The World Bank: http://www.worldbank.org/
World Health Organization (WHO): http://www.who.int/

JOURNALS

U.S. Journals

Age & Ageing: http://www.ageing.oupjournals.org/
Ageing International: http://alidoro.catchword.com/vl=10950634/cl=6/nw=1/rpsv/catchword/tranpub/
    01635158/contp1.htm

American Journal of Epidemiology: http://www.aje.oupjournals.org/ or http://www.jhsph.edu/Publications/
   JEPI
American Journal of Health Behavior: http://131.230.221.136/ajhb/
American Journal of Health Promotion: http://www.healthpromotionjournal.com
American Journal of Health Studies: http://education.nyu.edu/hepr/resources/journals/3.html
American Journal of Preventive Medicine: http://www.elsevier.com/locate/ajpmonline
American Journal of Public Health: http://www.ajph.org/
American School Board Journal: http://www.asbj.com
Annals of Behavioral Medicine: http://psychweb.syr.edu/sbm/abm.html
Annals of Epidemiology: http://www.elsevier.com/locate/annepidem
Consumer Reports: http://www.consumerreports.org/cro/index.htm
Emory University: http://www.gen.emory.edu/MEDWEB/alphakey/electronic_publications/a.html
Evaluation and the Health Profession: http://www.sagepub.co.uk/journals/details/c001.html
Global Health Promotion: http://www.iuhpe.org/?page=19&lang=en
The Hastings Center Report: http://www.thehastingscenter.org/Publications/HCR/Default.aspx
Health Education and Behavior: http://www.sph.umich.edu/group/hbhe/heb
Health Education Research: Theory and Practice: http://www.oup.co.uk/healed or http://her.oupjournals.org
The Health Educator: The Journal of Eta Sigma Gamma: http://www.etasigmagamma.org/healtheducator
Health Promotion International: http://www.oup.co.uk/heapro or http://heapro.oupjournals.org
Health promotion journals: http://www.ki.se/phs/hprin/hprin_journals.html
Health Promotion Practice: http://www.sagepub.co.uk/journals/details/j0309.html
Health science journals: http://www.mco.edu/lib/instr/libinsta.html
Journal of American College Health: http://www.heldref.org
Journal of the American Medical Association (JAMA): http://www.ama-assn.org/public/journals/jama/
   jamahome.htm
Journal of the American Medical Informatics Association: http://www.jamia.org
Journal of Community Health: http://www.plenum.com/title.cgi?1018
Journal of Epidemiology and Community Health: http://www.bmjpg.com/data/ech.htm or http://www.jech.
   com or http://ije.oupjournals.org
Journal of Health Communication: http://www.emerson.edu/JHealthCom/
Journal of Health Education: http://www.aahperd.org/johe/johe.html
Journal of School Health: http://www.ashaweb.org
New England Journal of Medicine: http://nejm.org
Online health journals: http://www.thomson.com/brookscole/health/journals/html
Public Health Reports: http://www.publichealthreports.org/
Social Marketing Quarterly: http://www.socialmarketingquarterly.com/

International Journals and Reports

African Studies: http://alidoro.catchword.com/vl=10950634/cl=6/nw=1/rpsv/catchword/carfax/00020184/
   contp1.htm
British Medical Journal: http://www.bmj.com

Bulletin of the World Health Organization: http://www.who.int/bulletin/volumes/en/
Canadian Journal of Aging: http://www.cmpa.ca/canjourag.html
Canadian Journal of Public Health: http://www.cpha.ca/Periodicals/Period.home.html
Canadian Medical Association Journal: http://www.cma.ca/cmaj
Critical Public Health: http://www.tandf.co.uk/journals/CARFAX/09581596.HTM
Eastern Mediterranean Health Journal: http://www.emro.who.int/Publications/EMHJ/index.asp
European Journal of Public Health: http://www3.oup.co.uk/eurpub
International Council for Health, Physical Education, Recreation, Sport and Dance (ICHPERD-SD) Journal:
    http://www.ichpersd.org/index.php/journal
The International Classification of Diseases: http://www.who.int/classifications/icd/en/
International Electronic Journal of Health Education: http://www.aahperd.org/aahe/publications/iejhe/
International Health Regulations: http://www.who.int/ihr/en/
International Journal of Environmental Health Research: http://www.carfax.co.uk/ije-ad.htm
International Journal of Epidemiology: http://www3.oup.co.uk/ije/contents or http://ije.oupjournals.org
International Journal of Rehabilitation and Health: http://www.plenum.com/journals_list.cgi?434
International Journal of Medicine Online: http://www.priory.com/journals/med.htm
Internet Journal of Health Promotion: http://www.monash.edu.au/health/IJHP
Pan American Journal of Public Health: http://journal.paho.org/
Social Science and Medicine: http://www.elsevier.com/wps/find/journaldescription.cws_home/315/
    description
World Health Organizations Weekly Epidemiological Record: http://www.who.int/wer/en/
The World Health Report: http://www.who.int/whr/2008/en/index.html

TECHNOLOGY PRIMARY SOURCES FOR STATISTICAL DATA

United States

Centers for Disease Control and Prevention: http://www.cdc.gov/
Combined Health Education Database: http://chid.nih.gov/
Data resources: http://www.abag.ca.gov/abag/overview/datacenter/popdemo/datamine.htm
EBSCO: http://www.ebscohost.com/
Epidemiologic Data Resource: http://cedr.lbl.gov/index.html
Epidemiology resources: http://chanane.ucsf.edu/epidem/epidem.html
ERIC searches on educational research: http://www.ericfacility.net/extra/index.html
Google Scholar: http://scholar.google.com/
Google Uncle Sam: http://www.google.com/unclesam
Government Printing Office: http://www.gpoaccess.gov/databases.html
Health A to Z search engine: http://www.healthatoz.com/
Health information database: http://chid.nih.gov/
Index Medicus (journal abbreviations): http://www.nlm.nih.gov/tsd/serials/lji.html
Institute of Medicine: http://www2.nas.edu/iom/
Morbidity and Mortality Weekly Report: http://www.cdc.gov/epo/mmwr/mmwr.html
National Center for Health Statistics: http://www.cdc.gov/nchs/about.htm

National Institutes of Health: http://www.nih.gov/
National Library of Medicine (Medline, MeSH, PubMed): http://www.nlm.nih.gov/
Public Health Shareware: http://www.jhsph.edu/People/Org/DeltaOmega/software/
U.S. Bureau of the Census: http://www.census.gov/

International

Bio-Med Central (BMC) International Health and Human Rights: http://www.biomedcentral.com/
bmcinthealthhumrights/
Biosciences resources: http://golgi.harvard.edu/htbin/biopages
International health resources: http://www.pitt.edu/HOME/GHNet/GHKR.html
Organisation for Economic Co-operation and Development (OECD): http://www.oecd.org/home/0,298
7,en_2649_201185_1_1_1_1_1,00.html
The State of the World's Children (UNICEF) Annual Report: http://www.unicef.org/sowc/
UNESCO Statistical Yearbook: http://www.uis.unesco.org/en/stats/statistics/yearbook/YBIndexNew.htm
United Nations Demographic Yearbook: http://unstats.un.org/unsd/demographic/products/dyb/dyb2.htm
United Nations Yearbook: http://unyearbook.un.org/
United States Agency for International Development (USAID): http://www.usaid.gov/
The World Bank Atlas: http://web.worldbank.org/WBSITE/EXTERNAL/DATASTATISTICS/0,,content
MDK:20798108~menuPK:64133152~pagePK:64133150~piPK:64133175~theSitePK:
239419,00.html
World Development Report: http://econ.worldbank.org/WBSITE/EXTERNAL/EXTDEC/EXT
RESEARCH/EXTWDRS/0,,contentMDK:20227703~pagePK:478093~piPK:477627~theSitePK:
477624,00.html
World Health Organization's Weekly Epidemiological Record: http://www.who.int/home-page/
World Health Organization's Global Infobase: https://apps.who.int/infobase/report.aspx

U.S. CAREER OPPORTUNITY AND ADVOCACY SITES

American University job site: http://www1.american.edu/academic.depts/cas/health/nchf/jobs/ftjobs.
html
Career Builder: http://www.careerbuilder.com/JobSeeker/Jobs/JobDetails.aspx?Job_DID=J8A11R656
MHPK75XG87&cbRecursionCnt=1&cbsid=1a290377e88144318635bc4f041e1a42-324242230-
wc-6&ns_siteid=ns_us_y_Health_Educator_Jobs
Chico State University, California, Career Opportunities in Health Education: http://www.csuchico.
edu/hcsv/hejobs.shtml
FirstGov (official U.S. government portal): http://permanent.access.gpo.gov/lps1393/firstgov.gov/index.
htm
International City/County Management Association (ICMA): http://www.icma.org/main/sc.asp?t=0
Jobvolume: http://www.jobvolume.com/q-health-educator-p-usa-jobs.html
Library of Congress: http://www.loc.gov/index.html
Monster.com: http://jobsearch.monster.com/Search.aspx?cy=US&brd=1&q=Health+AND+eduator

National Association of Counties: http://www.naco.org/

National Governor's Association (NGA): http://www.nga.org/portal/site/nga/menuitem
.b14a675ba7f89cf9e8ebb856a11010a0

National League of Cities: http://www.nlc.org/

New York State Department of Labor Career Zone: http://www.nycareerzone.org/text/profile.jsp;jsessi
onid=755471072197038645?onetsoc=21-1091.00

U.S.A. Recruit: http://usa.recruit.net/search-public+health+educator-jobs

U.S. Conference of Mayors: http://www.usmayors.org/

U.S. House of Representatives: http://www.house.gov/

U.S. Senate: http://www.senate.gov/

U. S. White House: http://www.whitehouse.gov/

SPECIFIC RESOURCES AND ADDITIONAL SITES FOR HEALTH CAREERS

Academy for Educational Development: http://www.aed.org

American Alliance for Health, Physical Education, Recreation and Dance: http://www.aahperd.org (see
career link)

American Public Health Association CareerMart: http://www.apha.publichealthjobs.net/

APHA Student Assembly Resource: http://aphastudents.org/opportunities.php

APHA Career Development Center: http://careers.apha.org/careerdev/

Association of Schools of Public Health: http://www.asph.org/

American College Health Association–Jobline Classifieds: http://www.acha.org/prof_dev/classifieds.cfm

American Association for Health Education/AAHPERD–Career Link: http://www.aahperd.org/careers/
careerlink.cfm

American Evaluation Association: http://www.eval.org

Association of Schools of Public Health: http://www.publichealthjobs.net/

CareerBuilder.com: http://msn.careerbuilder.com/jobs/keyword/health+educator

Career Development: http://www.mlanet.org/jobs/index.html

U.S. Center for Disease Control and Prevention (CDC): http://www.cdc.gov/employment/

Chronicle of Higher Education Jobs: http://chronicle.com/jobs/

Health and Wellness Jobs: http://www.healthandwellnessjobs.com/joblist.cfm

Healthcare Source Job Board: http://www.healthcaresource.com/findajob.cfm

Higher Ed Jobs: http://www.higheredjobs.com/

HP Career Net: http://www.hpcareer.net/index.jsp

Idealist Guide to Nonprofit Careers: http://www.idealist.org/careerguide

INDEED: http://www.indeed.org

Inside Higher Ed: http://www.insidehighered.com/careers

International Job Finders: http://www.internationaljobfinders.com/

International Jobs: http://www.intljobs.org/

International Jobs Center: http://www.internationaljobs.org/

Job Hunt.Org: http://www.job-hunt.org/international.shtml

Jobs Abroad: http://www.jobsabroad.com/search.cfm

Jobs World: http://www.jobs-world.biz/

Juju–Job Search Engine: http://www.juju.com/keyword/wellness-health-promotion

National Association of City and County Health Officials: http://www.naccho.org/careers/

National Commission for Health Education Credentialing: http://www.nchec.org/news/docs/jobs.htm

National Commission for Health Education Credentialing (NCHEC): http://www.nchec.org/seekers/seekers.htm

Public Health Employment Connection: http://cfusion.sph.emory.edu/PHEC/phec.cf

Public Health Jobs.net: http://publichealthjobs.net/

Public Health Jobs Worldwide: http://www.jobspublichealth.com/

Partners in Information Access for the Public Health Workforce: http://phpartners.org/jobs.html

Society of Public Health Educators (SOPHE): http://www.sophe.org

The Riley Guide: http://www.rileyguide.com/internat.html

U. S. Department of Health and Human Services Division (USDHHS): http://www.hhs.gov/careers/

U.S. Federal Department of Agriculture: http://www.fda.gov/AboutFDA/WorkingatFDA/default.htm

U.S. National Institute of Health: http://www.jobs.nih.gov/

USAJOBS: http://www.usajobs.gov/

WHO Employment: http://www.who.int/employment/vacancies/en/

GLOSSARY

A Competency-Based Framework for Health Educators–2006: The undergraduate and graduate standards of the health profession adopted by many universities and associations/organizations that outline the basic responsibilities and competencies for health educators.

A Competency-Based Framework for Graduate-Level Health Educators: The ten unique roles and services of graduate-prepared health educators adopted by many universities, associations/ organizations, and state certification and accreditation agencies as graduate health program standards. It was replaced by Competencies Update Project (CUP) of 2006.

Acculturation: The process of adapting to another culture.

Axiology: One of the four criteria of philosophy; it works with goodness and studies values, ethics, and aesthetics.

Bachelor of Arts (BA): A degree granted in the humanities, requiring general education courses, along with a foreign language; it is sometimes considered a more traditional education.

Bachelor of Science (BS): A degree that requires more major courses, fewer electives, and often a formal minor and/or a research paper.

Bacteria: Groups of microorganisms, some of which are pathogenic and cause infectious diseases including fatal bacterial diseases.

Barriers: Obstructions that participants believe they may have to overcome to practice beneficial health behaviors or bring about environmental change.

Behavior change/modification: A philosophy that concerns individual modification of habits, but can include group/community changes.

Behavior science/health education: A focus on ways to encourage healthy choices in humans by developing communitywide education programs that promote healthy lifestyles to prevent disease and injury, and by researching health issues.

Behavior modification: This philosophy is the same as behavior change and concerns individual modification of habits, but can include group/community change.

Behavioral objectives: Changes in the individual participant's health behavior(s) in a program.

Benefits: The positive effects that participants believe a particular behavior or environmental change will bring about.

Best practices: The ideal approach to help planners manage strategies and methods for particular circumstances for a program.

Biostatistics: A discipline that identifies health trends through the application of statistical procedures, techniques, and methodology that lead to life-saving measures.

Bioterrorism threats: A public health threat to deliberately release infectious or chemical agents; such threats have heightened the risk of epidemics today.

CDCynergy: An interactive, comprehensive communication plan that allows for planning, implementing, and evaluating program strategies to address the health problems using health communication involvement.

Certification: When a professional organization identifies a person who completes a competency-based curriculum and predetermined standard of performance and can practice the given profession.

Certified Health Education Specialist (CHES): A specific credentialing available to qualified health educators requiring academic qualifications and testing requirements administered by the National Commission for Health Education Credentialing, Inc.

Chain of Infection Model: A model that shows how diseases are spread as pathogens enter the human reservoir, exit, transmit through the portal of entry, and establish the disease in a new host.

Chemical Incident Alert and Response System: An alert and response system for communicable diseases and other environmental health emergencies.

Code of Ethics for the Health Education Profession: A document outlining the ethical standards of conduct and rights and protection of human subjects in health research, teaching, and programs.

Cognitive-based and healthy decision making: A philosophy that espouses increasing the knowledge base and skills of individuals so they can make wise choices and decisions in life.

Communicable Disease or Infection Model: A triangle depicting how the agent (disease), host, and environment interact to cause an infectious disease in a new person.

Communicable diseases: Infectious diseases caused by some specific biological agent or toxic product that are transmitted from an infected person, animal, or inanimate reservoir to a susceptible host.

Community models: Models that cover institutional, community, and public policy factors.

Community Organization Theory: A theory that emphasizes active participation and development of communities that can better evaluate and solve health and social problems.

Community theories: Theories that include institutional, community, and public policy factors that influence health in programs.

Comprehensive School Health Education: The identified content areas that are recommended as part of the core curriculum in health education in the schools K–12.

Concepts: The primary elements of the theory.

Constructivist: A philosophy that concerns the formulation of knowledge; a learning premise used mainly in the educational setting.

Constructs: The key concepts developed for a theory.

Consumer Information Processing: A theory that an individual's behavior is determined by behavioral intention, or the result of attitudes toward the behavior, and subjective perception of norms adjacent to the behavior. This theory uses the process by which consumers acquire and use information for decision making.

Coordinated School Health Program: The eight components determined as part of a planned, sequential, and integrated school health program that meets the health/safety needs of students grades K–12 according to the National Center for Chronic Disease Prevention and Health and the Centers for Disease Control and Prevention.

Credentialing: A process by professional organizations that involves individual and/or programs and includes processes of licensure, certifications, and/or registration.

Cultural competence: The ability to work with other cultures with sensitivity, effectiveness, and respect for their differences.

Cultural components: The behavioral components of lifestyles and learned experiences (socialization) that determine how people see and interpret their environment.

Cultural models: Models that address embedded cultural factors and attempt to change those negative ones detrimental to health.

Cultural theories: A community theory that addresses the embedded cultural traditions, beliefs, and practices that are detrimental to health in the population.

Cultural Transformation Theory: A theory that proposes that the diversity of human culture is founded on two basic social models and advocates for the partnership linkage model.

Culture: The learned experiences (socialization) and knowledge people gain through their environment.

Demographic trends: Statistics collected on population size and geographic distribution including population growth, fertility and contraception, mortality, migration, ageism, and urbanism.

Determinants of health (or health determinants): The personal, social, economic, and environmental factors that determine health status, focusing on the basics of health maintenance.

Diffusion of Innovations: A theory that delineates the process of how new products and messages are introduced and widely distributed to the audiences.

Disease trends: Disease patterns that determine increased health risks in humans.

Doctor of Education (EdD): A terminal degree that is normally practice-focused and includes specific education requirements.

Doctor of Philosophy (PhD): A terminal degree encompassing a broad spectrum in public health emphasis.

Doctor of Public Health (DrPH): A terminal degree that focuses on one specific aspect of public health and emphasizes research and administration.

Ecological Model: A model that comprehensively addresses public health problems at multiple levels of influence, combining behavioral and environmental components.

Education: Formal knowledge training and skills provided in grades K–12 and higher education settings.

Education setting (K–12 and higher education): A setting for health education that includes teaching and faculty positions and administrative positions in educational settings.

Education standards: The basic skills a person should possess after a period of education.

Egalitarian philosophy: A philosophy that involves cooperation and support to change society's infrastructure for the betterment of all.

Electronic portfolio or hard copy portfolio: A selective and specific collection of work made available in hard copy format or on a Web site. It documents abilities and records and provides evidence of achievements.

Empirical review: A review of relevant research literature for identifying similar programs, replicable programs, and multiple interventions and levels.

EMPOWER: An interactive technological tool system, based on the PRECEDE–PROCEED program planning model, to support professional planners in developing programs to meet the unique needs of a particular local group or community.

Empowerment: A concept in theory that involves the ability of participants to gain mastery and power over themselves and their community to produce change.

Empowerment Model: A theory that suggests that a problem-proposing process can help participants feel more powerful, thus freeing them to make healthier behavioral and life choices. This concept involves the mastery and power of participants in a community to produce change.

Empowerment philosophy: This is a philosophy of enablement or shared power in which groups/communities are given the skills and knowledge to continue positive change on their own.

Enabling factors: Factors that allow people to act on their own inclinations due to support, resources, assistance, and services.

Endemic rates: Large numbers of disease cases that occur in a population regularly.

Epidemic rates: Large numbers of disease cases not normally expected in a population.

Epidemiology: The study of disease transmission in humans including descriptives, statistics, causes, rates, risks, trends, and problem solving.

Epistemology: One of the four criteria of philosophies; known as the study of knowledge, it is based on observation of the known and uses evidence-based practice for determining the most effective solutions to problems.

Environmental change: The differences in any ecological element during a health promotion program.

Environmental health: The impact of our surroundings on our health.

Environmental objectives: Changes in a program such as prevention and promotion factors and removing barriers in a program.

Ethics: The values or standards of professional conduct.

Etiology: The study of disease causes.

Evidence-Based planning, programs, and practice: These are detailed programs that are based on research with proven empirical verification of effectiveness.

Existentialism: An extension of the pragmatist philosophy; it is about emotions and humanism.

Explanatory theory: Change theory that when combined with strategic planning models is crucial in the success of a health behavior change program.

Fleming, Alexander: A Scottish medic, pharmacologist, and bacteriologist who discovered the antibiotic penicillin in 1928.

Formalist: A philosophy of concepts that are explained in terms of intellectual intuition concerning rights, duties, and obligations.

Formative evaluation: Evaluation that includes information collected during the process evaluation and pilot program evaluation of a program.

Functional/utilitarian philosophy: A philosophy concerned with the change to a productive infrastructure in communities that leads to better and healthier lives.

Genetic determinants: These are inherited health traits that play a great role in risk factors for certain diseases in humans.

Global health: Health initiatives that involve worldwide cooperation and interaction across national borders. It extends to relations beyond governments to include individuals and groups within societies advocating for the protection of communities, countries, and the globe to deter health and disease risks through preventive medicine, health education, communicable disease control, sanitary measures, and environmental controls.

Global health problems: Ecological conditions caused by global integration across boundaries that can positively or negatively affect the health of countries as well as the environment, health prevention, planning, and services, healthcare access, socio-economic conditions, political structures, and socio-cultural patterns.

Global health security: Monitoring and preventing acute public health events that endanger the collective health of populations living across geographic regions and international boundaries.

Global networks: Electronic intelligence-gathering tools that provide a safety net for detection of events not otherwise reported.

Global problems: All influences affect the global structure. Environments, politics, infrastructures, and social/cultural patterns vary in many different countries and parts of the world. Recognizing these differences and working with supportive laws, policies, regulations, and norms can support environmental changes and communities.

Goal: A broad statement of the program's aim; the objective for the community and participants to achieve.

Governmental/public health agency: A setting for health education that includes the country of origin or unilateral, bilateral, and/or multilateral agreements among governments to form organizations that influence the well-being and health of a population.

Greatest public health achievements in the world: Three achievements cited by WHO in 2007 that have influenced public health in the greatest capacity, including plague and quarantine, cholera and sanitation, and smallpox and immunization.

HABIT Model: A model that takes the health educator through the stages of a health program using strategic planning; the acronym HABIT stands for hiring, assessing, building, implementing, and testing.

Health: "A state of complete physical, mental, and social well-being and not merely the absence of infirmity" (WHO, 1947).

Health Behavior Change Program: A program that uses explanatory theory and the strategic planning model for altering performance or behavior patterns.

Health Belief Model: A medical model that helps establish the factors that affect a person's ability to perform preventive health behaviors.

Healthcare access or Access: The availability of quality health care and disease control tools including clinics, medical personnel, drugs, vaccines, and diagnostics; it is a critical health determinant of populations.

Health disparities: Discrimination against certain people concerning their health needs, limiting prevention, promotion, protection, literacy, and access for all.

Health education: A combination of planned learning experiences based upon proven research theories and models that provide individuals, groups, and communities the needed skills, knowledge, and opportunities to make informed and meaningful health decisions.

Health educator: A professionally prepared health educator who develops, implements, and evaluates policies, procedures, interventions, systems, and appropriate educational strategies conducive to the health of individuals, groups, and communities for prevention of disease and adverse health conditions.

Health enhancement: Extraordinary measures taken above and beyond the norm to continuously improve one's health.

Health indicators: The statistics or health data that describe health problems and identify trends that help decision makers set priorities and improve global health when designing, implementing, and evaluating health education programs used as health indices.

Health indices: The statistics collected to compare international, national, state, and local health data as a way to describe health problems.

Health literacy: The capacity of an individual to obtain, interpret, and understand basic health information and services.

Health maintenance: The everyday way that people attempt to stay well, including such considerations as proper clothing, food, shelter, healthcare access, healthful environment, and social support.

Health prevention: The practice of beneficial health behaviors, actions, and interventions designed to identify risks and reduce susceptibility or exposure to health threats before the onset of disease.

Health Program Strategic Plan: A targeted program plan with an identified scope and sequence of the program's focus to target the identified problems.

Health promotion: The process of enabling people to improve their health by increasing control over the determinants of health.

Health protection: Health shields or traditional beliefs that a person or community has in place to provide physical and mental protection and spirituality, enabling a high quality of life.

Health statistics: The data collection techniques used for health indices or indicators in groups.

Health status categories: Healthy, nonhealthy, afflicted, and death.

Healthy People 2010 and 2020: A continuous government program led by health experts to present a vision for the future and bring change, prevent disease, and promote improved health to all people in the United States.

Holistic: Relating to the physical, mental, spiritual, emotional, and social components that influence human well-being.

Home page of a Web site: The first page of the Web site with basic contact information and a menu bar or table of contents that links to other elements.

Human subjects review boards: These are governments, agencies, universities, medical centers, and other institutional review boards that monitor all programs and research involving human subjects.

Immunization: The active exposure of a certain disease element in a person to illicit an immune response; it is commonly given in the form of a vaccination.

Impact evaluation: An assessment of the behavioral and other positive changes of the participants of a program.

Incidence rates: The new case numbers of people infected with a disease or illness in a specified time.

Individual credentialing: A process that involves the regulation of a professional by requiring predetermined, specific professional preparation and practice, academic standards, and achievement of standards of performance.

Informatics: Information availability and accessibility via technology.

Institutional/organizational factors: The organizational factors that address rules, regulations, policies, and informal structures that can restrict or support the behaviors recommended.

Institutionalization: The organizational factors that address rules, regulations, policies, and informal structures that can restrict or support the behaviors recommended.

Institutionalized: The state of informal rules and policies becoming embedded in communities.

Integrative plans: Multiple theories and multiple resources combined to address a single problem.

Intergovernmental organization: A setting for health education that includes regional and global organizations with an interest in international health and working in conjunction with a government agency.

International Health Regulations: Global rules adopted and enforced by WHO in 2005 that provide a framework for member states to respond to events that threaten national, state, and global security.

International Sanitary Regulations: Worldwide regulations on the containment of epidemics within territories.

Interpersonal models and theories: Models and theories that address individual factors as they relate to individual needs, environment, and personal characteristics.

Intrapersonal models and theories: Individual models and theories that impact individual knowledge, attitudes, beliefs, and behaviors.

Jenner, Edward: An English physician who successfully gave the first cowpox vaccination against smallpox in 1796.

Koch, Robert: A German physician who advanced the theory of specific disease agents or the relationship between a microorganism and a disease. His first demonstration was with the anthrax bacillus in 1876.

Learning objectives: Changes in the participant's knowledge, attitudes, and behaviors in a program.

Leeuwenhoek, Anton van: A Dutch scientist who discovered and identified bacteria in 1674.

Licensure: Certified permission given by a governmental body to a person to practice a given profession after the person has produced documented evidence and achieved a specified competence level.

Logic: One of the four criteria of philosophies; it involves the use of scientific methods and research as the programmatic focus.

Maintenance: The everyday way that people attempt to stay well, including proper clothing, food, shelter, healthcare access, healthful environment, and social support.

Maslow's Hierarchy of Needs: A theory that human needs are arranged in a hierarchy according to their relativity and that each step needs to be approached successively.

Master Certified Health Education Specialist (MCHES): An advanced credential and practice level available for CHES health professionals, passed by the National Commission for Health Education Credentialing in 2009 by the Board of Commissioners.

Master of Arts (MA): A degree focused on one area and awarded in the liberal arts to prepare students for the application of theory to health issues.

Master of Public Health (MPH): A degree that provides a generalized preparation for public health work.

Master of Science (MS): A degree focused on one area and awarded in sciences to prepare students for the application of theory to health issues.

Master of Science in Public Health (MSPH): A degree that tends to focus on one particular public health topic.

MATCH Model: A multilevel ecological model that provides a way to establish connections between the health outcomes, intervention objectives, and approaches.

Meaningful learning: A concept that describes how participants recognize and link concepts.

Media advocacy: A theory that uses the mass media as a resource to advance a social or public policy initiative.

Medical care setting: A setting for health education that includes working along with the medical professionals in assisting the organization and the patients in education, information, advocacy, and health communications.

Metaphysics: One of the four criteria of philosophy; called ontology, it includes the study of reality and change.

Mission statement: A statement of what you will achieve and a reason for applying your program to this objective.

Morbidity rates: The number of persons infected with a disease or illness.

Mortality rates: Measures of deaths due to disease or injury; most are expressed in populations per 100,000.

Multicausation Communicable Disease Model: A model that describes when diseases are caused by more than one factor or a combination of factors such as behavior choices, lack of medical care, exposure, environment, or social circumstances.

Multiple interventions: The use of many different types of strategies across all levels of influence for more effective and proper program planning.

Multiple levels: The use of many levels of influence drawing from evidence-based practice for more effective and proper planning.

Multiple levels of influence: The use of multiple theories with programs to offer many different experiences, strategies, and multiple solutions for program implementation and evaluation.

National Health Education Standards: Model standards written by the Joint Committee on National Health Education Standards for the health education core curriculum in grades K–12 and adopted and adapted by many states as the evaluation criteria for health instruction.

Needs assessments: Research and investigative tools used to determine the root cause(s) of a health problem(s).

Noncommunicable diseases: Chronic diseases caused by behavior, lifestyles, and inherited predispositions and not transmitted from an infected host to a susceptible host.

Nontraditional health setting: A setting for health education that includes sales, marketing, or other sales-related jobs marketing health and health products.

Objectives: The specific, measurable written statements of achievements for the program and/or participants; this collected information ensures accurate testing or evaluation during and after the health program.

Organizational Development Theory: A theory that describes the organizational social processes and structures that influence the behavior and motivation of participants and identifies problems that obstruct that function.

Outcome evaluation: The final evaluation conducted; it assesses the total program results on health-related quality of life.

Pandemic rates: Disease outbreaks over a very large geographic area.

Pasteur, Louis: A French chemist and microbiologist who in 1862 proposed the germ theory or biogenesis theory disproving the spontaneous generation theory. He is also credited with pasteurization of milk for sanitary purposes.

PATCH Model: A community-based model used by communities to plan, conduct, and evaluate health promotion and disease prevention programs.

Philanthropic foundation: A setting for health education that includes privately funded foundations with a specific health interest contributing to solving health-related problems in international health work and other causes.

Philosophy: A logical reasoning and solution about the meaning and importance of life and actions to promote it.

Point prevalence: The number of active disease cases existing in a defined population at a defined point in time.

Pragmatism: A philosophy about humanity and social justice.

PRECEDE–PROCEED: A program planning model that covers many different situations and causations. PRECEDE stands for predisposing, reinforcing, and enabling constructs in educational/ecological diagnosis. PROCEED stands for policy, regulatory, and organizational constructs in educational and environmental development.

Predisposing factors: Factors that provide a reason or motivation to perform a behavior, including knowledge, attitudes, readiness, and beliefs.

Prevalence rates: The number of community disease cases existing at a given time.

Prevention types: The four types of prevention: primordial prevention, primary prevention, secondary prevention, and tertiary prevention.

Primary data collection techniques: Techniques in which evidence is collected by the program team; it is firsthand information.

Principles of ethics: The eight values that include ethics: autonomy, nonmalfeasance, beneficence, justice, utilitarianism, respect, and paternalism.

Private industrial company: A setting for health education that includes commercial industries providing investments, employment, and market access in international health enterprises for altruistic enterprises with multinational and/or transnational approaches.

Private voluntary or nonprofit organization: A setting for health education that includes working in organizations founded by citizens and/or groups to fulfill a need, education, and/or public information and involves advocating for a particular health condition.

Process evaluation: An assessment of the administration of the health program.

Process objectives: The administrative tasks for a program.

Profession: A type of employment requiring specialized learning and training.

Professional or technical association/organization/society: A setting for health education that includes organizations and nonprofits that consist of professionals who meet for professional development, advocacy, and promotion of the profession, certification, licensure, and other reasons.

Professional standards: The specific academic and other requirements that must be met for individuals in a profession in the form of certification and licensure.

Program credentialing: A process that involves the regulation of professional programs by requiring specific standards.

Program plan: Structured outlines that are documented and describe what works to achieve a specific purpose and produce the intended outcome.

Program or community objectives: Changes in the overall health statistics (quality of life) of the participants/community/group in a program.

Protection: A person or community's health shields or traditional beliefs that provide physical and mental protection and spirituality, enabling a high quality of life.

Public policy factors: Local, state, and federal policies and laws that regulate and support healthy actions, practices, and resource distribution for prevention, early detection, control, and management of diseases.

Qualitative assessment techniques: Data collections acquired from conversations, direct observations, and interviews.

Quality of life: A person's sense of satisfaction with his or her life and environment. This concept includes all aspects of life that affect health, including rights, values, benefits, beliefs, and conditions.

Quality of Life: Program Goal: The final aim of a health program that raises the level of health in communities and groups as evidenced by the data collection, epidemiological statistics, and/or statistical computations.

Quantitative assessment techniques: Data collections using numbers.

Quarantine: The mandatory isolation of people infected with a disease or arriving from countries with certain diseases.

Rates: The epidemiological measures and monitoring of an event, disease, or condition that determine health or health status in a unit of population along with time specification based on surveillance data collected, recorded, and documented.

Rationale: The reason a program is necessary, supported by relevant data.

Registration: A process involving less formal requirements for a person to become registered and accepted within a profession.

Reinforcing factors: Factors that continually encourage certain behaviors due to social support, rewards, and praise.

Relative risk: A measure of the association between exposure and outcome.

Research organization: A setting for health education that includes health research conducted at medical centers, universities, hospitals, private companies, and medical-based companies.

Resume or vita: A written document of what you have achieved in your career; it displays your credentials when searching for employment or for professional development.

Risk factors: Inherited, environmental, and behavioral influences capable of provoking disease and health risk factors. Health disease risk factors can be modifiable, semimodifiable, and nonmodifiable.

Salk, Jonas: An American medical researcher who developed the first safe and effective polio vaccine in the 1950s.

Sanitation: A health prevention measure concerned with international trade and cross-border health risks that led to measures for disease notification and handling of infected travelers and goods. It resulted in the first International Sanitary Regulations.

Secondary data collection techniques: Techniques in which evidence is collected by someone else or accessed from another source.

Settings for health education: The 11 diverse settings for career options for health educators: education settings (K–12 and higher education), research organizations, medical care settings, worksite healthcare settings, nontraditional health settings, private voluntary or nonprofit organizations, philanthropic foundations, professional or technical associations/organizations/ societies, private industrial companies, governmental/public health agencies, and intergovernmental organizations.

Six generic tasks of program models: Assess the needs of the target population, identify the problem, develop appropriate goals and objectives, create an intervention that is likely to achieve desired results, implement the intervention, and evaluate the results.

Snow, John: A physician who discovered the waterborne transmission of cholera in 1854.

Social-behavioral epidemiology: The study of biological, cultural, and social phenomena for analysis.

Social Cognitive Learning Theory: A theory based on reciprocal determinism that helps identify the personal factors, environmental influences, and behaviors that continually intermingle.

Social determinants: Positive or negative conditions in life that influence behavior and health in positive and negative ways.

Social Marketing Model: A model that assesses the needs, analyzes the problems, selects channels and materials, develops materials and pretesting, implements methods, assesses effectiveness, and uses feedback to segment and improve target populations.

Standard Occupational Classification (SOC) for health educators: A designation of health education as an occupation with a description of the skills necessary according to the U.S. Department of Labor, Bureau of Labor Statistics (2001); identified as SOC 21-1091.

Summative evaluation: Evaluation that includes information collected from the impact and outcome evaluations. This collected information determines the conclusions and benefits of the program.

Surveillance: This is the epidemiological collecting, monitoring, recording and documenting of rates of both communicable and noncommunicable disease rates in humans.

Theory: The conceptual frameworks that coordinates with evidence-based health promotion plans and gives credibility to a program.

Theory of Planned Behavior: A theory that helps explain an individual's behavioral intention, the result of attitudes toward the behavior, and perceptions of subjective norms.

Timetable plan: A description of how the activities relate to the other program components and the scope and sequencing of the program.

Transtheoretical Model or Stages of Change: A theory that involves an individual's readiness to change to healthy behaviors.

Utilitarianism: A philosophy advanced by John Stuart Mill concerning individual civil liberties that should not be impeded unless the individual causes extreme harm to another person.

Variables: The operational forms of constructs that help delineate the way a construct is measured.

Vision statement: A forecast of where you hope the community/group will be in the future; a predictive statement or the future focus for a program.

Wellness: An active process of positive health choices, decisions, and lifestyles by individuals that affects the quality and years of human life.

Worksite healthcare setting: A setting for health education that includes corporate fitness centers in many different settings and involves creating and managing wellness centers and programs for employees in a company.

World Health Assembly: The decision-making body for WHO on health issues, budget, management, and administration.

World Health Organization (WHO): The directing and coordinating authority on health for the United Nations that promotes health development, security, systems, research, partnerships, and performance.

Youth Risk and Behavior Surveillance Survey (YRBSS): A telephone survey of randomly selected adolescents about risk factors, preventive health, and access to services and insurance; it monitors priority health-risk behaviors and the rates for young people and adolescents in the United States. These behaviors are identified by continued nationwide surveys of U.S. youth by the CDC and Health Promotion Data and Statistics.

PHOTOGRAPHY CREDITS

Chapter 1
Opener: © Christopher Futcher/ShutterStock, Inc.

Chapter 2
Opener: © FLariviere/ShutterStock, Inc.; 2–1 Reproduced from Bartholin, Thomas. *Historiarum anatomicarum rariorun centuria I {-VI}.* Hafniae, 1654–1661. Photo © National Library of Medicine; 2–2 Courtesy of Library of Congress, Prints & Photographs Division [Reproduction number LC-USZC4-3147]; 2–3 Courtesy of USDHHS-HRSA-BPHC, Division of National Hansen's Disease Museum, Carville, Louisiana, http://www.hrsa.gov/hansens/museum. Used with permission; 2–4 Courtesy of the Al and Gwen Knehr family; 2–5 Courtesy of the Jared and Hollie Wagner family.

Chapter 3
Opener: © Dmitriy Shironosov/ShutterStock, Inc.

Chapter 4
Opener: © Rob Marmion/ShutterStock, Inc.; 4–5 Courtesy of USDHHS-HRSA-BPHC, Division of National Hansen's Disease Museum, Carville, Louisiana, www.hrsa.gov/hansens/museum. Used with permission.

Chapter 5
Opener: © Andresr/ShutterStock, Inc.; 5–3 Courtesy of USDHHS-HRSA-BPHC, Division of National Hansen's Disease Museum, Carville, Louisiana, www.hrsa.gov/hansens/museum. Used with permission.

Chapter 6
Opener: © Dmitriy Shironosov/ShutterStock, Inc.; 6–2 © Zatletic/Dreamstime.com; 6–3 © Craig Hanson/ShutterStock, Inc.; 6–4 Courtesy of family members of the author; 6–5 Courtesy of Judith Ottoson; 6–6 Courtesy of Dr. Collins Airhihenbuwa, Professor and Head, the Department of Biobehavioral Health, College of Health and Human Development, The Pennsylvania State University; 6–7 Courtesy of Dr. Bob Blackburn, Former Executive Director, North Carolina AAHPERD.

Chapter 7
Opener: © Dennis Owusu-Ansah/ShutterStock, Inc.

Chapter 8

Opener: © Christopher Futcher/ShutterStock, Inc.; 8–1 Courtesy of Dr. Mohammad Antaki, Amman, Jordan; President, Jordaniana Gaucher Association, Chairman, CBRC Marka. Used by permission; 8–2 Courtesy of Cassandra Harris, MS, CHES, MD. Anderson Cancer Center. Used by permission; 8–3 Courtesy of Kelly Bishop, MA, CHES, FASHA, of CDC. Used by permission.

Unless otherwise indicated, all photographs are under copyright of Jones & Bartlett Learning.

INDEX